The 100

Healthiest

Foods to Eat During

Pregnancy

The Surprising, Unbiased Truth About Foods You Should
Be Eating During Pregnancy but Probably Aren't

Jonny Bowden, Ph.D., C.N.S., and Allison Tannis, M.S., R.H.N.

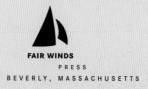

FAIR WINDS
PRESS
BEVERLY, MASSACHUSETTS

Text © 2009 by Jonny Bowden and Allison Tannis

First published in the USA in 2009 by
Fair Winds Press, a member of
Quayside Publishing Group
100 Cummings Center, Suite 406-L
Beverly, MA 01915

13 12 11 10   4 5

ISBN-13: 978-1-59233-400-1
ISBN-10: 1-59233-400-8

Library of Congress Cataloging-in-Publication Data
Bowden, Jonny.
  100 healthiest foods for pregnancy : what, when, how, and why
you should eat these fabulous foods for a healthy pregnancy and a
healthy, happy baby / Jonny Bowden and Allison Tannis.
      p. cm.
  Includes index.
  ISBN-13: 978-1-59233-400-1
  ISBN-10: 1-59233-400-8
1. Pregnancy—Nutritional aspects—Popular works. 2. Pregnant women—
Health and hygiene—Popular works. I. Tannis, Allison. II. Title. III. Title:
One hundred healthiest foods for pregnancy.
  RG559.B68 2009
  618.2—dc22
                                                2009028322

Text by Jonny Bowden and Allison Tannis
Edited by Ellen Phillips
Book design by Rachel Fitzgibbon, studio rkf
Cover design by Mattie Reposa

Printed and bound in China

dedication

To everyone who strives to give their baby the healthiest possible start.
—Jonny and Allison

For my little bundle of joy—may this help you grow big and strong.
—Allison

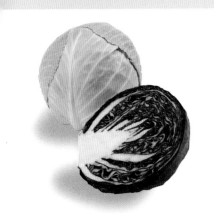
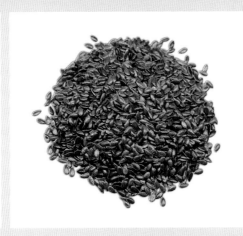
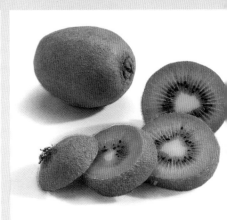

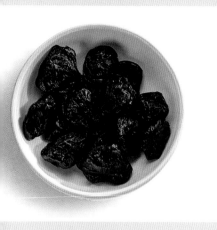
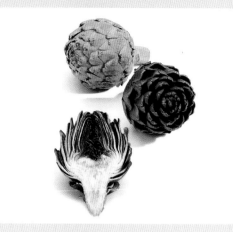
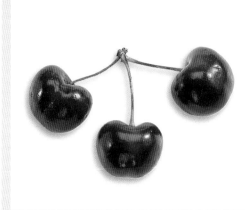

CONTENTS

INTRODUCTION	Eating Your Way to a Healthy Pregnancy	8
CHAPTER 1	Foods for a Healthy First Trimester	18
CHAPTER 2	Foods for a Healthy Second Trimester	78
CHAPTER 3	Foods for a Healthy Third Trimester	124
CHAPTER 4	Foods that Quiet Complaints	173
CHAPTER 5	Tricky Foods and Herbs	210
CHAPTER 6	Best Foods for Breast-Feeding	240
CHAPTER 7	Bite Back against Postpartum Depression	265
CHAPTER 8	Foods for Fertility and a Healthy Pregnancy from the Get-Go	285

AFTERWORD	314
ABOUT THE AUTHORS	315
INDEX OF THE 100 HEALTHIEST FOODS	316
GENERAL INDEX	317

Preface

WHY YOU (AND YOUR BABY) NEED THIS BOOK

Years ago, I asked my friend Robert Crayhon, M.S., the great nutrition educator and director of the Boulderfest nutritional medicine conference, the following question:

"If you could wave your hands and make one single dietary change that would benefit the world the most, what would it be?"

Here's what he said: "I'd put every pregnant woman on fish oil supplements."

Now, what's interesting about this response is not just the fact that Crayhon picked fish oil as the most important supplement for pregnancy (which it may well be). What's also interesting is the implication that a *pregnant woman's diet has such a profound effect on the health and well-being of her baby* that multiplied many times over it might actually translate into betterment for the whole planet.

That's how important your diet during pregnancy and postpartum really is.

Look, I know I'm a guy and I've never experienced it, but hundreds of women have told me that pregnancy and birth are the most life-altering, profound experiences they've ever had. I believe profoundly that what you eat influences everything you do and everything you experience, and that is never more true than during pregnancy and postpartum. "Birthing a baby runs the gamut from the intensity of the physical to the sublime of the spiritual, whether it is your first baby or your fifth," write my friends Dean Raffelock, D.C., L.Ac., C.C.N., DACBN, DIBAK, and Robert Rountree, M.D., authors of the terrific *Natural Guide to Pregnancy and Postpartum Health.* Your diet (and lifestyle) during pregnancy not only deeply affects your own experi-

ence but has a great influence on your baby's health, vitality, and well-being.

Hence this book.

In a previous book, *The 150 Healthiest Foods on Earth,* I discussed the health and nutrition benefits of many foods that—not surprisingly—are also in *this* book. After all, if a food benefits your health, it stands to reason it's probably good for your baby as well. But during pregnancy, your needs for certain nutrients change—your need for iron, for example, doubles during pregnancy, and that increased amount can't really be met by diet (which is why iron supplements are nearly always recommended during pregnancy). Your need for protein is higher, as is your need for vitamin E, vitamin C, niacin, riboflavin, thiamin, B6, B12, magnesium, iodine, zinc and selenium, and—most especially—folate (folic acid).

Bottom line: Some foods (and supplements) are even *more* important during pregnancy than they are at any other time of life.

There's more. Pregnancy and birth may be a wonderful, exciting journey, but it's probably going to have more than a few bumps along the road. (Okay, forget the "probably"—I was being gentle.) Morning sickness comes to mind, as does the possibility of postpartum depression. Weird food cravings are common, not to mention nausea.

To make matters worse, the amount of information about what to do about all these things is overwhelming—and while some of the information out there is high-quality stuff, much of it is not, some of it is really bad, and an awful lot of it is just plain confusing. Just for fun, I looked on the Internet and "researched" what advice was available on how to have a great pregnancy and a healthy baby. Even this trial run left me feeling overwhelmed, and I'm not even pregnant! I can only imagine how overwhelming and confusing it might be to someone who really needs to act on the best information available but doesn't know how to separate the good stuff from the downright silly.

In *The 100 Healthiest Foods to Eat During Pregnancy*, we've broken it down for you into manageable chunks of information that you can actually use. You'll discover the right foods for a number of common problems, from morning sickness through postpartum depression. You'll discover what's happening to your baby at each stage of pregnancy and how your food choices can directly support his or her growth and development. Equally important, you'll learn what foods to avoid and why.

One of the things I've tried to do in all my writing is to cut through confusion and misinformation and put to bed common myths about food and nutrition that have actually hurt us more than they've helped us (like the wholesale avoidance of fat, for example). And pregnancy and postpartum is an area ripe for what my grandmother used to call "old wives' tales." Perfect example: "You're eating for two!" This "advice" has led more than a few mothers to consume twice the calories they'd normally consume. Actually, the truth is that you only need to eat about 300 extra calories a day to fuel your baby's growth, and that isn't even till the second and third trimester! But choosing those calories wisely—which is what this book is about—is of critical importance. The payoff: a healthy mom, healthy baby, minimal weight gain, and easy postpregnancy weight loss!

Choosing foods wisely also affects your ability to conceive, so if you're reading this in anticipation of becoming pregnant, you've come to the right place! And choosing foods wisely can make a huge difference when it's time to bounce back from pregnancy and delivery. Even understanding your cravings may help—for example, as you'll learn in the book, that pickles-and-ice-cream craving just might be your body's way of telling you to get more calcium and sodium in your diet!

Speaking of cravings, one concept you'll find in the book that many people have found particularly useful is the Art of the Nutrition Shift: healthy substitutions for commonly craved foods (we'll give you a ton of examples). We'll also tell you the results of the most up-to-date research regarding such pregnancy dilemmas as how to get more omega-3s from fish in your diet while avoiding mercury. Or how to stay properly hydrated when you're feeling nauseous and can't face the thought of another glass of water (ice chips, anyone?). We'll give you tips on how to choose, store, and prepare each food we discuss, as well as when and how much of it to eat!

Here's what this book is *not* meant to be: a source of anxiety. As an expectant mother, the last thing you need is a stern taskmaster telling you what you *must* do if you want your pregnancy to be successful and your baby to be healthy. We *know* you want those things—so do we. But we also know that each person—and each pregnancy—is completely unique and that a perfect set of "must-follow" rules does not exist. We want you to look at this book as a tool, a partner in a collaboration that has you (and your baby) at the center. If some of the information we present makes sense to you, please act on it. If some of it doesn't feel right, feel free to amend or adapt it.

Your body has its own innate wisdom, even if some of its messages tend to get drowned out in a sea of noise. We want to help you listen for that innate wisdom and to provide the nourishment needed to make that inner voice more audible. Remember, women have been making babies since the beginning of time. You don't need us to tell you how to do it.

But if we can help you do it in a way that will increase the odds that this journey will be an astonishing one and that you and your baby will have all the raw materials you need for a fabulous experience together, then this book will have more than served its modest purpose.

Enjoy the journey.

Jonny Bowden, Ph.D., C.N.S.
Woodland Hills, California

Introduction: Eat Your Way to a Heathly Pregnancy

Eating for yourself and a baby can be more complicated than it sounds. But with the right information, you can eat your way to and through a healthy pregnancy. We all know that food and your health are tightly linked, but in pregnancy, what you eat is more important than ever. It's not so much "you are what you eat" but "your baby is what you eat."

Your baby relies entirely on you for nutrients, so what you choose to put on your plate is now affecting two of you. And scientists have discovered that what you choose to eat now can affect the health of your baby for years to come. So grab a fork and let's dive into these pages filled with the secrets of food for a healthy, happy pregnancy.

WHAT'S FOOD GOT TO DO WITH IT?

Can you imagine being able to eat your way through pregnancy-related complaints like morning sickness? Or that making the right choice from the dinner menu may improve your chances of becoming pregnant in the first place? It's all true. What you eat has a profound effect on your body and how well it will endure the adventure of motherhood. Certain nutrients that you can find in foods can help your body with the various stages, discomforts, and joys of pregnancy.

Luckily, becoming pregnant will not require you to stand on your head to eat your food. The principles for a healthy diet during pregnancy are very similar to the ones you've used for most of your life. In a nutshell, focus on natural foods that are not processed and avoid foods that are covered with fat or salt. Eat lots of leafy green vegetables, whole grains, nuts, beans,

and fruit. And particularly when you are pregnant, don't forget to reach for the fish course and a glass of milk to wash it all down.

During pregnancy, you need to focus on particular nutrients so you and your baby can enjoy the best of health. Let's look a little more closely at some of these super-important pregnancy nutrients.

KEY NUTRIENTS

Many nutrients are of particular importance as you enter into pregnancy and motherhood. You probably already know about folate and calcium. But many women aren't aware of the importance of other nutrients like iron, DHA, and vitamin B6. In fact, there are more than a dozen nutrients that you need more of in your diet during pregnancy than you have ever needed before.

Some experts suggest that during pregnancy you'll need 100 percent more iron, 60 percent more vitamin A, 50 percent more vitamin B6 and folate (folic acid), and 30 percent more vitamin C, niacin, vitamin B12, and vitamin B2. Nutrients can do more than simply prevent deficiencies. Certain nutrients can enhance fertility, ease nausea, boost your energy, relieve breast engorgement pain, or prevent postpartum depression. Let's see what these important pregnancy nutrients have to offer.

To Eat or Not to Eat?

If you search for your favorite foods on the Internet, you'll probably find someone telling you why pregnant women shouldn't eat them. How do you know if it's true or false? Get the facts. Here are two simple "Do Eat" and "Don't Eat" lists to get you started. Then just wait till you read about all the fabulous foods you can enjoy during pregnancy as you dig into the chapters ahead. You'll find a buffet of delicious meals with endless possibilities. For more on the bad guys, check out chapter 5, beginning on page 210, where we take a detailed look at those foods on the "Don't Eat" list.

THE DO EAT LIST:
- WHOLE GRAINS
- FRUITS AND VEGETABLES
- LOW-FAT PROTEIN SOURCES
- GOOD FATS (PLANT OILS, FISH)

THE DON'T EAT LIST:
- TRANS FAT OR LOTS OF SATURATED FAT
- SWEETENED, CAFFEINATED, OR ALCOHOLIC BEVERAGES
- CANDY AND OTHER SWEETS
- IMPROPERLY COOKED OR HIGH-RISK FOODS

FOLATE FIGHTS BIRTH DEFECTS

Folate (folic acid) has been associated with a decrease in some birth defects, including neural-tube defects, anencephaly, myelomeningocele, meningocele, oral facial cleft, structural heart disease, limb defects, urinary tract anomaly, and hydrocephalus. You may not be familiar with all of these, but trust me, they're a really great reason to make sure you get plenty of folate in your pregnancy diet! Foods that are a good source of folate include grains, spinach, lentils, chickpeas, asparagus, broccoli, peas, and Brussels sprouts.

Folate

You need to start getting more folate (folic acid) before you even conceive. This B vitamin plays a vital role in the growth and division of cells, a process that occurs at an astounding rate in your developing baby. Experts now suggest that women take a folic acid supplement at least three months before conception to give their baby the best start in life. During pregnancy, your folic acid needs are double that of an average woman (increasing from 500 mcg to 600 to 1,000 mcg per day). Not having enough of this essential vitamin in your diet can lead to problems with your baby's development. Deficiencies in folic acid during pregnancy have been linked to increased incidence of neural-tube defects and lower birth weights in research studies.

Folate also plays a role in the formation of red blood cells and aids in forming proteins in the body. Many foods in this book are excellent sources of folate, including leeks, asparagus, tahini, and pinto beans. And each food is packed with other nutrients that help support your health and the health of your baby. You'll find these foods featured in the chapters on the stages of pregnancy where they can offer you the maximum benefit. But don't let that stop you from enjoying these foods at all stages of pregnancy! Every food in this book is a healthy choice any day.

Iron

Pumping iron—This phrase may conjure pictures of large, muscular men in a weight room doing biceps curls, but it's useful to keep in mind when it comes to understanding how iron works in your body and during pregnancy. Women of childbearing age and pregnant women are at risk of having low iron levels in their blood.

Iron is an essential part of your red blood cells, which are responsible for carrying oxygen (the body's main source of fuel) from your lungs to the rest of your body. Suffering from low iron levels will slow the movement of oxygen around your body, making you feel fatigued and preventing you from pumping iron. Anemia, the clinical term for low iron levels, is associated with fatigue. During pregnancy, you may feel fatigue caused by the immense energy demands of this new baby-making venture your body has embarked on. By including lots of foods in your diet that are high in iron, you can prevent anemia and keep your energy levels up.

During pregnancy, your iron requirements increase to support your new blood volume (which can be almost double what it was before) and the development of your baby's blood cells. In the next four chapters, we've included the healthiest foods for pregnancy, many of which provide you with iron, including lamb, apricots, spinach, and pumpkin seeds. If you are a vegetarian, you are particularly susceptible to iron deficiency, but as you can already see, there are lots of vegetarian-friendly foods that are packed with iron to keep you pumping iron too. A healthy diet that contains a mixture of iron-rich foods is a great way to ensure that your pregnancy is a healthy and happy experience.

Calcium

You'll be trading in that glass of wine for a glass of milk during pregnancy. Your calcium requirements double during pregnancy; in fact, you will need about 1,000 mg of calcium a day. That's about the amount of calcium in 3–4 glasses of milk.

It's well known that calcium is important for healthy bones, and your baby is trying to grow 300 of them. But many women don't appreciate what a medical marvel calcium is. Keeping your calcium levels up can help decrease your risk of developing preeclampsia, a condition that can develop during pregnancy in which a mother's blood pressure becomes too high. Eating calcium-rich foods like yogurt, Cheddar cheese, tofu, and chia seeds (all featured in this book) can help you ensure that your body has enough calcium. Vegetarians will find the wide variety of leafy green vegetables and other calcium-rich foods, like tahini and figs, highlighted in the next few chapters helpful, because if you're a vegetarian, you're particularly susceptible to low calcium levels in your diet.

But skip the glass of milk if you're having steak for dinner. Calcium interferes with iron absorption. Some prenatal vitamins are divided into two separate pills to help you separate your iron and calcium intake to improve absorption. Do the same with your meals: Let one of your main meals be calcium-focused and another iron-focused to ensure that you and your baby are getting enough of both of these super-important pregnancy vitamins.

Vitamin D

Vitamin D is calcium's right-hand man in the body. Vitamin D improves the absorption of calcium in your body and improves your ability to use calcium to make bone. It also plays a role in nervous system function and heart health.

The importance of vitamin D in our diets, especially during pregnancy, is becoming more apparent thanks to new research. British researchers have found that giving pregnant women vitamin D supplements could reduce the risk of their children developing multiple sclerosis later in life. Plus, researchers from the University of Aberdeen in the United Kingdom reported that women who consume more vitamin D during their pregnancy have children with a lower risk of developing asthma symptoms.

Unfortunately, many women are vitamin D-deficient, particularly if they live in climates that don't receive a lot of sunlight or their days are spent mostly indoors. You need about 400 IU of vitamin D a day, which you can get from sunlight and most dairy products. Including foods like salmon, sardines, milk, and eggs in your diet is a great way to get your vitamin D. You'll find more about these healthy pregnancy foods in the next few chapters.

Calcium Food Sources

Offering 300 mg per serving

Milk (1%, 2%, homogenized, chocolate, organic, goat)	1 cup (235 ml)
Plain and flavored yogurt	³/₄ cup (175 g)
Cheese (firm—Cheddar, mozzarella, Colby, Swiss)	1.5 oz (45 g)
Soy beverage (fortified with calcium 28-30%)	1 ½ cup (355 ml)
Almond/rice beverage (fortified with calcium)	1 cup (235 ml)
Orange juice (fortified with calcium)	1 cup (235 ml)
Salmon with bones	½ can (7.5 oz)
Sardines with bones	1 can (7 oz)
Tofu—firm or regular (calcium sulfate or chloride)	½ cup to 1 cup
Soybeans, cooked	2 cups (200 g)
Soynuts	1 cup (145 g)
Collards, cooked	1 cup (190 g)
Bok choy, cooked	1 cup (190 g)
Turnip greens	1 ½ cups (83 g)

Offering 150 mg per serving

Almonds	½ cup (70 g)
Hazelnuts	½ cup (60 g)
Sesame seeds	²/₃ cup (90 g)
Tahini	3 tbsp (45 g)
Beans, baked	1 cup (253 g)
Beans, navy	1 ¼ cups (125 g)
Beans, pinto	2 cups (200 g)
Figs, dried	6
Orange, fresh	3
Broccoli, cooked	2 ½ cups (170 g)
Brussels sprouts	2 ½ cups (220 g)
Ice cream, regular	1 cup (140 g)
Macaroni and cheese	1 cup
Waffles	2

Source: USDA National Nutrient Database SR 16 2003; Bowe & Church's Food Values

Vitamin B6

Also known as pyridoxine, this vitamin helps keep your energy levels up. Plus, it's well known to quell the nausea and vomiting that some women experience during their first trimester (or longer) of pregnancy. Studies suggest that between 25 mg and 75 mg of vitamin B6 is needed to stop this queasy pregnancy complaint. Including foods like paprika, red bell peppers, basil, and leeks, all of which are featured later, can help you enjoy colorful meals and get the vitamin B6 you need to stay energized and free from queasy mornings.

DHA

Docosahexaenoic acid (DHA) is an essential fat found primarily in fish. This little fat has received a lot of attention thanks to its amazing ability to improve brain health. Babies whose moms consume more fish have been found in clinical trials to have higher IQs, better sleep patterns, and greater visual acuity.

They're also better at communicating. A study called *The Children of the 90s* is looking at links between diet during pregnancy and the health of the baby through childhood and beyond. The study involves 14,000 British children who have been followed from development in the womb through their early teens. Results so far indicate that eating higher-fat fish like mackerel, sardines, anchovies, salmon, and tuna (about 300 mg of DHA a day, or 2 to 4 servings of fatty fish servings a week) during pregnancy leads to better language and communication skills. The full results of this research are likely to show us more about the importance of diet and pregnancy.

There's more: Moms who enjoy fish more than a few times a week have a reduced risk of developing postpartum depression. There are many great food sources of DHA, including mackerel, coho salmon, tuna, and even lamb. Read more about this amazing fat in the next few chapters and you just may find yourself craving a little fish for dinner.

WHAT YOU EAT NOW CAN HELP YOUR CHILD LATER

Scientists have discovered that a mother's diet during pregnancy has lasting effects on the health of her baby. Eating a healthy diet during pregnancy may help your child avoid or reduce his or her risk of many diseases, including some of the most deadly diseases in the world, like heart disease, cancer, and diabetes. Clinical studies are starting to discover how important a mother's diet is to her child's future development through population comparisons.

For example, a group of researchers from the National Institute of Public Health reported in 2007 that fish intake during pregnancy may reduce the risk of a child's developing atopy-related diseases such as asthma and eczema later in life. The study involved 462 women whose fish consumption during pregnancy was compared with their children's health at the age of 6. The researchers found that children of mothers who ate 2.5 servings of fish per week versus 1 serving had a 37 percent lower risk of having eczema at age 1. And the mother's fish intake during breast-feeding reduced a child's risk of having asthma-related symptoms.

A group of researchers at the University of Crete in Greece found that if a woman adhered strictly to a Mediterranean diet during pregnancy, it also reduced her child's risk of having asthma and eczema. A Mediterranean diet is rich in olive oil, vegetables, antioxidants, and fish, which are all indisputably healthy foods to include in any diet.

More Crucial Nutrients

Many more nutrients play a crucial role in your health before, during, and after pregnancy, including zinc, vitamin A, selenium, fiber, and protein. As you read about the 100 healthiest foods for pregnancy in the following pages, you'll discover the important links between nutrition and pregnancy.

The Weight Thing

One of the hardest aspects of pregnancy when it comes to food is the fear of weight gain. Almost every pregnant woman worries about gaining too much weight during her pregnancy. Horror stories of women who cannot shed those baby pounds years after giving birth can leave some women hesitating to reach into the refrigerator and eat.

But not eating enough food can put you and your baby at risk. You'll have to learn to live with the extra pounds that will form on your hips and thighs during pregnancy: They are there for a reason. Your body has taken inventory of your current state and decided how much fat it needs to add to your body in order for you to be able to produce a baby and breast-feed him or her for a few months after birth. Plus, the weight you're gaining is not all fat. Your breasts enlarge, your uterus is growing, and the baby himself adds weight.

So when the scale starts to tip and your pants become too snug, don't let the years of societal pressure to have a supermodel body stop you from eating. It will take about 80,000 calories to carry your baby to term. Dig in! Using the healthy foods in this book can help ensure that you get the nutrients you and your baby need in a way that will help reduce any unnecessary weight gain during your pregnancy.

What's the Right Weight?

Weight plays an important role in a healthy pregnancy. Women whose weight is below normal for their height are at a greater risk for premature delivery and having a smaller-than-average baby. Overweight or obese women are at a higher risk for having complications during pregnancy, a difficult delivery, and a baby who weighs more than average. In addition, their babies are more likely to have weight problems later in life. Extremes in a mother's weight can lead to stunted growth and development in the womb.

Do *not* diet! Babies who experience growth restriction in the womb have a higher risk of developing chronic disease as adults. Instead, eat a well-balanced diet that meets your daily caloric needs (only about 300 calories more per day) during pregnancy to help ensure that your weight doesn't reach either extreme.

FOOD VERSUS SUPPLEMENTS

Current research supports the use of prenatal vitamins by pregnant women regardless of their dietary practices. Your nutritional needs are great during pregnancy, and as we have seen, the impact of your diet on your baby is immense. Eating a diet rich in healthy foods, such as the 100 foods we highlight in this book, can help ensure that your body has the nutrients it needs to support you and your baby through pregnancy, after delivery, and during breast-feeding.

But we know that it's easier to read about a perfect diet than to actually eat one. Use the information in this book to guide you in the right direction and help you choose the healthiest foods for you and your baby. But be sure to follow your obstetrician's prenatal vitamin recommendations. Even if you intend to make every meal a healthy one, you can never control what life might throw at you, occasionally throwing your nutritious meal plans out the window. Better safe than sorry!

Calculating a Healthy Weight

BODY WEIGHT (POUNDS)

	Ideal Weight					Overweight					Obese				
58	96	100	105	110	115	119	124	129	134	138	143	148	153	158	162
59	99	104	109	114	119	124	128	133	138	143	148	153	158	163	168
60	102	107	112	118	123	128	133	138	143	148	153	158	163	168	174
61	106	111	116	122	127	132	137	143	148	153	158	164	169	174	180
62	109	115	120	126	131	136	142	147	153	158	164	169	175	180	186
63	113	118	124	130	135	141	146	152	158	163	169	175	180	186	191
64	116	122	128	134	140	145	151	157	163	169	174	180	186	192	197
65	120	126	132	138	144	150	156	162	168	174	180	186	192	198	204
66	124	130	136	142	148	155	161	167	173	179	186	192	198	204	210
67	127	134	140	146	153	159	166	172	178	185	191	198	204	211	217
68	131	138	144	151	158	164	171	177	184	190	197	203	210	216	223
69	135	142	149	155	162	169	176	182	189	196	203	211	216	223	230
70	139	146	153	160	167	174	181	188	195	202	209	216	222	229	236
71	143	150	157	165	172	179	186	193	200	208	215	222	229	236	243
72	147	154	162	169	177	184	191	199	206	213	221	228	235	242	250
73	151	159	166	174	182	186	197	204	212	219	227	235	241	249	257
74	155	163	171	179	186	194	202	210	218	225	233	241	249	256	264
75	160	168	176	184	192	200	208	216	224	232	240	248	256	264	272
76	164	172	180	189	197	205	213	221	230	238	246	254	263	271	279

BODY HEIGHT (INCHES)

WHERE THE POUNDS GO

A typical newborn weighs about 7 pounds, but you will probably put on anywhere between 25 and 40 pounds during your pregnancy. Here's where those pounds are going:

baby	7 pounds
breasts	2 pounds
maternal fat stores	7 pounds
placenta	1.5 pounds
uterus	2 pounds
amniotic fluid	2 pounds
blood	4 pounds
body fluids	4 pounds

As you can see, the changes happening in your body require lots of nutrients. Don't let the scale prevent you from eating during pregnancy—just eat right and any extra baby weight will disappear in due time.

EATING DISORDERS AND PREGNANCY

Women of reproductive years have a high rate of eating disorders. Anorexia nervosa and bulimia can complicate pregnancy. Babies rely on their mothers to provide them with nutrients to grow and survive. Be sure your diet is full of healthy foods, and consult your obstetrician or midwife immediately if you think you may be suffering from an eating disorder during pregnancy. Your baby's health depends on it!

WHAT'S ON *YOUR* PLATE?

Do pregnant women make the grade? Are you eating the right foods? According to a group of Russian researchers, women do not eat enough of the right foods during pregnancy. In 2005, a study involving 100 pregnant women (ages 23 to 32) looked at the diets they consumed. The researchers found that the pregnant women did not eat enough vegetables, fruit, dairy products, or protein. Plus, they consumed alarmingly low levels of folic acid (only 27 percent of the recommended amount) and iron (only 17 percent of the recommended amount), two of the most important pregnancy nutrients.

Meanwhile, researchers around the world are finding that the connection between diet during pregnancy and the health of the mother and baby is strong and linked at many levels, as we'll see in detail in the chapters that follow. It's because the importance of nutrition during pregnancy is so great that prenatal vitamins are currently being recommended to pregnant women around the world. Proper nutrition during pregnancy can reduce the chances of birth defects, may reduce the risk of miscarriage, can quiet pregnancy complaints, improve birth weight and duration of pregnancy, and may improve development of the brains and eyes of infants.

Eating right during pregnancy really *is* important. This book will show you the best foods to reach for and even give you some tips on great, easy ways to prepare them. Enjoy!

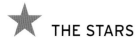 ## THE STARS

The foods that feature this red star are the foods that made the biggest impression during the writing of this book. They were chosen based on the strength of their safety profile, associated research, and their nutritional benefits. They are the "superfoods" that sit at the front of an already impressive class of healthy foods to eat during pregnancy.

TWINS, TRIPLETS, AND MORE

If you're having twins, triplets, or any multiple-gestation pregnancy, your nutrition needs are even greater than a single-birth mom's. Your babies need the same nutrients as every other growing baby in the world, but because there are more than one, you'll need to pay particular attention to your diet to ensure that it's packed with foods that will offer each of your babies enough nutrients to grow big and strong.

If you're carrying twins, you'll need to eat an additional 150 calories a day over the dietary recommendations for a mother carrying a single baby (that would be about 450 extra calories a day). It may seem strange that you aren't actually doubling your calories for each additional baby you're carrying, but many of the changes you're fueling in your body during pregnancy work for both of your babies, such as a growing uterus, increased blood volume, and breast growth. Your folic acid needs will increase to about 1 mg a day, and your iron and vitamin B6 needs will also increase to 27 mg and 1.9 mg a day respectively. And those numbers go up with each additional baby you're carrying. Luckily, by using the information in this book, you'll find it easy to include a variety of interesting and delicious foods in your diet that will support your babies' nutritional needs.

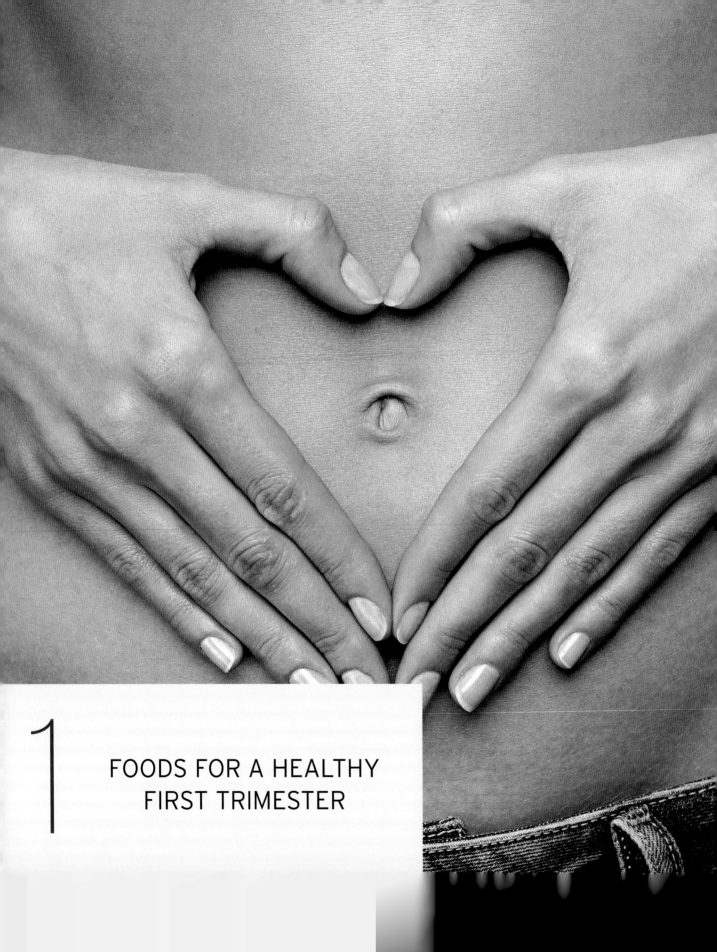

1

FOODS FOR A HEALTHY FIRST TRIMESTER

YOU'RE PREGNANT—CONGRATULATIONS!

If you're the mom-to-be or if you're a supporting part-ner reading this book, you deserve a serious pat on the back. That's because you've taken one of the first and most important steps as a new parent: learning about the food that will nurture both you and your baby as you embark on what is certainly going to be one of life's greatest adventures.

Over the next few chapters, we will discuss many factors of pregnancy. You'll see the many ways in which food and nutrition play a powerful role in this incred-ible journey, influencing everything from the health of your baby to the way that you feel during the next nine months (and beyond!). By becoming food-savvy, you'll be taking one of the most important steps toward a healthier pregnancy. And because every mother-to-be is different, you need to discover what foods are best for you and your baby. In *The 100 Healthiest Foods to Eat During Pregnancy*, we'll help you do just that!

In this chapter, we'll discuss the joys and pitfalls of the first trimester of pregnancy and the foods that can offer both mom and baby nutrients to help you stride through these next three months with ease.

FERTILITY IS A SIGN OF HEALTH

Many people think that it all begins when the sperm meets the egg. But think a minute about how much energy (and how many nutrients!) it took to make the egg in the first place, not to mention the millions of sperm. Fertility is a sign of a healthy body. Health *before* pregnancy is vital to a healthy baby. Researchers are discovering that the health of both mom and dad *before* conception is much more impor-tant than we ever realized. In fact, a healthy prepreg-nancy lifestyle is not only linked with healthy babies; it's also linked with a reduced risk of pregnancy problems!

EARLY SIGNS OF PREGNANCY

Look for these signs if you think you might be pregnant. Check with an obstetrician if you have even a few of these symptoms. Now's the time to start changing your diet to support your growing baby. This chapter will show you what you need.

- Implantation bleeding
- Missed period(s)
- Fatigue
- Swollen/tender breasts
- Nausea
- Vomiting
- Backaches
- Headaches
- Frequent urination
- Darkening of areolas
- Food cravings

FAST FACT

Fetal development begins before you even know you're pregnant.

Look, let's face it: Eating right is always important. But if you're thinking of conceiving or are already pregnant, there's no time to waste. Now's the time for you to *really* work on eating better. (And if you're struggling with infertility, be sure to read chapter 8 and get the inside scoop on foods that support fertility.)

IT BEGINS

The ability of an egg and sperm to unite and then divide, divide, and divide until they make hundreds and thousands of cells—and eventually a baby—has to be one of the most fascinating things on earth. Cell division is a *lot* of work. Just as it takes a village to raise a child, it takes an awful lot of nutrients to *make* one—particularly B vitamins, vitamin A, protein, and fat.

In the first few hours and days, the egg and sperm turn into a ball of cells called a zygote. The zygote eventually grows large enough to become the *fetus*. The rate of growth is amazingly fast and takes a whole lot of energy to accomplish. No wonder one of the very first symptoms of pregnancy is feeling tired all the time! Eating foods that are energizing, like oatmeal, and foods that contain B vitamins, like asparagus, brown rice, and salmon, can go a long way toward helping you battle these tired feelings.

OFF TO A GOOD START

Eating well is important throughout pregnancy, but the first few weeks of pregnancy are particularly important. That's when all the main features of your baby are being created and assembled: the spine, the organs, and the limbs. While certain nutrients, such as folic acid, iron, and calcium, are known to be of particular importance at this stage, the rapid growth of the zygote requires a wide variety of vitamins, minerals, protein, carbohydrates, and fats. Many healthy foods can provide these valuable nutrients to your baby, including nuts, seeds, vegetables, fruits, dairy, grains, and meat.

THE ZYGOTE: THE FIRST FOUR DAYS

The zygote, the developmental stage that begins with the fertilized egg and leads to the embryo and finally the fetus, contains 23 chromosomes from you and 23 from your partner. These chromosomes contain genetic material that will determine your baby's sex and traits such as eye color, hair color, height, facial features, and to some extent, intelligence and personality.

FAST FACT

During pregnancy, your body is working really hard, even if all the work it's doing is flying underneath your conscious radar. You may not know why your body is sending you such weird signals, but learn to pay attention.

Most women find out they are pregnant around the fifth week of pregnancy, by which time the baby's circulatory system and heart have already started to form. Why even wait till then? Start now, and get your baby off to a good start by eating lots of healthy foods. Even before conception, fueling your body with the best possible nutrition can make a difference, and it's equally—if not *more*—important in the first trimester as it is throughout your entire pregnancy.

THE GREAT DISCOVERY

The moment you find out you're pregnant is one of the most emotionally charged moments you may ever experience. It doesn't matter if it happened while you were hovering over that silly-looking plastic stick waiting to see if a second line appeared or if you were sitting impatiently waiting in the doctor's office for the nurse to give you the verdict on your test results.

Whether you were expecting it or not, finding out that you are actually pregnant may have felt completely overwhelming. If so, you're hardly alone.

THE HORMONAL ROLLER COASTER

Many moms-to-be will feel emotionally charged throughout the entire pregnancy. Don't worry: It's perfectly normal. Your body is working overtime producing hormones and chemicals that have a profound effect on your feelings, and many of your moods are a direct result of their action. Creating hormones is a tiring process. This is yet another reason (as if you needed one!) to eat lots of healthy foods: Think of them as the delivery system for the many nutrients your body needs to keep going through this challenging time.

Take protein, for example. Your body needs protein to produce all of the hormones that are causing your breasts to grow, your uterus to enlarge, and (of course) your emotions to fluctuate wildly. (Sorry about the last one; it just comes with the territory.) Beans, nuts, dairy products, seeds, and meat are all good sources of protein.

By eating the right foods, you can sit back and enjoy (or at least accept!) the excitement, joy, and occasional worries that come with the hormonal roller coaster of pregnancy. And all the while, you'll know that you *and* the baby are fueled and healthy and are going to make it through just fine.

NUTRITIONAL NEEDS FOR THE FIRST TRIMESTER

Because every woman's body is different, it's important to work closely with your obstetrician or midwife to develop a nutritional program that's ideal for you. Factors from your health, age, and weight to your activity level, heredity, and the amount of stress you're experiencing combine to create unique nutritional needs. This chart will give you nutritional guidelines for a healthy first trimester. You'll read about these nutrients in detail later in the chapter.

Key Vitamins

Thiamin: 1.4 mg daily

Riboflavin: 1.4 mg daily

Niacin: 18 mg daily

Biotin: 30 mcg daily

Pantothenic acid: 6 mg daily

Vitamin B6: 1.9 mg daily

Folate: 800 mcg daily

Vitamin B12: 2.6 mcg daily

Choline: 450 mg daily

Vitamin A: 2,700 IU daily

Vitamin C: 85 mg daily

Vitamin D: 400 IU daily

Vitamin E: 15 mg daily

Vitamin K: 90 mcg daily

Key Minerals

Sodium: 1,500 mg daily

Chloride: 2,300 mg daily

Potassium: 4,700 mg daily

Calcium: 1,000 mg daily

Phosphorus: 700 mg daily

Magnesium: 350 mg daily (360 mg/day for pregnant women 31–50 years of age)

Iron: 27 mg daily

Zinc: 11 mg daily

Iodine: 220 mcg daily

Selenium: 60 mcg daily

Copper: 1,000 mcg daily

Manganese: 2 mg daily

Fluoride: 3 mg daily

Chromium: 30 mcg daily

Molybdenum: 50 mcg daily

Baby Progression Through Gestation

AGE (WEEKS)	BABY LENGTH	DEVELOPMENTAL CHANGES
1	0.1 mm	Blactocyst implants in walls of uterus
3	1 mm	Early spinal cord and gut develop
4 to 5	2–3 mm	Arm and leg buds form
6	1.5 cm	Heartbeat can be detected with ultrasound
8	3.7 cm	Eyelids and ear canals form; head becomes more rounded; muscles grow, allowing small movements
12	8.8 cm	Body is more elongated; sex can be distinguished externally; hair and nails grow
16	14 cm	Head is held erect; lower limbs and more developed; movements can be felt
24	32 cm	Body is longer but very lean; alveoli (air sacs) in lungs form
28	38.5 cm	Brain forms its characteristic folds; eyelids open; testes descend for boys
32	43.5 cm	Body fat begins to accumulate; toenails form
36	47.5 cm	Nails have grown to fingertips; body is plump
38	50 cm	Brain cells become more efficient; chest grows more

FUELING THE EXPANSION

"Eating for two" may be the expression we all use to joke about how a pregnant woman should eat, but it sure isn't a very accurate statement. If you're looking at pregnancy as an opportunity to finally eat everything you want and as much as you want of everything, listen carefully: Your goal is *not* to eat twice as much as normal!

You actually only need about 300 extra calories per day. What you *do* need to do is make sure that you're eating enough nutrients to support the growth of the fetus and to feel good through the process. A much better expression would be "quality over quantity." Maybe the new mantra for pregnancy should be, *Eat twice as healthy as before*!

Let's take a closer look at the key nutrients you'll need to kick off your healthy pregnancy.

Protein

Protein comes from the Greek, meaning "of prime importance," which is exactly what it is during pregnancy. Protein's actually one of the foods most underconsumed by women in Western society, and it's truly "of prime importance" for new moms. Every single cell in your new baby's body will need protein to form properly.

You may remember that protein is needed to create the hormones responsible for the miraculous changes happening in your body, but did you know that protein is also the raw material for enzymes? Enzymes instruct cells to divide, grow, metabolize, and more. They help your baby to grow and develop. And they give you energy, something you might be seriously lacking in that first trimester.

BODY CHANGES IN THE FIRST TRIMESTER

Even before you really start showing, your pregnant body undergoes dramatic changes. Here are some of the earliest:

- Blood volume can almost double.
- Heart rate increases.
- Muscle mass of heart can increase.
- Breasts may enlarge.
- High hormone production occurs.
- Mood swings are frequent.
- Nausea and/or cravings may occur.

FAST FACT

What's the right amount of weight to aim for? Women who are at a normal weight before pregnancy should aim to gain 25 to 40 pounds while pregnant, added gradually throughout the 40 weeks of pregnancy. Women who are overweight at the time of conception should aim to gain only 15 to 25 pounds.

Vitamin A

Vitamin A is another important nutrient that helps fuel your baby's growth. Vitamin A is a powerful antioxidant that can help protect the important process of cell division. When cells divide, they make a copy of their DNA—the cells' "blueprint"—and you don't want any mistakes to happen here.

Antioxidants neutralize damaging compounds called *free radicals* that attack your cells and are the enemy of your DNA. You want the powerful protection of vitamin A and other antioxidants working for you, *especially* during pregnancy. They protect not only your cells and your DNA but also your proteins and fats—all compounds that can be seriously damaged by free radicals.

Vitamin E

Another powerful member of the antioxidant SWAT team is vitamin E. Researchers from the University of Medicine and Dentistry of New Jersey found that a mother's blood level of vitamin E was positively associated with fetal growth. We suspect this may be due to vitamin E's ability to improve blood flow and nutrient supply to the fetus.

In fact, researchers have found that antioxidant levels in general may affect many pregnancy outcomes besides fetal growth, including birth weight, preterm deliveries, and preeclampsia. The bottom line: Eating foods rich in antioxidants is a smart strategy for promoting a healthy pregnancy.

Folate (folic acid)

Although it's been an accepted and uncontroversial fact for years, many women are still unaware of the vital importance of folate (folic acid) before and during pregnancy. In fact, *Dietary Guidelines for Americans* in 2005 suggested that all women of childbearing age take a daily folic acid supplement and eat folic acid-rich foods like spinach, liver, and fortified cereals.

Evidence shows that folate is important for preventing birth defects of the brain and spinal cord, specifically a disabling defect called spina bifida. And the time to start taking folic acid is before you get pregnant!

Here's why: The nervous system is one of the first body systems to develop in your baby. A few weeks after conception, the special cells in your embryo begin to take shape. A cylinder called the neural tube forms and will become your baby's spinal cord and brain. Folate is required for the neural tube to close. If the neural tube fails to close properly, fatal or greatly debilitating birth defects can occur, including spina bifida, lower limb paralysis, learning disabilities, and nerve damage.

Since folic acid is so vital to this early stage of development, taking folic acid early, even before conception, is very important. And since many women don't learn that they're pregnant till well into the first trimester, it's important to take folic acid supplements if there's even a chance you may become pregnant.

FOLIC ACID VERSUS FOLATE

While the two terms are often used interchangeably, folate is the form of this B vitamin that's found naturally in foods (like leafy green vegetables), while folic acid is the synthetic form found in vitamin supplements. Folic acid from supplements is actually better absorbed than folate from foods, but that doesn't mean you shouldn't also load up your diet with folate-rich foods like the ones in the chart below. Many of these foods are included here in this chapter's list of top foods for a healthy first trimester.

Foods That Contain Folate

Food	Micrograms (mcg)	% Daily Value (DV)
*Breakfast cereals fortified with 100% of the DV, ³⁄₄ cup	400	50
Beef liver, cooked, braised, 3 oz	185	23
Cowpeas (blackeyes), immature, cooked, boiled, ³⁄₄ cup (83 g)	105	13
*Breakfast cereals, fortified with 25% of the DV, ³⁄₄ cup	100	12
Spinach, frozen, cooked, boiled, ³⁄₄ cup (95 g)	100	12
Great Northern beans, boiled, ³⁄₄ cup (89 g)	90	11
Asparagus, boiled, 4 spears	85	11
*Rice, white, long-grain, parboiled, enriched, cooked, ³⁄₄ cup (88 g)	65	8
Vegetarian baked beans, canned, 1 cup (254 g)	60	8
Spinach, raw, 1 cup (30 g)	60	8
Green peas, frozen, boiled, ¹⁄₂ cup (65 g)	50	6
Broccoli, chopped, frozen, cooked, ¹⁄₂ cup (92 g)	50	6
*Egg noodles, cooked, enriched, ¹⁄₂ cup (80 g)	50	6
Broccoli, raw, 2 spears (each 5 inches [13 cm] long)	45	6
Avocado, raw, all varieties, sliced, ¹⁄₂ cup (73 g) sliced	45	6
Peanuts, all types, dry roasted, 1 oz	40	5
Lettuce, Romaine, shredded, ¹⁄₂ cup (28 g)	40	5
Wheat germ, crude, 2 tablespoons (14 g)	40	5
Tomato juice, canned, 6 oz	35	5
Orange juice, chilled, includes concentrate, ³⁄₄ cup (175 ml)	35	5
Turnip greens, frozen, cooked, boiled, ¹⁄₂ cup (86 g)	30	4
Orange, all commercial varieties, fresh, 1 small	30	4
*Bread, white, 1 slice	25	3
*Bread, whole wheat, 1 slice	25	3
Egg, whole, raw, fresh, 1 large	25	3
Cantaloupe, raw, ¹⁄₄ medium	25	3
Papaya, raw, ¹⁄₂ cup (70 g) cubes	25	3
Banana, raw, 1 medium	20	2

* Items marked with an asterisk (*) are fortified with folic acid as part of the Folate Fortification Program.
Note: Eating a variety of folate-rich foods and taking a prenatal vitamin/mineral supplement is the best way to ensure that you and your baby get adequate folate.

From the National Institutes of Health, Dietary Supplement Fact Sheet, Folate.

FOLATE AND CLEFT LIPS

Researchers from the United States National Institute of Environmental Sciences reported a study that looked at infants born between 1996 and 2001 in Norway. More than 1,300 infants were observed to see if folic acid supplements, dietary folates, and multivitamins prevented facial clefts. The study concluded that folic acid supplements during early pregnancy reduce the risk of cleft lip (with or without cleft palate) by about a third. Dietary folates and multivitamins may also offer this benefit.

FAST FACT

Your body's iron needs can *double* during pregnancy.

Iron

Iron deficiency is the most common nutritional deficiency in North America, and it's the most common nutritional deficiency in women of childbearing age. You lose iron every time you have your period, which can also contribute to low iron stores in women during their childbearing years—just when you need iron most. During pregnancy, your blood volume increases to meet the demands of your growing baby, increasing the need for iron even more.

Women who are iron deficient are at higher risk of having a preterm delivery or a baby with a low birth weight. At first, your body is okay: It has a small reserve of iron on hand for the time when your needs start to increase. But those reserves get depleted really quickly, and to fight off fatigue, irritability, weakness, and shortness of breath, you need plenty of iron-containing foods.

Vitamin C helps enhance the absorption of iron, so eating iron-rich foods in combination with foods that contain vitamin C is a really smart idea. For example; Have an orange with your iron-fortified multigrain cereal or accompany your burger with some sliced tomatoes.

GOOD FUEL, BAD FUEL

It's important to choose your fuel sources carefully during pregnancy. Fuel for your body comes in the form of carbohydrates. There's been a ton of confusion about carbohydrates in the last few years, so forget everything you've ever heard about "simple" versus "complex" carbs and listen up: There are only two types of carbohydrates—*good* carbs and *bad* ones.

There. Now didn't that clear it up for you?

Okay, we know what you're thinking: how do you know which is which? It is simple: *Good* carbohydrates are high in fiber and offer your body a slow, steady release of sugar to help keep you fueled over a few hours. *Bad* carbohydrates are high in sugar, tend to be highly processed, and have very little fiber. These "bad" carbohydrates are bad precisely because they cause your blood sugar levels to rise quickly, stimulating your body to produce a lot of a hormone called *insulin*. This isn't good for your body, and it *certainly* isn't good for your growing baby.

A common saying among midwives is "sugar makes big babies." This may sound like a good thing, but trust us—it's not. Babies over 9 pounds are very hard to deliver vaginally. The increasing amount of sugar consumption in our diets (170 pounds per year, as of this writing!) has caused women to have larger babies and may be a factor in the huge increase in Cesarean sections performed recently. Diabetic women tend to have higher blood sugar levels and as a result are at risk of having big babies. Big babies are a problem when it comes to delivery. Personally, I'd rather have a healthy baby (6 to 7 pounds) and skip the sugar! File that under the heading "Grandma was right." Be sure to limit your intake of sugary juices, sodas, candy, and other sugary processed foods.

Limiting sugar or foods that rapidly turn into sugar (like white bread) may also reduce the risk of a condition called *gestational diabetes*, a (usually) temporary condition that can develop during pregnancy. Gestational diabetes is a sign that your body is having a hard time balancing blood sugar. It's usually diagnosed around weeks 24 to 28, but making good food choices early on may reduce the risk. Foods high in fiber are helpful in keeping blood sugar levels low. Good fats, vegetables, nuts, and beans are also helpful in regulating blood sugar levels. As for artificial sweeteners, these are best avoided—definitely during pregnancy, but truth be told, you're better off without them permanently. We'll take a closer look at this tricky pregnancy food in chapter 5.

MORNING SICKNESS AND OTHER FOOD PROBLEMS

Get ready to rock and roll! The first three months of pregnancy may be the ones in which you experience the biggest highs and lows of the entire process. If you're finding this first trimester difficult, take comfort in knowing that you're not alone: It's almost always the hardest three months for everyone. The excitement of discovering that you're pregnant is certainly a high,

FAST FACT

Gestational diabetes is a temporary condition that a woman can develop during pregnancy. Limiting sugar and bad carbs can reduce the risk of developing gestational diabetes.

but unfortunately in just a few weeks it's likely to be matched with one of the all-time lows of pregnancy: morning sickness!

There is more bad news: "Morning sickness"—typically nausea and vomiting—isn't just something that happens in the morning. For more than a few women, it can be a day-long event. According to the Motherisk Clinic at the Hospital for Sick Children in Toronto, approximately 80 percent of pregnant women are affected to some degree. The good news is that some lucky women find the symptoms of morning sickness to be very mild: They may not even experience vomiting at all. And while morning sickness usually begins around week 7, it typically disappears around week 12. Remember, every pregnancy is different, and your experience may be completely different from what the textbooks say!

WHAT CAUSES MORNING SICKNESS?

Researchers are still unsure about the actual cause or causes of morning sickness. However, researchers from the University of Athens conducted a study involving more than 100 women and found that vomiting and nausea during the first trimester were correlated with an unsuitable diet and big and infrequent meals; poor communication with their husbands and/or obstetricians; and stress, doubt, and inadequate information about pregnancy, childbirth, and healthy fetal development. So maybe just reading this book is the first step to avoiding morning sickness!

MORNING SICKNESS TAKES ITS TOLL

Morning sickness—nausea and vomiting—is a hallmark of the first trimester of pregnancy. When about 600 pregnant women were questioned in a study done by researchers from the University of Adelaide in Australia, women complained that nausea was the most troublesome symptom, both in its duration and intensity. Women also reported problems with physical functioning, low energy, and social functioning due to morning-sickness symptoms. The researchers concluded that nausea and vomiting in early pregnancy has a profound impact on women's general sense of well-being and routine, day-to-day activities.

NUTRITION SHIFTS

Satisfy your cravings with healthier options and feel good about your food choices by using these smart switches.

CRAVING	NUTRITIOUS SUBSTITUTE
Ice cream	Low-fat frozen yogurt
Soda	Mineral water with fruit juice
Doughnuts	Whole-grain bread with jam
Cake	Banana or zucchini bread
Sugar-coated cereal	Oatmeal with brown sugar
Potato chips	Popcorn
Sundae toppings	Fresh berries

Luckily, when it comes to morning sickness, there are a few tricks you can do—and many foods you can eat—that can minimize the effects or even (if you're lucky) prevent it altogether! Here are some of the best:

- Don't allow yourself to get hungry.
- Eat smaller, more frequent meals.
- Don't overeat.
- Try not drinking fluids at mealtime.
- Eat something before you get out of bed in the morning.
- Identify any nausea triggers (foods, odors) and avoid them.
- Try taking a prenatal vitamin at a different time of day.
- Choose healthy foods.
- Avoid fatty, greasy, hard-to-digest foods.
- Eat high-fiber foods.
- Wear loose-fitting clothing.
- Sniff a lemon.
- Get the right nutrients by eating some of the foods outlined in this chapter.

MASTERING CRAVINGS THROUGH NUTRITION SHIFTS

Cravings can happen at any time during your pregnancy, and it's best to deal with them head on. The first and most important step in dealing with cravings is to identify their source. Is it because you're hungry, dehydrated, or low on protein? Is it because you're depressed, angry, or tired? Identification is the first step to mastery: Once you know where the cravings are coming from, you can develop effective strategies to deal with them.

Let's say you're craving ice cream. You might simply be craving the comfort of some sugar and fat (not a big stretch of the imagination), but it's also possible you might need some calcium. In any case, gritting your teeth and trying to will the craving away isn't likely to work for long. So we suggest what we call a "nutrition shift," which is basically a switch to a healthier food that still satisfies your craving.

In this case, here are some alternatives to ice cream: A piece of juicy fruit will give you a sugar fix. Some cheese may satisfy your craving for fat (and for calcium, for that matter). Frozen yogurt might also stop the ice cream craving and for a lot less calories. So might a bowl of frozen cherries covered with a little full-fat yogurt (Jonny's personal favorite "craving buster").

This nutrition shift works just as well when you're craving salt or crunchy things, like that jar of pickles that's just calling your name. It might be a signal that you're lacking sodium. While a cucumber might satisfy the need for crunch, if it's sodium you need, the cuke won't cut it. But a piece of Cheddar cheese with that cuke may be just what the doctor ordered, offering you and the baby a much more nutritious snack while knocking the cravings right out of the box. You'll find more examples of nutrition shifts on page 28.

FOOD AVERSIONS

Many women will find that during pregnancy, certain foods—even ones they used to like—will suddenly seem disgusting. There's a good reason for this: When you're pregnant, your senses are on high alert. You're extremely sensitive to smells, textures, sounds, and all sorts of other stimuli that may make even familiar foods seem terribly unappealing, while certain weird food combinations like pickles and ice cream suddenly seem like manna from heaven.

If certain foods make your stomach turn, then don't eat, cook, or hang out near them. It's more important that you eat something, even if it's just bland foods, than not eat at all or spend these weeks feeling miserable.

DIETING DURING PREGNANCY: JUST SAY NO!

Remember, you don't need to consume a ton of extra calories a day to have a healthy pregnancy—just 300 extra calories a day is all it takes. Those 300 calories will go to your baby, not your hips, so you don't have to agonize about gaining weight. And you certainly shouldn't be thinking about dieting!

It's just not worth the risk unless you're very overweight, and even then, you should work very closely with your obstetrician or midwife and aim for a very slow loss. Otherwise, dieting during pregnancy is a dangerous mistake. During a diet, you try to cut back on calorie consumption. The easiest ways to do that is to cut back on fat consumption. This can lead to a deficiency in fat-soluble vitamins like vitamin E and A, both needed for your baby's growth. Plus, diets tend to cut back on dairy products-your main source of calcium and vitamin D during your pregnancy. Dieting makes it hard to eat healthfully. Instead, focus on foods with a low glycemic load. And reach for healthy foods like vegetables, beans, grains, low-fat dairy products, and fish, and you'll find your weight will sort itself out.

Look at it this way: How many times are people telling you *not* to diet? Relax and enjoy the break. There'll be plenty of time to diet once your baby is weaned.

Top Foods for The First Trimester

The first trimester is a time of rapid growth and change, and you need to support that growth and change with nutrient-packed foods. At the same time, it's a time when many women find it difficult to eat, especially if nausea, food aversions, and (for some) vomiting dominate their dietary choices.

Lucky for you, many of the top foods for the first trimester are both nutritious and easy on the stomach. There's no need to be stuck with a diet of soda crackers and flat ginger ale! You can eat bland foods and still get nutrients. Almonds, brown rice, applesauce, and oatmeal are just a few examples of foods that are good for you and easy to digest.

Folate is king during the first trimester and should be at the top of your list when considering which foods to eat during these months. Many of the top foods for the first trimester are packed with folate and other nutrients that support fetal growth and development. But they're also fairly bland and aren't hard to keep down.

Remember that these foods are just the beginning! Eating a well-balanced diet with a wide variety of foods is always a healthy choice.

HERE ARE THE 23 TOP FOODS FOR THE FIRST TRIMESTER:

- ALMONDS
- ANCHOVIES
- APPLESAUCE
- BANANAS
- BROTH
- BROWN RICE
- CHIVES
- CREAM CHEESE, PASTEURIZED
- GINGER
- ICE CHIPS AND WATER
- LAMB
- LEEKS
- LEMONS
- MINT TEA
- MULTIGRAIN CEREAL
- OATMEAL
- PEANUT BUTTER
- PINTO BEANS
- POPCORN
- SWEET POTATOES
- TAHINI
- TILAPIA
- WATERMELON

Let's look at each of these first-trimester favorites and see what makes them so great. And please, don't be afraid to try them! Even if foods like tahini and tilapia haven't yet made it onto your food radar, check out "Jonny's Tasty Tips" to find great ways to enjoy them.

★ Almonds

ALMONDS ARE A GREAT SOURCE OF FOLATE, one of the most important nutrients for you in the first trimester. Folate is the natural form of folic acid, and folic acid supplementation is recommended for prevention of birth defects. Eating foods such as almonds that contain folate can help boost you and your baby's folate levels, supporting a healthy pregnancy. In your handful of almonds (20 to 25 nuts) you'll find 10 mcg of folate. It's worth noting that if you're having more than one baby at a time—let's say twins—you probably need even *more* folate/folic acid.

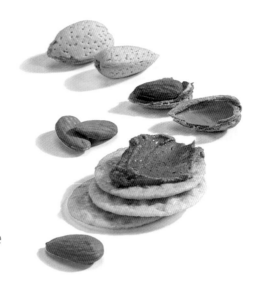

ALMONDS AT A GLANCE

Serving Size: 1 oz (85 g or 20-25 almonds)	**Calcium:** 8%
Calories: 169	**Vitamin A:** 0%
Saturated Fat: 1 g	**Vitamin C:** 0%
Protein: 6 g	**Iron:** 5%
Fiber: 3 g	

Note: The nutritional facts data provided in this book are approximations based on the foods' nutrient value and a pregnant woman's RDA.

Snack Light

Ignore the silly rumors that almonds are fattening. A study in the *British Journal of Nutrition* reported that eating up to two 1-ounce (20 to 25 almonds) servings of almonds per day helps you feel full and satisfied and also helps promote a healthy weight. When you eat this satisfying, nutritious, baby-supporting snack, feel good about choosing almonds!

Go Low

Research on nutrition in pregnancy suggests that reducing the glycemic load of foods may improve pregnancy outcome. *Glycemic load* is a phrase used to describe the impact that foods have on your blood sugar. Generally, low-glycemic-load foods are best (though there are exceptions). Foods with a low glycemic load, such as vegetables, nuts, and berries, are easy for your body to use. High-glycemic foods like sugar, white bread, and mashed potatoes break down into sugar very quickly, presenting a big sugar rush for your body to deal with. This is not good!

Research suggests that diets with a low glycemic load during pregnancy may reduce the risk of gestational diabetes and may also reduce the risk of having a baby that is considered large for his or her gestational age. Scientists aren't suggesting that you restrict your food intake during pregnancy, but that you should simply try to make healthier choices (nuts, seeds, fruits, vegetables, and high-fiber whole grains rather than processed foods, crackers, and cookies) to optimize your health and your baby's during pregnancy.

Jonny's Tasty Tips

One ounce of almonds (or a smear of almond butter) together with a piece of fruit like an apple makes a great snack. It's one of my favorites! The almond butter also tastes great smeared on a few sticks of celery. Either snack has only about 250 calories for guilt-free goodness!

Fighting Nuts

Almonds are a source of antioxidants, which are natural compounds that help you and your baby fight free radicals. A Canadian study found that compounds in almond skins have strong antioxidant activity. The researchers found high levels of four different types of flavonol glycosides, known to have positive antioxidant effects. The glycosides in almonds work together to fight free-radical damage, keeping you and your baby healthy.

Heart-Healthy Almonds

Studies have connected almond consumption with heart-healthy effects. Almonds elevate the good cholesterol in the blood (high-density lipoproteins, or HDL) and lower the levels of bad cholesterol (low-density lipoproteins, or LDL). Since almonds improve your blood circulation, more oxygen and nutrients can reach your baby, so he or she is sure to get all of the building blocks he or she needs to grow big and strong.

Grab a Handful

Almonds are one of the easiest foods to add into your diet. It's easy to carry a bag of almonds in your purse as a convenient snack to help ward off hunger, one of the main causes of nausea during the first trimester. Sprinkle some almonds on salads, eat them as a snack, or include them in your favorite trail mix or muesli. Or try some almond butter—it's delicious.

Buy almonds that are uniform in color and not withered or limp. Raw almonds are delicious, but if you prefer yours roasted, read the label and choose "dry roasted" almonds over "roasted"; dry-roasted almonds have not been cooked in oil. And check that the label doesn't include sugar, preservatives, or syrups, all of which counteract the healthy aspects of this baby-healthy food. Eat whole rather than peeled or blanched almonds, since the skin contains most of the baby-nourishing nutrients.

When storing almonds, remember that air, heat, and humidity can affect them. Almonds in the shell have the longest shelf life, but they're also less convenient. Storing your shelled almonds in a sealed bag in the fridge keeps them fresh longer. Almonds should smell nutty and sweet—a sharp or bitter odor suggests that they've turned rancid.

Anchovies

SURE, ANCHOVIES MAY NOT BE your most desired food right now if your first trimester is full of bouts of nausea and mad dashes to the toilet to vomit. However, some of you may actually be craving anchovies! (Yes, cravings are common during the first trimester.)

ANCHOVIES AT A GLANCE

Serving Size: 3 oz (85 g)	Calcium: 12%
Calories: 111	Vitamin A: 1%
Saturated Fat: 1 g	Vitamin C: 0%
Protein: 17 g	Iron: 13%
Fiber: 0 g	

Anchovies are a tasty, naturally salty snack. And they're full of protein that can help you feel full, a great strategy for avoiding feelings of nausea. So if these tiny fish don't make your stomach turn, order some on your pizza or crack open a can and enjoy them with some whole-grain crackers.

Good Fish Fat

The fats in anchovies are extremely healthy for both you and your baby. Anchovies and other small fish contain high amounts of omega-3 fatty acids called eicosapentaenoic acid acid (EPA) and docosahexaenoic acid (DHA). In a 3-ounce serving of anchovies, you'll find about 450 mg of EPA and 775 mg of DHA, which makes it a great source of these healthy fats. There is no recommended daily allowance (RDA) for EPA or DHA, but there is an RDA for linolenic acid, a precursor of these fats that is found in plants. The RDA for linolenic acid is 1.4 g. Researchers think pregnant women and their infants could benefit from 250 to 400 mg of DHA a day and maybe even more. Scientists have been discovering the amazing health benefits of these good fats and the devastation that occurs when you don't eat enough of them, including an increased risk of heart disease and mood-related problems. Omega-3 fatty acids are vital to brain cells, and during this first trimester, your baby's brain is forming at an amazingly fast rate. It needs a lot of omega-3s to develop optimally.

Check Out the Choline

You'll also find a lot of choline in your anchovies. You probably won't be breaking down your anchovies under a microscope to try to find this nutrient, but you should know that about 24 mg of choline can be found in half a can of anchovies. Choline may not be a vitamin by definition, but it is an essential nutrient. The body can only produce a small amount, so you need to get it from foods.

Most of the choline in your body is found in special fat molecules called phosphatidylcholine, lecithin, and sphingomyelin. (Don't worry—you'll never be asked to pronounce them, let alone spell them!) These fats are involved in cell signaling (communication between

FOLATE MAY NOT BE ENOUGH

Folate's ability to prevent neural-tube defects such as spina bifida is well known. Now researchers are discovering that choline may also play an important role in the proper formation of the neural tube in the fetus. In a case-control study involving more than 880 pregnant women, researchers found that women who consumed higher amounts of choline had up to a 72 percent lower risk of a neural-tube defect in their babies. Eating choline-rich foods like anchovies or eggs can help you lower your risk.

cells). Plus, choline is needed to make acetylcholine, an important neurotransmitter that is involved in controlling muscles, memory, and many other functions. Pregnant women need about 450 mg of choline daily to ensure that they are getting adequate amounts. Anchovies may not be the best source of choline, but there are others in this book like eggs (choline is in the yolks!), turkey, and salmon that can help you meet your needs.

If these little fish are tasty to you, then you should definitely dig in. Packed with calcium and iron, two nutrients your body is in higher need of these days, and full of good fats to support your mood and proper brain development in your baby, anchovies are an excellent food to include in your pregnancy diet. There is one warning though: There's a lot of sodium in anchovies, which is great for satisfying those salty-food cravings, but be sure to reduce your sodium intake in other areas of your diet and drink enough water to compensate.

Jonny's Tasty Tips

Anchovies are a classic ingredient of Caesar salad, which is a great way to add some anchovies to your menu. They're delicious with feta cheese and kalamata olives on Greek salads. Or try them in a Caesar variation with romaine lettuce, red onion, mandarin oranges, yellow or orange bell peppers, and shredded Asiago or Swiss cheese. A simple dressing of extra-virgin olive oil and balsamic vinegar is all you need to make this salad irresistible!

Applesauce

APPLESAUCE IS A GREAT FOOD FOR EVEN THE
pickiest eaters. But it's a perfect food for any
mothers-to-be who are suffering from morning
sickness! Applesauce is gentle on your stomach. It's packed with valuable nutrients for you
and your baby. And it's a good source of fluid
to help you stay hydrated. Grab a spoon and dig
into some applesauce—it's one of the very best
foods for your first trimester.

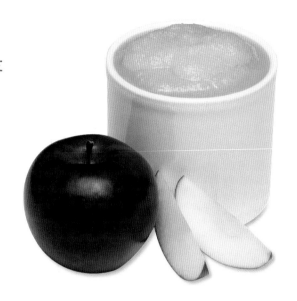

APPLESAUCE AT A GLANCE

Serving Size: 1 cup (244 g)	Calcium: 1%
Calories: 102	Vitamin A: 1%
Saturated Fat: 0 g	Vitamin C: 80%
Protein: 0 g	Iron: 2%
Fiber: 3 g	

Color Me Healthy

Flavonoids in the skin of apples are great antioxidants.
Flavonoids can help keep your body healthy by fighting
off damaging free radicals, and they help support your
immune system so you don't catch a cold or the flu.
And guess what? Apples are one of the best source of
flavonoids in the North American diet! Out of ten varieties of apples commonly consumed in the United States,
Fuji apples have the greatest amount of phenolic and
flavonoid compounds, and they are very high in antioxidant activity. Red Delicious apples are a close second.

Getting sick while you're pregnant can make you
feel even more exhausted than the pregnancy itself.
And you can't even turn to many common cold remedies to ease your symptoms, since they may not be
safe for your developing baby. So make sure you reach
for fruits and vegetables that are packed with vitamins
and other antioxidants like flavonoids to help you stay
healthy. Applesauce is a great place to start. If you are
making it from scratch, be sure to leave that skin on
since it's where you'll find a lot of the apple's healthy
compounds. And remember that the best way to eat
all of your applesauce—homemade or store-bought—is
to choose organic. Organic fruits and vegetables are
grown without pesticides and herbicides, which means
they are healthier for you. Plus, researchers have
found that organically grown fruits and vegetables
have higher amounts of flavonoids and other nutrients
than conventionally grown food, making an organic
apple or applesauce a super-healthy choice. When you
choose apples for their flavonoid content, remember:
the redder, the better!

Jonny's Tasty Tips

Believe it or not, it's super-easy to make your own applesauce! And when you make it yourself, you know it's healthy. But there are a few tricks that will help you make applesauce that's more delicious than any you can buy.

Here's all you have to do: Buy a mix of organic apples, including some red-skinned apples for those all-important antioxidant flavonoids and some tart, crisp apples like Granny Smith. (Look for apples like McIntosh and Rome that are recommended for cooking, rather than the famous fresh-eating apples like Red Delicious and Golden Delicious.)

Once you get your apples home, wash, slice, and core them and then toss the slices into a deep, heavy pot. Cook them covered on very low heat, stirring frequently to prevent sticking, until they soften and can be stirred into the thick but soupy consistency of applesauce. (Note: You can compost the cores or feed them to your dog—mine actually likes them, but then again she likes anything edible.)

Want to up the ante? Add even more antioxidant oomph by tossing in some fresh cranberries or a little pure cranberry juice. (Cranberry juice will turn your applesauce a beautiful, appetizing pink as well.) You can also stir in a little spice in the form of cinnamon or ginger to add antioxidants and help quell morning sickness.

Store your homemade applesauce in the fridge in a sealed container or can it for long-term storage. Besides eating it plain, you can use it as a topping for pancakes, yogurt, or frozen yogurt. Yum!!!

FRESH APPLE FACTS

If you enjoy getting your antioxidants from whole apples rather than applesauce, make sure your apples are fresh. Store apples in the refrigerator, and don't buy more than you can eat in a week. Fresh apples not only taste better, they have the highest antioxidant content. If you live in a northern climate, you may wonder how to find fresh apples out of season. But luckily, apples are one fruit that's grown year-round in various parts of the world, making fresh apples readily available most of the time.

Energy-Saving Practices

Fatigue is a major symptom of the first trimester and can leave some women feeling really lethargic. Saving your energy for important projects like getting to work and growing a baby is important, and antioxidants like the ones found in organic applesauce can help.

Quercetin is a powerful flavonoid found in apple skin and other produce like citrus fruits and onions. Quercetin battles with free radicals to prevent them from damaging the cells in your body—not to mention your baby's developing cells. Your body has to spend a lot of energy repairing the damage caused by free radicals. So eating foods that are packed with antioxidants can save your body energy, which is already in short supply during this very tiring first trimester.

Skip the Spray

You should know that apples are among the most heavily sprayed produce in North America. According to the Environmental Working Group's 2006 report "Shopper's Guide to Pesticides in Produce," apples are among the twelve foods on which pesticide residues have been most frequently found. Pesticides are toxic to your body and are even more damaging to your vulnerable growing baby.

Purchase organic applesauce or apples whenever possible to avoid pesticide consumption. If organic is not available (it should be, and it's definitely worth the extra expense!), use water or a special fruit and vegetable wash to wash the wax off the peel of your apple, since most of the pesticides end up in or just beneath the peel. But don't peel your apples, because the skin contains a lot of the good antioxidants and vitamins in the fruit. That's why we recommend buying organic! Make your apple crisps, apple pies, and applesauce with the whole apple and enjoy maximum goodness for both you and your baby.

THE RICHEST ANTIOXIDANT FOODS

The United States Department of Agriculture conducted a comprehensive study of the antioxidant content of more than 100 commonly consumed foods in 2004. Not surprisingly, the top of the list was dominated by fruits and vegetables. Some of the highest-ranking antioxidant-rich vegetables and fruits on the list were wild blueberries, cultivated blueberries, cranberries, artichoke hearts, blackberries, Red Delicious apples, Granny Smith apples, raspberries, prunes, strawberries, black plums, cherries, russet potatoes, plums, and Gala apples.

Bananas

PEEL A BANANA AND TAKE A BITE

or slice or mash it into your diet. Why? Because there are so many fabulous nutrients in bananas, plus they're easy on your stomach. One large banana contains 4 g of fiber and about 20 percent of your daily vitamin C and vitamin B6 needs.

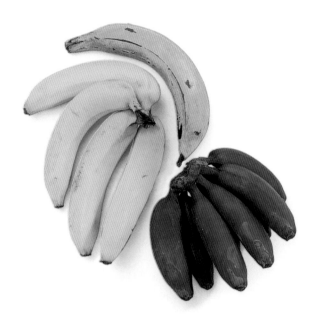

BANANAS AT A GLANCE

Serving Size: 1 large banana	Calcium: 1%
Calories: 121	Vitamin A: 2%
Saturated Fat: 0 g	Vitamin C: 20%
Protein: 1 g	Iron: 2%
Fiber: 4 g	

FAST FACT

Vitamin B6 helps alleviate morning sickness.

We've all heard that bananas are potassium-rich—a large banana contains about 480 mg of potassium, nearly one-fourth of your daily requirement. Plus, it contains close to 40 mcg of folate which as we've seen is a very important nutrient for your baby's neural-tube development. (The neural tube forms and closes in your first trimester, by the way, making it even more important to get plenty of folate right now!)

An "A-Peeling" Balance

Vitamin B6 helps regulate your sodium/potassium levels, which can be imbalanced if you're vomiting. Your large banana includes 0.5 mg of vitamin B6. For addi-tional help, bananas are also a good source of magnesium (37 mg) and potassium (480 mg), minerals needed for healthy fluid balance. Perhaps this combination of fluid-balancing nutrients is why eating bananas after vomiting is a common "old-wives'" home remedy.

Monkey Business

If you think bananas are for monkeys, listen up: Researchers have found that there is certainly no monkey business behind the healthy benefits of eating bananas. People who consume diets rich in potassium are 50 percent less likely to have a stroke compared to their non-potassium-consuming peers, according to a study recently published in *Neurology*. Potassium also fights high blood pressure. And researchers at the

University of California, San Francisco, found that bananas may prevent osteoporosis in postmenopausal women.

True, these studies aren't about pregnancy, but they do show some pregnancy-related health benefits to eating bananas:

1) Adding bananas to your diet during pregnancy can help you keep your blood pressure at a healthy level. High blood pressure in later pregnancy can lead to complications such as eclampsia.

2) Getting plenty of calcium is vital if you're pregnant because your growing baby is pulling this mineral from your bones. If bananas can help postmenopausal women keep their bones healthy, they can help you, too.

Bananas Go Low

Bananas are also bursting with phytochemicals such as myricetin (a potent antioxidant that is thought to help lower blood sugar) and beta-sitosterol (may help lower bad cholesterol levels). Low blood sugar levels and healthy cholesterol levels are part of a healthy pregnancy.

Morning-Sickness Approved

If you're pregnant, morning sickness can be the worst part of your first trimester. Morning sickness doesn't affect all pregnant women, but if it strikes, you can experience a feeling of nausea at particular times or even throughout the whole day. For some women, it may include vomiting.

Especially if your morning sickness makes you vomit, try to eat foods that are bland, acceptable to an upset stomach, and packed with minerals that help restore your body's fluid balance, which is disrupted during vomiting. Bananas are just what the doctor ordered: They're bland, good on a queasy stomach, and packed with potassium to help you get your fluid balance back quickly.

With all of these healthy reasons to eat bananas, it's no surprise that they're the leading fresh fruit sold in North America.

BANANAS FOR GOOD BLOOD PRESSURE

Healthy blood pressure is important for a healthy pregnancy. In the DASH (Dietary Approach to Stop Hypertension) Study, consuming 8 to 10 servings of vegetables and fruit per day, along with an overall healthy diet, was associated with a decrease in blood pressure normally only achieved with the use of medication. Potassium, found in good quantities in bananas, is just one of the nutrients found in fruits and vegetables that help maintain normal blood pressure.

Jonny's Tasty Tips

Bananas and rice are a famous home remedy for an upset stomach, but if you're not feeling sick, try these instead: Slice a banana lengthwise and smear a little peanut butter (and/or sprinkle peanut pieces) on each cut side; or slice a banana into plain or vanilla yogurt; or add strawberries to make your own version of strawberry-banana.

You can make a great smoothie by blending a cup of yogurt, a sliced banana, and a cup of crushed ice until thick and smooth. Try it with plain yogurt and a handful of fresh or frozen strawberries, a banana, and a splash of orange juice for a luscious, refreshing treat!

Craving ice cream? Make a healthy banana split with a banana cut lengthwise and topped with frozen yogurt, fresh berries (any combination of strawberries, blueberries, cherries, and/or raspberries), and sliced almonds. It is both decadent and delicious!

Broth

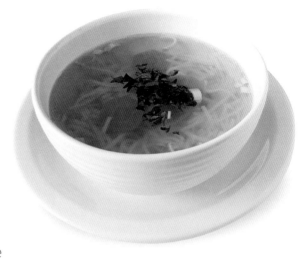

IT'S DEFINITELY NOT THE HEALTHIEST FOOD on earth, but broth can be a godsend in your first trimester. It contains nutrients that are vital if you're suffering from vomiting due to morning sickness, including sodium and potassium. These two minerals help your body retain the proper water balance, something you'll have knocked out of balance if you've been vomiting. Broth is also a great antidote to morning sickness because it's mostly water, and vomiting can lead to dehydration, a very unhealthy state for a growing baby. Another plus: Broth is bland and easy to swallow, even for the most nauseated of pregnant women.

BROTH AT A GLANCE

Serving Size: 1 cup	Calcium: 0%
Calories: 12	Vitamin A: 0%
Saturated Fat: 0 g	Vitamin C: 9%
Protein: 0 g	Iron: 0%
Fiber: 0 g	

Note: Chicken, beef, and fish broth will contain more saturated fat, protein, and iron.

FAST FACT

Nausea and vomiting are the most common symptoms experienced in early pregnancy, with nausea affecting 70 to 85 percent of women. About half of pregnant women experience vomiting.

Salty Soup

Some brands of broth are much higher in sodium than others, so make sure you read the labels when you choose a broth. Look for a brand that has low sodium and other healthy features, such as being organic and/or MSG-free. Remember, "low sodium" is not "no sodium." Some sodium can be helpful if you're vomiting regularly, since vomiting can cause your body's natural fluid balance to become disrupted. But too much sodium can cause your blood pressure to rise, a state that is not healthy for your growing baby. Your broth can have various amounts of sodium, but a commonly used canned chicken broth (reduced sodium) contains about 550 mg of sodium per cup.

Three Kinds of Broth

There are three types of broth: chicken, beef, and fish. Chicken broth offers niacin, riboflavin, selenium, and protein. Beef broth contains some protein, riboflavin, and niacin. Fish broth offers niacin, protein, and some omega fatty acids. One is not particularly healthier than the others, but if your stomach allows you, try adding all three to your diet. As with all foods, variety and moderation are always best.

Hidden Nutrients

In each mouthful of this clear and watery liquid are some healthy nutrients for you and your baby, including the B vitamins niacin and riboflavin. These vitamins play an important role in your body's energy metabolism. They can help both you and your baby use fats, carbohydrates, and proteins to make energy needed for growth, health, and happiness. Plus, you'll find some protein in broth (about 3 g per cup of chicken broth and 1 g per cup of beef broth from boullion cubes). As we've mentioned earlier, protein is typically lacking in women's diets, yet it not only plays a vital role in energy production, it's essential for the healthy development of your baby's organs, which are forming in your first trimester.

Jonny's Tasty Tips

Broth is bland, and that can be really good if you're feeling nauseated. But there are ways to kick it up a bit if you really don't want another mug of plain, clear liquid. How about a one-two-three anti-nausea punch? Add a little cooked brown rice (see the next entry) and some peeled, minced fresh gingerroot to chicken broth. All three will help settle your stomach.

Sound appealing? If you're not fighting morning sickness, you can make an even more wholesome and flavorful soup by adding some sliced shiitake mushrooms and chopped chives or sliced green onions (scallions) to the basic broth, rice, and ginger. Cubed tofu or chicken will make it even more satisfying.

Here's another tip: If plain broth doesn't appeal to you and you're not much of a soup person, you can always add the benefits of broth to your meals by sneaking it in: Cook your brown rice in broth instead of water. Simmer meat in broth and then reduce it to make gravy. Replace water with broth when you're cooking pasta (or pasta sauce) or making dishes like stew and chili. Broth is also a good replacement for oil in stir-fries and other sautéed dishes.

★ Brown Rice

MORNING SICKNESS, THE BEST-KNOWN symptom of the first trimester of pregnancy, can have many women looking for bland and nutritious foods. Brown rice is a great option. If you're a white-rice girl, don't panic: Brown rice has come quite a way from the days of all-brown health foods. Now you can enjoy brown rice that's as good as it is good for you!

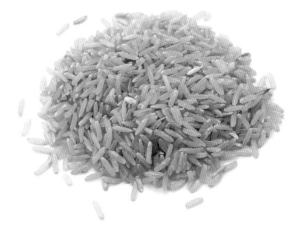

BROWN RICE AT A GLANCE

Serving Size: 1 cup (195 g) of medium-cooked brown rice	Calcium: 2%
Calories: 218	Vitamin A: 0%
Saturated Fat: 0 g	Vitamin C: 9%
Protein: 5 g	Iron: 5%
Fiber: 4 g	

Brown rice may seem bland, but inside those mild-mannered grains lurk a powerhouse of nutrients. Brown rice is packed with many minerals and a wide variety of B vitamins. Brown rice contains niacin, magnesium, manganese, phosphorus, and selenium. Niacin is a coenzyme needed for energy production, a process you'll want to have working at top speed to help combat the fatigue commonly experienced during the first trimester. There are 2.5 mg of niacin per cup of brown rice. More important, many studies have found that vitamin B6 plays a role in combating first-trimester morning sickness. Ensuring that your diet contains sufficient vitamin B6 can alleviate this undesirable symptom.

Studies have found that getting 25 mg of vitamin B6 every 8 hours for 72 to 96 hours decreases nausea and vomiting in pregnancy. But that's a lot of brown rice to eat (about 75 cups every 8 hours)! So in these studies, they used supplements of vitamin B6 to combat morning sickness. If you just want relief from nausea associated with morning sickness, as little as 10 mg of vitamin B6 may work. Other sources of vitamin B6 in your diet include breakfast cereals, which are fortified with this vitamin in North America. You can also load up on sweet peppers, sunflower seeds, and wheat bran—all of which are featured in *100 Healthiest Foods for Pregnancy*.

Fiber-rific

Brown rice is also a good source of fiber. Fiber is a real workhorse in your healthy pregnancy diet: It helps keep blood pressure, cholesterol, and sugar levels low, while helping you feel full. One strategy for battling back against morning sickness is to not get hungry—fullness can help nausea symptoms subside.

WHITE VERSUS BROWN

White rice accounts for most of the rice eaten worldwide, but brown rice is the nutritional champion. Brown rice is the whole grain of rice, while white rice has had the bran layer removed. Stripping the grain of its bran layer strips it of a majority of its vitamins, minerals, and fiber. Check it out: A cup of brown rice contains about 4 g of fiber, about four times more than in the same amount of white rice. It's way better for you!

The glycemic index is a measurement of how quickly a food you eat will turn into sugar in your body and how quickly your blood sugar levels will rise in response. Foods that cause your blood sugar to rise to high levels quickly are called high-glycemic foods, like white rice. These high blood sugar levels are hard on your body and can be toxic, leading to damage of the small blood vessels in your eyes and kidneys. During pregnancy, some women are at risk of developing gestational diabetes. This is usually a temporary problem, when your body can't control your sugar levels properly. But it can lead to damage to your body's small blood vessels and a big or overweight baby. Plus, high-glycemic foods promote fat storage! It's best to go brown when it comes to rice, and reach for other low-glycemic foods (these tend to be high in fiber).

Jonny's Tasty Tips

Bland, sweet, delicious–brown rice pudding is all that and more! It's also nutritious and packed with fiber. Search online for a good brown rice pudding recipe or experiment with substituting brown rice for white in your favorite recipe. (Remember that brown rice takes longer to cook and absorbs more liquid than white rice, so you might want to start with a recipe developed specifically for brown rice.)

Brown rice pudding is a great comfort food, and it's also a good way to satisfy your sweet tooth, especially if you toss in some raisins and/or cranberries. But please keep an eye on those calories! If your recipe calls for a lot of cream and sweetener, they can add up fast. Try substituting the cream for skim milk and the sweetener for a bit of honey or your favorite dried fruit. Remember portion control: An ice-cream-scoop-size serving is about right. Fortunately, brown rice pudding keeps well in the fridge and also reheats well if you like yours hot.

Craving a savory rice dish instead? Topping brown rice with a stir-fry, curry, ratatouille, or bean or lentil dish will give you great flavor, and it's filling. But stick to that ice-cream-scoop serving of rice! Even brown rice is fairly high on the glycemic index.

As for white rice, especially instant white rice, I have one thing to say: It makes a much better packing material than a food!

Chives

SPRINKLE SOME CHIVES ON YOUR NEXT meal and enjoy their pregnancy-healthy nutrients, including vitamin K, folate, and iron. In fact, these small, mild-tasting green onions may be seriously nutritionally underestimated. Seen as a garnish, chives tend to get overlooked. Chives are a source of thiamin, niacin, panthothenic acid, phosphorus, and zinc. And they're also a source of fiber, vitamin A, vitamin C, riboflavin, vitamin B6, calcium, magnesium, potassium, copper, and manganese.

CHIVES AT A GLANCE

Serving Size: 2 Tbsp (3 g) chopped	Calcium: 1%
Calories: 2	Vitamin A: 4%
Saturated Fat: 0 g	Vitamin C: 4%
Protein: 0 g	Iron: 1%
Fiber: 0.2 g	

A Tasty Way to Get Folate

Folic acid may be the most important nutrient of the first trimester. As we've discussed earlier in this chapter, folate is required for your baby's neural tube to close. Without it, the fetus is likely to have structural defects that could be fatal. This may explain why studies have found that women with low levels of folate have been more likely to suffer from recurrent miscarriages. Today, folate is recommended as a supplement to all women of childbearing age, and the laws of many countries require that it be added to many foods, including cereals and breads. Just a sprinkle of a few tablespoons of chives on your dinner can help increase your folate consumption—there are 6.4 mcg per 2 tablespoons of chopped fresh chives.

Two for the Price of One

One of the most exciting nutritional facts about chives is that they contain both vitamin C and iron. For proper iron absorption, your body needs vitamin C, and this delicious herb gives you both (about 3.5 mg of vitamin C and 0.1 mg of iron per 2 tablespoons). Sure, it may not be a lot, but it's a tasty way to boost the nutritional value of your meal. For a food with more vitamin C, check out acerola cherries, and look at apricots for iron; both are stars in *100 Healthiest Foods to Eat During Pregnancy*.

Mega Mineral

Don't be one of the women who doesn't understand the importance of getting plenty of magnesium during her pregnancy! In bone health, magnesium receives a lot of attention, but in pregnancy, its role is forgotten. Magnesium can help alleviate constipation, a common symptom during pregnancy. It also helps regulate blood pressure and insulin/blood sugar levels. Plus, magnesium is useful in preventing leg cramps, a common complaint in later stages of pregnancy. Your sprinkle of chives has about 12 mg of magnesium in it. Researchers have found that magnesium may even help alleviate pregnancy-related leg cramps (luckily not a symptom suffered by a majority of pregnant women). In fact, magnesium is involved in more than 300 cellular reactions, making it very important to your health and the health of your growing baby. A pregnant woman needs about 350 mg of magnesium a day.

Pass Them Around

Chives are easy to find at your local market, and they're also easy to grow at home. With their very mild taste and vibrant green color, chives are a fun addition to almost every meal. Sprinkle some on your salad or soup. Or go with the all-time favorite and sprinkle them on your potato. They're also a great addition to salsas, salad dressings, and pasta dishes.

Jonny's Tasty Tips

Here are more great ways to eat chives: Mix chopped chives into softened cream cheese before you spread it on a bagel, cracker, tortilla chip, or slice of bread. Stir them into dips. Add them to hummus. If you like cheese spreads, top that cracker with some cheese and chives. Mix them into low-fat cottage cheese, or top a sliced tomato with a scoop of cottage cheese and a colorful sprinkling of chives. I also enjoy chives topping a sliver of Cheddar or other flavorful cheese on a mini-slice of hard whole-grain rye or pumpernickel bread.

Cream Cheese, pasteurized

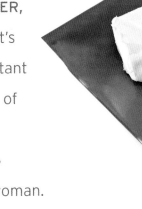

A PERFECT FOOD FOR THE FIRST TRIMESTER, cream cheese is both bland and nutritious. It's packed with calcium, one of the most important nutrients for pregnant women. Just 1 ounce of low-fat cream cheese (about 2 tablespoons) contains about 50 mg of calcium, which is 5 percent of your daily needs as a pregnant woman. Calcium plays a role in almost every system in your body.

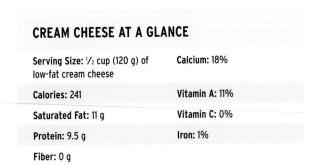

CREAM CHEESE AT A GLANCE

Serving Size: ½ cup (120 g) of low-fat cream cheese	Calcium: 18%
Calories: 241	Vitamin A: 11%
Saturated Fat: 11 g	Vitamin C: 0%
Protein: 9.5 g	Iron: 1%
Fiber: 0 g	

Grow Big and Strong

Every mother wants her child to grow up to be big, strong, and healthy. This is only possible if you and your baby both get plenty of calcium. As early as the first trimester, calcium is playing an important role in your pregnancy. It is involved in the release and uptake of hormones, which have been raging in new ways since you conceived to make sure your body is ready to support the needs of pregnancy. (This role in supporting hormone metabolism may explain why calcium is known to help alleviate PMS symptoms).

Calcium also plays a vital role in your baby's bone formation. Fetal bone mineralization can only take place if there's enough calcium present. Your baby's source of calcium is your blood. If your blood levels of calcium aren't high enough due to a calcium-poor diet, then your own bones will give up calcium to help maintain your blood levels. Over the 40 weeks of pregnancy, your bones could be giving up a lot of calcium if your diet is lacking in calcium. Fortunately, eating calcium-rich foods like cream cheese is an enjoyable way to add more calcium to your diet (which is more than you can say for those horse-pill-size calcium supplements).

Ten Fingers, Ten Toes

"She's healthy: She has ten little fingers and ten little toes." It's funny that many people describe the health of their newborn by the number of fingers and toes they have; but it's true, and calcium found in dairy foods like cream cheese can help ensure that all of these digits are properly formed. Even though the bones are just beginning to form toward the end of the first trimester, calcium is as important during the first trimester as during later stages of pregnancy. In fact, your baby's fingernails and toenails are beginning to form around the twelfth week of pregnancy.

Fast Firing

Calcium also plays a role in nerve transmission, the passing of a message from your brain to parts of your body. In the first trimester, your baby's brain is developing into its lobes. By the end of the first trimester, it will be developing more than 250,000 new neurons every minute! Cream cheese contributes to your baby's brain through its calcium content, of course, but it also contains choline (3.5 mg per 2 tablespoons or 1 ounce), an important nutrient for brain development.

Cream cheese is a good first-trimester food because of its calcium content, bland flavor, and gentleness on a nauseated stomach. It also contains riboflavin, vitamin B12, folate, and phosphorus. Try to choose low-fat varieties of cream cheese and even then eat it in moderation, since it's high in saturated fat and cholesterol.

SKIP THESE CHEESES!

National health agencies around the world advise pregnant women not to eat soft, mold-ripened cheeses, such as Brie and Camembert, and blue-veined cheeses, such as Danish blue and Stilton, if they're made from unpasteurized milk. This is because these cheeses are more inclined to allow the growth of bacteria, such as listeria, which can harm your unborn child.

Jonny's Tasty Tips

A smear of cream cheese on multigrain toast makes a great on-the-go breakfast. Craving something sweet? Add a dab of apple butter or marmalade. For a healthy snack, spread a little cream cheese on carrot slices or Belgian endive leaves or try it instead of peanut butter or pimiento cheese on a celery stalk. Celery and cream cheese pack a one-two punch for your bones, since the cream cheese is loaded with calcium and celery is a great source of silicon, another important nutrient for bone, skin, and joint health.

Ginger

A 2001 SURVEY OF PREGNANT WOMEN FOUND that the most common reason for using a natural health product was to relieve nausea and vomiting. The most frequently cited herb was ginger.

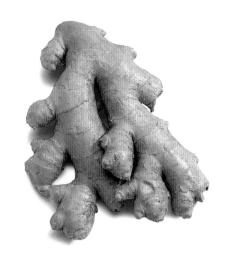

GINGER AT A GLANCE

Serving Size: 1 oz (28 g) raw root	Calcium: 0%
Calories: 22	Vitamin A: 0%
Saturated Fat: 0 g	Vitamin C: 2%
Protein: 1 g	Iron: 1%
Fiber: 1 g	

FAST FACT

Ginger is the most commonly recommended herb for morning sickness, according to surveyed certified midwives.

Nixing the Nausea

The efficacy of ginger against morning sickness has been clinically evaluated in five randomly controlled trials. At a daily dose of 500 mg, ginger reduced nausea but not vomiting in these studies. However, 1,000 mg of ginger given in four 250-mg doses throughout the day did significantly reduce frequency of vomiting in four clinical trials.

What's in It?

Ginger is a root with a hot and pungent flavor that's a great addition to stir-fries and salad dressings. The active nutrients in ginger include gingerol, gingerdione, shogaol, sesquiterpene, and monoterpene volatile oils. Ginger's anti-nausea abilities are likely caused by gingerol. Ginger's ability to help fight nausea is related to its ability to increase motility in the intestinal tract.

Ginger also has anti-inflammatory properties and may interact in a positive way with the central nervous system (it acts on serotonin receptors, your feel-good trigger).

Safety First!

Taking ginger orally for medicinal purposes at appropriate dosages is considered generally safe for pregnant women. You may read in some places that using ginger during pregnancy could be risky. But you can have confidence in the safety of ginger, knowing that a study done at one of the leading children's hospitals in the world found it safe. The Hospital for Sick Children in Toronto, Canada, reported that their study, involving 187 women, found no increase in the rate of malformations, and the ginger had a positive effect on reducing nausea and vomiting during pregnancy. In the clinical studies done on ginger, no adverse effects have been reported. Yet caution is still indicated when ginger is taken in larger quantities (as a high-dosage supplement) since in high doses ginger may act as an abortifacient (a substance that causes miscarriage) and emmenogogue (promotes menstrual bleeding). Another good reason to stick with the actual food during pregnancy!

Ginger versus Vitamin B6

Researchers from the University of Adelaide in Australia reported the results of a randomized study in 2004 that involved 291 pregnant women. Half of the women took 1.05 g of ginger or 75 mg of vitamin B6, and they found that ginger was as effective as vitamin B6 at reducing morning sickness. On the other hand, a study done by researchers at the University of Naples reported in 2005 that when six trials were reviewed, involving a total of 675 women, ginger was considered to be more effective than vitamin B6, and both were superior to a placebo. It may not be clear which of these two are best for combating morning sickness, but what *is* clear is that they're both effective.

Jonny's Tasty Tips

Don't forget that you can drink your ginger, too! I enjoy hot ginger tea with lemon. And I love the pungent, delicious taste of ginger ale. Remember one thing, though: If you're drinking it to reduce the symptoms of morning sickness, make sure the brand you buy contains real ginger as one of the ingredients!

Ice Chips and Water

SMALL ICE CHIPS ARE WET, COLD, AND PERFECT for your first-trimester needs. Nurses offer ice chips to patients after surgery if they are suffering from nausea. You can try the same practice to help soothe your stomach after vomiting. Or simply suck on ice chips throughout the day to help keep yourself hydrated.

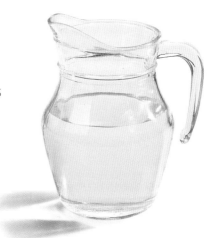

WATER AT A GLANCE

Serving Size: 1 cup of generic bottled water	Magnesium: 1% (4.7 mg)
Calories: 0	Sodium: 0% (5 mg)
Calcium: 2% (24 mg)	

Note: There are no calories, fats, proteins, fiber, iron, vitamin A, or vitamin C in generic bottled water.

FAST FACT

Feeling thirsty is a sign that you're already dehydrated.

Chip Away at Dehydration

Hydration is extremely important during pregnancy and can help you feel better. Constipation, preterm labor, fatigue, and miscarriage can be related to dehydration. Chewing on some ice chips can help you quench your feeling of nausea and fight dehydration. It is very important that you have enough water in your body. Water flushes waste products from the cells in your body and helps your liver and kidneys function better. It does the same things in your baby too. During pregnancy, your blood volume increases significantly, and water is needed for this additional volume. Thus, your needs for water are greatly increased during pregnancy. Water is also very important after labor to support milk production and flow.

Three Ways to Stay Hydrated

Most women know that staying hydrated during pregnancy is very important, but it can be hard to make sure you're getting enough fluids. One trick is to work with ice chips. Besides being a great way to ward off nausea and to calm your stomach after vomiting, ice chips are a fun, crunchy snack on hot days. And, if you're like many women who complain that they just don't like drinking water, you may find ice chips a good alternative.

Don't feel like eating? It's common when your stomach is queasy to avoid eating. But you and your baby need water and nutrients. If you simply can't eat, work with ice chips to help restimulate your appetite and calm your stomach. Once you're feeling better, try to increase your water intake to make up for any dehydration you may have suffered while queasy. One way is to fill a pitcher each morning with the amount of fluid you want to drink and keep it near your desk or on the counter. It will be a visual reminder to keep on drinking, and you can monitor your progress by watching the water level drop in the pitcher. Or set a timer to remind you to stop, get a drink, and stretch your legs.

How Much?

Pregnant women typically need between eight and twelve 8-ounce glasses of water per day. You can get this in with ice chips if you prefer. Simply fill a glass with ice chips and start nibbling on them. One glass of ice chips is about the same as one glass of water. If the weather is warm or you are exercising, you'll need even more. Ice chips are also a great food for pregnant women during the heat of summer. You can find it hard to cool off in the summer when you're pregnant. Ice chips are a cool way to munch your way to health. Dry environments, such as deserts, airplanes, and heated buildings in cold climates, will also cause your body to dehydrate faster. How do you know if you've had enough water? Many people think they are drinking enough if they aren't thirsty. But it's important to know that feeling thirsty is a sign that you are already dehydrated.

FAST FACT

Feeling tired? Dehydration can cause fatigue. Try increasing your water consumption for a few days and then see if you feel better.

Jonny's Tasty Tips

Water, water everywhere—But is it too boring? Then why not squeeze some fresh lime or lemon juice into your water or even give it a splash of your favorite 100 percent pure fruit juice. (Choose fresh juice, not juice made from concentrate.) Try ice chips or freezing juice in your ice cub tray. Juice, milk, and some herb teas are also good hydrating choices. (See the Mint Tea entry on page 58 for one of the best herb teas.)

Lamb

MARY HAD A LITTLE LAMB, WHICH SHE ATE during her first trimester because her cravings were so bad she was eating everything that wasn't secured to the wall with bolts. Plus, her lamb offered her and her baby an abundance of healthy nutrients to make them strong and healthy. Yes, lamb is not only very tasty, but it's packed with pregnancy-healthy nutrients like vitamin B6, iron, and protein.

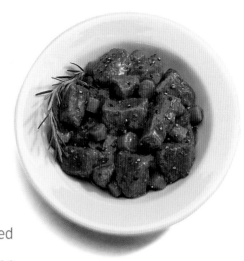

LAMB AT A GLANCE

Serving Size: 100 g fresh, lean lamb	**Calcium:** 2%
Calories: 165	**Vitamin A:** 0%
Saturated Fat: 4 g	**Vitamin C:** 0%
Protein: 19 g	**Iron:** 6%
Fiber: 0 g	

Feel-Good Food

Most women simply don't get enough protein in their diets. And since protein is needed for cell growth and blood production, when you're pregnant you need to be eating even more protein—a *lot* more. In fact, in your first 2 months of pregnancy, your blood volume increases by 40 to 50 percent. You need plenty of protein to produce that much blood.

If that isn't a good enough reason to up your protein intake, then consider this: The symptoms of protein deficiency are common symptoms associated with pregnancy—fatigue, vomiting, and loss of appetite. If you're feeling fatigue, vomiting, or experiencing a loss of appetite, try to eat more protein—it just might do the trick and kick these symptoms right out the door!

Smart Choice

Would you believe it if we told you lamb is a source of the essential fatty acid DHA (docosahexaenoic acid)? It's true. It isn't the most potent source of DHA available, but it's still pretty good. In a small serving of lamb (about 100 g), your body—and your baby—will receive 120 mg of DHA. That's close to half of the recommended daily dosage for growing brains, and as we've seen, during the first trimester, your baby's brain is hard at work forming lobes and creating hundreds of thousands of neurons.

Good Value

Just look at what a great nutritional value lamb is! Lamb is a good source of vitamin B6, pantothenic acid, phosphorus, manganese, riboflavin, niacin, vitamin B12, iron, zinc, copper, and selenium. Vitamin B6 can help fight morning sickness. Vitamin B12 is one of the most difficult vitamins to get in your diet since it is only available from animal sources. This is one of your key energy vitamins, and eating 100 g of lamb can offer your body 50 percent of your daily intake (3 mcg) of vitamin B12 to help you kick those first-trimester fatigue symptoms.

Lamb is rich in minerals, too. You need plenty of iron to support your drastic increase in blood volume and to help your baby create red blood cells. A serving of lamb contains about 1.4 mg of iron. Zinc helps support your immune system, which might help you avoid the common cold. Lamb offers 5.2 mg of zinc per 100 g—that's about 50 percent of your daily needs. And selenium is a potent antioxidant that also helps your skin maintain its elasticity while your belly grows. With 8 mcg of selenium and all of these other healthy nutrients, your serving of lamb is packed with many of the resources your body needs to stay strong, look great, and grow a healthy baby.

Spring Shopping

Since lamb is available in late spring, an event that occurs twice a year (once in the Northern Hemisphere, and once in the Southern Hemisphere), there is usually fresh lamb available. If the price of a rack of lamb scares you, than look for lamb shanks, which can turn out beautifully if left in a slow cooker for a few hours with your favorite vegetables and some liquid. Or, try mild-tasting lamb chops, which are easy to substitute in your diet for a pork chop or chicken. You can even cook them the same way if you like. Frozen lamb is also a healthy option if fresh is not available.

Jonny's Tasty Tips

Wait, you say you've never eaten lamb! Isn't lamb and rice the stuff they put in dog food? Yes, it is, because it's easy to digest and high in protein and other essential nutrients. And if you've ever seen a dog scarfing down a lamb-and-rice dinner, you might get the idea that he knows something you don't: Lamb is actually delicious. That's the reason it's a traditional Easter treat and is savored in Mediterranean cuisines, and it's also the reason why rack of lamb will cost you the big bucks at gourmet restaurants. Yum!

So give lamb a chance. If you love pork chops, you'll be in heaven when you try lamb chops. Or try lamb Greek-fashion, cubed and grilled on kebabs with chunks of sweet onion and mushrooms and served up in a warm minted yogurt sauce with lemon over brown rice. Talk about healthy and satisfying!

Leeks

LEEKS ARE THE VEGETABLE EQUIVALENT OF A SUPER

multivitamin-mineral tablet. Leeks are a great source
of vitamin A, vitamin C, and iron. Plus, leeks
contain fiber, B vitamins, iron, and
other minerals.

LEEKS AT A GLANCE

Serving Size: 1 cup (89 g)	Calcium: 5%
Calories: 54	Vitamin A: 28%
Saturated Fat: 0 g	Vitamin C: 15%
Protein: 1 g	Iron: 8%
Fiber: 2 g	

Not Your Ordinary Onion

Leeks look like huge green onions (scallions), which
is no surprise since they're both in the onion family.
But leeks have a very mild, sweet flavor, making them
especially appealing if you're suffering from morning
sickness in the first trimester. You can slice them up
and add them to your stir-fry or use them to make a
warm, soothing leek and potato soup. Packed with fiber
and water, leeks are a great vegetable to include in
your first-trimester diet.

What's in a Leek?

Let's take a closer look at the nutrients found
in leeks and why they're so important for you
and your baby during the first trimester. First
of all, leeks are a nondairy source of calcium (55 mg
per cup). As you know, calcium is essential for the
development of your baby's bones, fingernails, and
toenails, all of which are forming toward the end of
your first trimester. Calcium's important for you, too.
Besides keeping your own bones and teeth strong and
healthy, it may help combat some common symptoms
of pregnancy, including irritability, insomnia, and back
and leg pains.

Leeks are a good source of folate. There is close
to 60 mcg of folate in a cup of leeks—that's about
8 percent of your daily needs as a pregnant woman.
And as we've seen, folate helps ensure that your
baby's spinal cord forms and closes properly. Leeks
are also high in vitamin B6 (pyridoxine), which is
necessary for your body to metabolize energy from
the carbohydrates, fats, and proteins in your diet.

There's also evidence that vitamin B6 can help alleviate morning sickness. A cup of leeks contains 0.2 mg of vitamin B6 (about 10 percent of your RDA).

There's more: Leeks are a good source of iron and magnesium and an even better source of vitamin K and manganese. Vitamin K is needed for proper clot formation and healthy bone growth. You'll need plenty of iron to help produce the millions of red blood cells forming in your baby. Manganese is not as well known, but it is an important mineral in your body since it helps support normal skeletal development, which is vital to your growing baby. In a cup of leeks there are 40 mcg of vitamin K, 2 mg of iron, 25 mg of magnesium, and 0.4 mg of manganese.

Healthy Brains

Choline is an important nutrient for the growth and development of your baby's brain and nervous system. It is not commonly discussed in nutrition books on pregnancy, but it should be! You should aim for 450 mg of choline a day during pregnancy. You can get a bit of that through leeks, which contain a small amount of choline, about 9 mg per cup.

Jonny's Tasty Tips

Leeks are so delicious that once you start using them in food, you'll never want to stop. But here's a tip: As leeks grow, they act like magnets for sandy grit. And since you're not a chicken, you want to leave that part out of your meals! When I prepare leeks, I like to cut off the fibrous green tops (save the delicious green part of the stems) and the base (the bottom part with the roots, though I know one nutrition expert who actually washes and cooks the roots for their nutrient content) and slice the stem in half. Then I rinse it thoroughly to wash out any hidden grit before placing each half-stem cut-side-down on a cutting board and slicing it.

Now I'm ready to add those sliced leeks to soups, sauces, and stir-fries. Yum! If your stomach's a little sensitive but you can't face plain broth, try adding sliced leek and shiitake mushrooms with some finely minced fresh ginger. (For even more body, add a half-cup of brown rice to the pot or a tablespoon per bowl.) Now that's good eating!

Lemons

THESE SUNNY CITRUS FRUITS MAY NOT be sweet, but they're packed with healthy nutrients for you and your baby. And while you might not feel like sucking on a lemon as an afternoon snack, they're wonderful at accentuating the flavors of other foods and make a great addition to a boring glass of water.

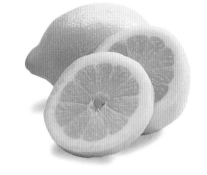

LEMONS AT A GLANCE

Serving Size: 1 fruit without seeds (108 g)	**Calcium:** 7%
Calories: 22	**Vitamin A:** 1%
Saturated Fat: 0 g	**Vitamin C:** 125%
Protein: 1 g	**Iron:** 3%
Fiber: 5 g	

SNIFF A LEMON

One simple strategy for staving off morning sickness is to sniff a lemon. The fresh, crisp smell of a fresh lemon can ward off nausea and vomiting for some women. You can even try carrying around a zipper-lock bag of cut lemons while you're at work or out doing errands. Take a sniff and feel better!

Packed with C

Mostly water and vitamin C, lemons offer moms-to-be some serious health benefits. Here's why: Vitamin C is one of the most important antioxidants in nature. This water-soluble vitamin travels around your bloodstream and neutralizes free radicals, preventing them from damaging the inside and outside of your body's cells. Vitamin C protects your baby's developing cells, too. And lemons have about 20 mg of vitamin C in each ounce of juice!

Vitamin C also plays an important role in supporting your immune system. The immune system's main goal is to protect you from illness. A little extra vitamin C in the form of a squeeze of lemon into your glass of water may be useful in preventing and fighting conditions like the common cold.

Long-Lasting Nutrition

There are two other nutritional gems hiding in lemons: flavonol glycosides and limonin. Flavonols are great antioxidants, like vitamin C, and may have some antibiotic-like effects as well. Scientists from the United States Agricultural Research Service have shown that our bodies can absorb and utilize limonin, a very long-acting antioxidant. And limonin is thought to help lower bad cholesterol levels. That squeeze of lemon offers you a lot more than you think!

Skin Support

The first trimester may seem early to think about stretch marks—you may not even be showing yet!—but the baby growing inside your uterus is going to get bigger and bigger, and eventually your belly will start to grow too. In your second and third trimester, the skin around your belly will be asked to stretch...and stretch...and stretch. Ouch! Now's the time to get your skin ready with the help of vitamin C. Vitamin C helps your skin create collagen, the skin's structural scaffolding. Keep your skin strong, elastic, and ready for the big stretch by including foods like lemons in your diet throughout your pregnancy.

Jonny's Tasty Tips

Who doesn't love a refreshing glass of lemonade? Next time you're in the mood for one, try one of my favorite tricks: Make your lemonade out of the whole fruit, including the peel! Those peels can add a lot of cancer-fighting oomph to your lemonade. Just make sure you buy organic lemons if you plan to use the peels.

Here are some of my other favorite ways to add lemon juice to my meals. Replace the vinegar in your oil and vinegar dressing with fresh-squeezed lemon juice. Easy and delicious, especially on a crisp Greek salad. You have to try it! If you make fresh orange juice, add a lemon (or two). It's less sweet and more refreshing! Lemon juice brightens the flavor of salsas like you wouldn't believe. (That goes for tomato-based soups and sauces, too.) Ditto for fresh fruit, like berries, melon slices, and fruit salads. And I never serve broccoli, broccoflower, or asparagus without a squeeze of fresh lemon juice on top. Mmmmm!

Mint Tea

HOT OR COLD, MINT TEA IS A GREAT WAY TO hydrate your body and soothe your stomach. The water in a glass of mint tea (peppermint, spearmint, or a combination) is hydrating, unlike some other teas—including black and green tea—that can have a diuretic effect. Herb teas like peppermint, spearmint, raspberry, ginger, chamomile, lemon balm, citrus peel, and rose hip are soothing and refreshing during pregnancy (and are safe in moderation, which means a maximum of 2 to 3 cups a day).

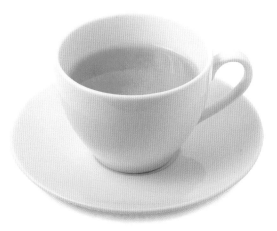

MINT TEA AT A GLANCE

Serving Size: 8 fl oz (1 glass)

Calories: 0

Note: There are no calories, fats, proteins, fiber, iron, calcium, vitamin A, or vitamin C in mint tea.

FAST FACT

Instead of extra coffee or tea, drink herb teas, milk, or pure fruit juices. And don't forget that you still need to drink six to eight glasses of water each day to stay hydrated.

And they don't contain caffeine. In addition, mint teas are known for their soothing effect on your gastrointestinal lining.

Minty and Refreshing

Peppermint oil has been used to treat irritable bowel syndrome with some success. And postoperative studies have found that the smell of peppermint can help alleviate nausea and vomiting, so maybe taking a deep breath of your freshly brewed cup of mint tea can help fight morning sickness too.

During your first trimester, when your digestive system is wreaking havoc on your well-being, it's nice to know that mint can help soothe and relax your stomach. But if you've started getting heartburn as a result of your pregnancy, you should be aware that peppermint may worsen its symptoms. It's also believed that peppermint may promote the flow of bile from the gallbladder and aggravate gallstone symptoms.

At the Market

When shopping for peppermint tea, look for 100 percent peppermint tea leaves. Watch for other hidden ingredients like green or black tea. Green and black teas contain caffeine, which—based on recent research—you should be trying to avoid. The concern is that caffeine can cross the human placenta: In other words, it can end up in your baby's blood. Studies show that your baby's blood and tissue levels of caffeine are similar to yours.

Thank goodness, caffeine is not considered a teratogen (a substance that causes malformations in fetal development). But the use of caffeine during pregnancy is still controversial. To date, moderate consumption (less than 200 mg a day) has not been associated with adverse effects on the fetus (baby). However, consuming over 200 mg/day is associated with a significantly increased risk of miscarriage. Mothers-to-be need to keep a close eye on their caffeine consumption and keep it below 200 mg/day, which is about the same as 2 cups (8-ounce measuring cups, not coffee mugs) of coffee. Check out the chart "Caffeine Content of Popular Foods" on page 221 for an inside scoop on the amount of caffeine found in common beverages, including decaf versions of your favorites.

Jonny's Tasty Tips

Did you know that when the Amish offer their families and guests iced tea, they're serving up iced mint tea? This hardworking group finds iced mint tea more refreshing than any other beverage. Try it—you will, too! And you can add even more health benefits by squeezing a fresh lemon into your iced tea.

Fresh mint is becoming readily available in the produce section of supermarkets nationwide. Take advantage by adding fresh mint leaves to your salads—the taste is incredible!—or mincing those leaves to add to plain yogurt, feta cheese, even artichokes. They're one of the best-kept secrets of Mediterranean cuisine!

Multigrain Cereal

STORE SHELVES ARE PACKED WITH cereals claiming to be "High in Fiber!", "Whole Grain!", and more. It can be hard to sift through the hype to find out what's really in your cereal. During your first trimester, a healthy choice is a cereal that contains multiple types of grains. In other words, puffed rice and cereals with marshmallows in them don't count as a healthy choice. Luckily, these days you have lots of options. Just remember: The sweeter it tastes, the more sugar it contains, so stay away from the sweetest of the bunch.

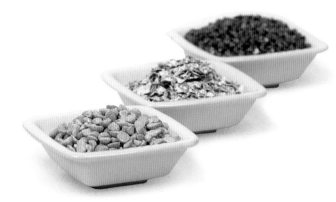

MULTIGRAIN CEREAL AT A GLANCE

Serving Size: 1/3-1/2 cup of cereal	Calcium: 1-3%
Calories: 100-175	Vitamin A: 0-10%
Saturated Fat: 0 g	Vitamin C: 0-10%
Protein: 2-5 g	Iron: 5-25%
Fiber: 4-12 g	

Read the Box

To help you decipher the aisle of cereal boxes, let's define *whole grain* and *multigrain*. If a package says it contains whole grains, that means the entire grain was used to make the product. Sometimes parts of the grain are stripped away to produce a white, sweet-tasting flour. This is a problem, because the bran and germ of a grain that are stripped away are the main source of nutrients. Going with the whole grain is always a better choice for any grain-based product. But you can go a step further and choose a multigrain product. Multigrain products contain more than one type of grain, offering you an even bigger diversity of nutrients—as long as the grains are whole. So read those labels carefully!

Protein Power

Whenever possible, look at the Nutritional Facts panel on the side of your multigrain cereal box and see if the cereal offers you any protein. In the "At a Glance" section we've highlighted ranges for each nutrient that you should strive for when picking your breakfast cereal. Starting the day with protein is a great way to help you boost your daily protein intake. And that breakfast protein boost can help you fight off hunger better throughout the morning and make the craving for a chocolate-coated doughnut easier to deal with. Remember that letting yourself get hungry can bring on morning sickness. Keeping nausea at bay is another great reason to start your day with some protein. Of course, you can pump up the protein content even more by adding milk or yogurt to your cereal.

Whole-Grain Goodness

Grains are a good source of chromium. This mineral is important in your first trimester, since chromium plays a role in stimulating protein synthesis in your growing baby's tissues. Chromium is also a regulator of blood sugar levels, a healthy bonus during pregnancy for you and your baby. High blood sugar levels can be damaging to your body and can increase your risk of developing gestational diabetes.

GOOD GRAINS = GOOD HEALTH

Harvard's Nurses' Health Study, involving more than 75,000 women, found that those who ate the most whole grains decreased their risk of heart disease by 25 percent, stroke by 30 percent, and diabetes by 40 percent. There's more: They were almost 50 percent less likely to experience weight gain over a 12-year period. Diets heavy in refined grains (like white breads, white rice, and cereals made from refined grains rather than whole grains) were linked to an expanded waistline as well as an almost 60 percent greater risk of diabetes. Yikes! Go for that whole-grain cereal, brown rice, and oatmeal. You—and your baby—will be glad you did!

Jonny's Tasty Tips

Breakfast cereal is so convenient, and when you've got a million things to do before rushing out the door in the morning, it can be a godsend. But even tasty multigrain cereal can get a little, well, boring. So I like to liven it up with mixed fruit and nuts: Try adding a sliced banana and fresh blueberries and/or raspberries and then sprinkling on sliced almonds. Add milk or yogurt for a yummy nutritional powerhouse.

Tempted to just skip it? Here are two other easy ways to make multigrain cereal part of your day: Fill a zipper-lock bag with multigrain cereal, tossing in dried cranberries (Craisins), raisins, and almonds. You can snack on this homemade "trail mix" when the munchies strike at work. Ready for lunch? Skip the croutons and sprinkle unsweetened multigrain cereal on your salad for some extra crunch.

★ Oatmeal

A WARM BOWL OF OATMEAL IS A SOOTHING feel-good meal. It's also bland and easy for queasy mothers in their first trimester to eat. Plus, oatmeal is packed with healthy nutrients: fiber, protein, vitamins, and minerals like iron. Oatmeal not only helps you feel good, it helps ensure that you and your baby are well nourished.

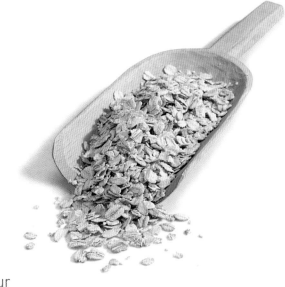

OATMEAL AT A GLANCE

Serving Size: 1 packet of instant oatmeal, fortified (28 g)	**Calcium:** 10%
Calories: 105	**Vitamin A:** 18%
Saturated Fat: 0 g	**Vitamin C:** 0%
Protein: 4 g	**Iron:** 40%
Fiber: 3 g	

Serving Size: 50 g of oats, uncooked (about ⅓ cup)	**Calcium:** 3%
Calories: 200	**Vitamin A:** 0%
Saturated Fat: 0 g	**Vitamin C:** 0%
Protein: 8 g	**Iron:** 10%
Fiber: 3 g	

Iron-Packed Packets

Wow! Just one packet of plain instant oatmeal contains about 40 percent of your daily iron needs. This bland, morning-sickness-friendly food is one of the all-time best foods for the first trimester. Iron is essential for making hemoglobin, the compound in red blood cells that carries oxygen from your lungs to your body and to your baby's tissues. Your growing baby, placenta, and rapidly increasing blood volume have increased your body's needs for iron. A pregnant woman needs about 27 mg of iron a day, but your nonpregnant girlfriends only need about 18 mg. If your iron levels become low, you'll become anemic. Anemia can lead to fatigue and fainting spells and can make it hard for you to fight off infections. If you find plain instant oatmeal too boring, try sprinkling in some cinnamon, raisins, or other dried fruit to make it more exciting. Definitely skip the instant oatmeals with all of the added sugar and flavoring in them. Better yet, prepare steel-cut oats as the ultimate healthy version of oatmeal.

The Fullness Factor

Oatmeal is gaining popularity as a weight loss food. That's because it's high in fiber and protein, two filling foods. The "stick-to-your-ribs" feeling you enjoy after eating a bowl of oatmeal is thanks to about 6 g of fiber and 8 g of protein in a bowl of oatmeal. Fiber is bulky, so it fills your belly and makes you feel full and satisfied. This is a great thing if you're trying to avoid cravings or simply trying to keep your nausea to a minimum. Protein is a valuable addition to any breakfast, because it can make it easier for you to get through your morning feeling fuller and calmer, digestively speaking.

"B" Happy

Oatmeal has a lot more to offer you and your baby. Oatmeal contains vitamin A, the B vitamin riboflavin, folate, and phosphorus. It also is a very good source of three other B vitamins: thiamin, niacin, and vitamin B6. Loading up on B vitamins can help boost your energy levels, and a bowl of oatmeal has about 3 to 10 percent of your Daily Value of these B vitamins. Plus, B vitamins aid in nervous-system functioning, help maintain muscle tone in your digestive tract, and play an important role in keeping both your and your baby's hair, eyes, and liver healthy.

Brain Food in a Bowl

Your bowl of oatmeal also contains a little choline—about 11 mg. During pregnancy, you should try to consume about 450 mg of choline a day. A lesser-known nutrient involved in proper brain and nervous-system development, choline is a good nutrient to watch for when choosing foods to includein your pregnancy diet.

Jonny's Tasty Tips

Those packs of instant oatmeal may be convenient, but I think they're not as nutritionally worthy as old-fashioned oatmeal. First of all, instant oatmeal is usually full of sweeteners and additives—which they need to cover up their lack of taste and pasty texture. Yuck! I like my oats with lots of rich flavor and body, so I usually go for steel-cut (aka Irish or Scottish) oatmeal or old-fashioned rolled oats. (You know, the ones in the round carton.) I usually just pour some milk, juice, or hot water on my oats, let them sit a few minutes, then throw on the berries and nuts and go to town!

Yup, you read that little secret right: You don't have to cook oatmeal to enjoy it. For the best "instant" oatmeal you ever ate, pour boiling water to just barely reach the top of the old-fashioned oats in your cereal bowl. Give it about five minutes for the oats to absorb the water, add a little milk and your favorite topping, and eat! You will be amazed and delighted by how much texture and sweet flavor those "instant" oats have!

Watch the Sugar

Be wary of some packaged instant oatmeals: They can be teeming with extra sugar, something neither you nor your baby needs. Remember the saying "sugar makes big babies," and big babies are hard to deliver. So cut out unnecessary sugar where possible. For example, choose oatmeals with lower amounts of added sugar or make plain oatmeal and add maple syrup, honey, or berries for a sweet touch.

Peanut Butter

PEANUT BUTTER MIGHT NOT MAKE IT onto your healthiest foods list—maybe you ate a few too many PB&Js when you were a kid—but we beg to differ. Peanut butter is packed with protein, niacin, manganese, choline, and folate. Plus, it's delicious and it usually agrees with even the most nauseous pregnant women. But not all peanut butters are created equal, and some are certainly more nutritious than others.

PEANUT BUTTER AT A GLANCE

Serving Size: 1/3-1/2 cup of cereal	Calcium: 1-3%
Calories: 100-175	Vitamin A: 0-10%
Saturated Fat: 0 g	Vitamin C: 0-10%
Protein: 2-5 g	Iron: 5-25%
Fiber: 4-12 g	

Picking Mr. Right

We always advise reading the labels before you choose your foods, but it really pays in the case of peanut butter. Conventional peanut butters—the ones you usually find on grocery shelves—can contain trans fats. And trans fats are considered the worst fats on earth. These giant, useless molecules are created when certain foods are processed, including peanut butter, hot chocolate mix, cookies, and other packaged foods. They're considered so harmful that some researchers are even lobbying their governments to ban trans fats from store shelves, because they're thought to play a major role in cardiovascular disease risk.

But not to worry: Since trans fats are now shown on most food labels around the world, you can easily tell if your peanut butter of choice contains this nasty little ingredient. (Sometimes it's called hydrogenated or partially hydrogenated vegetable oil on the Nutrition Facts label instead. But it's still trans fat.) If it does, that jar is not Mr. Right. The best choice is all-natural peanut butter with no added sugar, salt, or other ingredients because the nutritional value of peanut butter comes from the peanuts themselves.

Smooth or Chunky?

For some women, this debate is pointless, since they'll stick with their favorite type of spread—smooth or chunky—no matter what. But if you enjoy both, then reach for the chunky peanut butter. The pieces of peanuts in the spread are still in their natural state, offering you higher amounts of nutrients.

A Spoonful of Nutrients

Grab a spoon and take a scoop out of your peanut butter jar. It's packed with good nutrients like protein, niacin, folate, manganese, and choline. In fact, your spoonful of peanut butter also contains some polyunsaturated fats (close to 5 g), which can help your skin, heart, and joints stay healthy. In your baby, polyunsaturated fats helps maintain the cells' resilience and lubrication. And we know it's hard to believe, but researchers have found that peanuts are as high in antioxidants as strawberries and blackberries!

Have a Folate Sandwich

Peanut butter is another of the best foods for the first trimester that's rich in folate. This is important, because most women don't get sufficient folate in their daily diet. Used in red blood cell formation, folate is important for your growing baby and for you, since as we've noted, your blood volume is increasing greatly during this first trimester. Plus, folate is necessary for the growth and division of body cells, including the rapidly dividing cells that are becoming your baby. While spreading your tablespoon or two of peanut butter on your multigrain bread or banana (my favorite), feel good knowing there are about 20 mcg of folate in there.

Get Your Zs

You'll also find zinc in your lip-smacking spoonful of peanut butter. Zinc is needed to produce DNA. (Remember those school biology lessons about how DNA is the genetic material or blueprint of your cells?) Each new cell being produced in your growing baby has a copy of that DNA "blueprint," so it needs zinc in order to be created. Rapid cell growth during the first trimester, as well as in subsequent trimesters, increases your need for this mineral. Zinc also plays a role in a healthy immune system and in wound repair. A spoonful of peanut butter has about 1 mg of zinc.

Jonny's Tasty Tips

I like to make sure my peanut butter's as fresh as it gets, so I grind whole peanuts into all-natural peanut butter in my local health food store. But you can also find store-ground peanut butter in plastic cartons in most health food stores, and health-conscious companies offer pure peanut butter in jars, so you can buy it in grocery stores, too. Check those labels! You want to see words like "pure," "natural," "organic," and "100 percent peanuts" before you buy.

If shoveling down spoonfuls of peanut butter isn't your idea of entertainment, think of peanut butter the way you'd think of your favorite dip or spread. Spread some on celery stalks or dip in carrot slices, bell pepper strips, Granny Smith apples, bananas, or even broccoli florets.

Craving that comfort-food favorite, a peanut butter and jelly sandwich? Up the healthy quotient by cutting a slice of multigrain bread in half, spreading peanut butter on one half, and spreading an all-fruit spread like apple butter or strawberry, blackberry, or blueberry fruit spread on the other half. Those berries will add even more antioxidants without overloading you with sugar.

Craving something really decadent? Top some low-fat frozen yogurt with a spoonful of peanut butter. If you let the frozen yogurt soften a bit, you can swirl the peanut butter in and then add some peanut or almond bits on top.

Pinto Beans

PACKED WITH ENERGIZING FIBER AND PROTEIN, as well as minerals that support healthy red blood cell levels, pinto beans are a great food to help you get up and go! These little beans are packed with baby-healthy nutrients like folate, choline, fiber, protein, and iron. In fact, beans are so rich in the important nutrients needed for your baby's health and development that beans like pintos are a must-eat addition to your weekly diet during this first trimester, as well as throughout pregnancy and during breast-feeding.

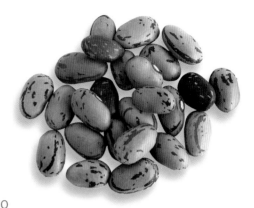

PINTO BEANS AT A GLANCE

Serving Size: 1/2 cup (100 g)	Calcium: 11%
Calories: 350	Vitamin A: 0%
Saturated Fat: 0 g	Vitamin C: 10%
Protein: 21 g	Iron: 25%
Fiber: 15 g	

Fill Up on Fiber

Eating foods that are high in fiber is healthy for everyone. High-fiber foods have been associated with low risk of heart disease and better digestive health. And did you know that beans are a great way to help control weight gain? For pregnant women, fiber can be an ally in your battle against morning sickness. One of the best strategies for helping women avoid the nausea and vomiting commonly experienced during the first trimester is to keep your belly feeling satisfied and full.

Not letting yourself get too hungry keeps your stomach busy digesting food and less involved in making your day miserable. Pinto beans are an excellent source of fiber, with a whopping 15 g in just 1/2 cup!

Pinto beans are packed with fiber. As a pregnant woman, you need about 28 g of fiber each day. If you are using canned pinto beans, be sure to rinse them well first to remove the extra sodium. The healthiest (and cheapest) way to eat beans, although not the most convenient, is to buy dried beans and soak them overnight before using.

Mineral Madness

Beans are one of the healthiest foods on earth. We should all eat more of them. Did you know that pinto beans contain a significant amount of copper, selenium, iron, phosphorus, and manganese? These minerals may not get you excited, but once you realize what they do for your growing baby, you may find yourself heading to the pantry to dig out a can of beans.

Copper aids in forming red blood cells, and you and your baby are making millions of red blood cells during this first trimester. Iron is important for making hemoglobin, the substance in your red blood cells that carries oxygen from your lungs to your baby. But it's also a great addition to your diet because it promotes growth and helps you metabolize protein. Did you know that during your first trimester, your baby's teeth have already started to form? Then you'll be glad to know that the phosphorus in foods like pinto beans works with calcium to ensure that your baby's bones and teeth are growing properly. There is 1 mg of copper (about 100 percent of your RDA), 5 mg of iron (about 19 percent of your RDA), and over 400 mg of phosphorus (that's more than half of your daily needs) in 1/2 cup of pinto beans!

Most Popular Bean

Pinto beans are the most widely produced bean in the United States, and they're one of the most popular beans in both North and South America. Pintos also contain the most fiber of all beans. One cup of pinto beans is your entire day's fiber needs! Pintos are great in refried beans and other Mexican dishes as well as in chili, soup, and pasta. And they're also great additions to salads!

KEEP ON KEEPING ON

Pinto beans and other energizing foods are great for giving you that extra oomph. And with the fatigue and low energy levels typical of the first trimester, you'll need it to help get yourself back in the gym or on the walking track or treadmill. Yes, we're talking about exercise.

Exercise during pregnancy is recommended for most women, but check with your obstetrician or midwife first. It's not a good time to start a rigorous new workout regime. Exercise during pregnancy can help boost your energy level, help keep weight gain in check, leave you feeling relaxed and positive, help keep your blood sugar levels stable, lower your blood pressure, and ward off pregnancy-related complaints like constipation and backaches.

Sounds like exercise can be your best friend during pregnancy, right? But it can do even more: Exercise can prepare your body for the rigors of labor. Studies have shown that women who are physically fit prior to labor experience faster labors and require fewer inductions, Caesarians, and forceps deliveries than their less-fit counterparts.

So reach for those pintos before you reach for your gym shoes, take a deep breath, and get going! You and your baby will be so glad you did.

Jonny's Tasty Tips

No time to make refried beans or chili from scratch? How about a delicious, decadent bean dip? Cream a can of pintos in your blender or food processor. Use a little veggie broth if you need to add liquid; you want a rich, thick dip consistency. Once you have it, pour the beans into a microwave-safe container and heat them. Then top them with salsa, a dollop of plain yogurt, and shredded Cheddar or Mexican cheese. Reach for healthy "chips" like celery stalks, carrot sticks, and strips of whole-wheat pita and dig in!

Popcorn

LIKE RODNEY DANGERFIELD, POPCORN gets no respect. Associated with movie watching, girls'-nights-in, and other events where junk-food consumption is a must, popcorn has been wrongly lumped in with junk foods. But there's nothing junky about popcorn (unless you drown it in melted butter and salt!). In fact, it's one of the healthiest foods for your first trimester.

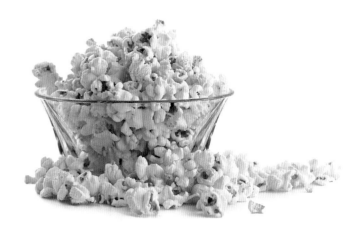

POPCORN AT A GLANCE

Serving Size: 1 cup, air-popped	Calcium: 0%
Calories: 33	Vitamin A: 00%
Saturated Fat: 0 g	Vitamin C: 00%
Protein: 1 g	Iron: 1%
Fiber: 1 g	

FAST FACT

Americans consume some 16 *billion* quarts of popcorn each year. That's 54 quarts for every man, woman, and child!

A Healthy "Junk" Food

Hard to believe but true, popcorn is a whole grain. Its white color has tainted our opinion of this healthy food. Remember that not *all* white foods are bad! Sure, white bread, white pasta, and white rice aren't healthy choices, but cauliflower and popcorn are white foods that are packed with nutrients.

To help you move popcorn off the junk-food shelf, let's break it down. Compared to most snack foods, popcorn is low in calories. Air-popped popcorn has only 31 calories per cup, and even oil-popped is only 55 calories per cup. Even natural microwave popcorn stacks up as a healthy snack. But remember buttered popcorn, particularly the "buttered" popcorn served at your local cinema, contains more calories, bad fat, and sodium than homemade popcorn. Some recent reports show that the typical large bucket of popcorn served at the movies weighs in at well over 1,000 calories!

Get Poppin'

The time-honored way to make popcorn requires a pot, oil, and popcorn kernels. Heat the oil (try coconut oil for a healthy and tasty option) in the pan with the lid on. Then add the popcorn kernels, making sure they're spread out evenly in the pan. Put the lid on and shake the pan every 10 to 15 seconds at first. When the kernels start popping, shake it every 5 or 6 seconds. When the popcorn is ready, add some brewer's yeast for an extra-healthy kick of B vitamins.

Healthy Snacking

Popcorn is not a dense food, so it isn't packed with nutrients. But it does contain an impressive amount of fiber (1 g per cup). And since I can easily eat 3 to 4 cups of air-popped popcorn during my favorite television show, it's a crunchy way to get about 15 percent of my daily fiber needs, as well as adding some protein, folate, manganese, and magnesium to my diet. More important, it's a great substitute when you're craving potato chips or other snacks that are high in bad fat, sugar, salt, and other nasties.

Morning-Sickness Hero

Popcorn in the morning may seem like a strange idea. But once the nausea kicks in, you may decide you like this idea. Air-pop some popcorn and keep it on hand in a sealed container beside your bed or in a zipper-lock bag in your purse. This bland munchie may do the trick if you need to fend off a bout of nausea. And you can eat it guilt-free, knowing that it's offering your body some healthy nutrients.

Jonny's Tasty Tips

Burned popcorn is nobody's idea of a good time, yet all too often, that's what happens when you microwave a bag. And that pervasive stench is horrible if you're not pregnant—I can't even imagine what it must smell like to a pregnant woman!

Standing over the stove shaking a heavy pan isn't exactly fun, either. But there's a great, inexpensive, compact alternative that will give you perfect, oil-free popcorn every time and requires no more than a quick wipe with a moist paper towel to clean up. It's an air-popper, basically a plastic milkshake-glass-size tube with a funneling hood. Fill the measuring-cup top with popcorn, pour it into the heating chamber, position the hood opening over a bowl, plug it in, and voilà! Talk about no fuss, no muss. It doesn't get easier than this!

Another great thing about air-popped corn is that, since it doesn't require oil or butter to cook, you can give yourself permission to add a few calories by way of healthy seasonings. We've already talked about brewer's yeast. Some of my other faves are a shake of oregano, a sprinkle of fresh-grated Parmesan, Asiago, or shredded Cheddar, a dash of lemon pepper, or (for a sweet treat) a very light powdering of cinnamon.

Sweet Potatoes

A BAKED SWEET POTATO (CALLED A YAM in some areas) is a tasty treat any time of year. And you can enjoy this delicious comfort food guilt-free. Just 1 cup of baked sweet potato contains an amazing 4 g of protein and 7 g of fiber, and it's a good source of vitamin B6, potassium, vitamin A, vitamin C, and manganese. All that and fantastic flavor, too!

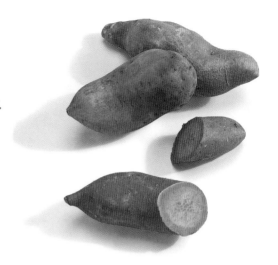

SWEET POTATOES AT A GLANCE

Serving Size: 1 cup (200 g) baked with skin on	Calcium: 8%
Calories: 180	Vitamin A: 750%
Saturated Fat: 0 g	Vitamin C: 60%
Protein: 4 g	Iron: 6%
Fiber: 7 g	

Grade A

Sweet potatoes are a great source of vitamin A. Just 1 cup of sweet potato contains more than 700 percent of your daily needs of vitamin A. Talk about a nutrient-packed mouthful! Vitamin A plays a part in eye, ear, heart, and limb development, and your baby's rapidly developing all of these during your first trimester.

Too Much of a Good Thing

There's some evidence that taking too much vitamin A during pregnancy may increase a woman's risk of giving birth to a baby with birth defects. But this refers to women who take massive doses of vitamin A in supplement form, not women who eat sweet potatoes, carrots, and other vitamin A-rich foods in moderation. Don't panic over your prescribed pregnancy supplements, either: Prenatal vitamins are naturally low in vitamin A.

The debate around vitamin A is based on research suggesting a link between high intakes of supplemental vitamin A by pregnant women and birth defects. A study was conducted at the Boston University School of Medicine that compared vitamin A intake during pregnancy in women who had given birth to healthy infants to women whose babies had defects of the head, face, nervous system, heart, or thymus. The study found that women who took about 10,000 IU or more of vitamin A every day during pregnancy were slightly more likely (1 in 57 births) to give birth to a child with these defects. Other studies have suggested that risk of defects doesn't occur until the vitamin A intake exceeds 25,000 IU. (For pregnant women the RDA for vitamin A is 2,700 IU, so you can see that these women were going overboard.) A sweet potato contains about 35,000 IU of vitamin A. Should you avoid sweet potatoes? Absolutely not! But, if you eat them every single day religiously, perhaps it's best you try mixing up your choice of vegetable to ensure you're getting other nutrients you need in your diet and not too much vitamin A.

As for megadoses of other vitamins, those aren't advisable during pregnancy either. Obviously, when you're pregnant, it's not a good idea to self-diagnose and load up on megadoses of vitamins unless they're prescribed by your obstetrician. At this point, using a prenatal vitamin to ensure that your nutrient intake is sufficient, combined with a healthy diet including foods like sweet potatoes, is a healthy choice for both mom and baby.

"B" Healthy

Vitamin B6 is vital for your baby's development, and sweet potatoes contain lots of this nutrient, about 0.6 mg per cup. Vitamin B6 is involved in red blood cell and antibody (immune-system compound) formation. It is also vital to the proper development of your baby's brain and nervous system.

HIDDEN NUTRITION

Having a hard time swallowing healthy foods? During your pregnancy, why not try a popular trick moms use to get their picky toddlers to eat: Hide healthy food in your favorite comfort food. Try hiding mashed sweet potatoes in macaroni and cheese. It's packed with nutrients but easy to swallow. (Believe it or not, it's great in chili, too!)

Remember pumpkin and zucchini bread? You can substitute mashed sweet potatoes to make luscious sweet-potato bread. (But substitute applesauce for all that oil, please!) Or swirl mashed sweet potatoes into your cornbread before baking for a delicious and traditional sweet-potato pone. Hiding mashed sweet potatoes in brownies is another great idea. (Believe it or not because brownies are so dense and flavorful you can even hide spinach in them!)

Jonny's Tasty Tips

Allison and I both love sweet potatoes. My favorite combo is to bake a sweet potato and enjoy it with grilled chicken. I find that if I bake a sweet potato in advance, wrap it in foil, and let it sit in the fridge for a day before eating, it gets even sweeter! Sometimes I'll bake a week's worth at a time and refrigerate them till I need them. Talk about convenient! By the way, I always eat the peel: It's the best part and has the most fiber.

One of Allison's favorite ways to eat sweet potatoes is to cut them into slices, toss the slices in some olive oil and rosemary, and lightly toast them in the oven to make sweet potato fries. (She cooks the slices at 400 °F for about 20 minutes, until the middle gets soft and then broils them quickly at 450 °F to make them crunchy.) She also loves to mash up a baked sweet potato for an elegant twist on mashed potatoes.

Tahini

IF YOU HAVEN'T YET DISCOVERED TAHINI,
give it a try. This savory Middle Eastern
spread is not only delicious; it's packed with
healthy nutrients, particularly nutrients important for a healthy pregnancy. Tahini is a made from
roasted or toasted sesame seeds, making a smooth, creamy, buttery spread.
It's great on crackers, in hummus and other dips, or as an ingredient in salad dressing.

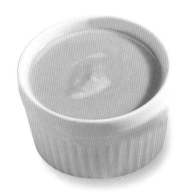

TAHINI AT A GLANCE

Serving Size: 1 oz (2 tbsp)	Calcium: 12%
Calories: 167	Vitamin A: 0%
Saturated Fat: 2 g	Vitamin C: 0%
Protein: 5 g	Iron: 14%
Fiber: 3 g	

FAST FACT

"Eating healthy" should be your mantra not
only during pregnancy but also if you are
actively trying to get pregnant. Your diet prior
to pregnancy plays an important role in your
maternal fatty-acid levels, which are key to
healthy reproductive development.

A Better Butter

Popular throughout the Middle East, tahini is a fun
twist on that old American favorite, peanut butter.
And it's just as healthy, offering you and your baby
a good source of thiamin, phosphorus, copper, and
manganese. These nutrients are key to your baby's
healthy development. A deficiency in these nutrients
can result in gastrointestinal disorders, weight loss and
loss of appetite, fatigue, dizziness, and even blindness
and deafness in children. We sometimes take health
for granted, but as you can see, what you eat plays a
major role in whether you and your baby are healthy
or not.

Up with Omega-6!

Made from sesame seeds, tahini contains all of sesame's nutrients, including healthy oils called omega-6
fatty acids. A few tablespoons of tahini contain more
than 6 g of omega-6 fats. Omega-6 fatty acids are an
essential part of any healthy diet. They play a role in

the healthy function of every cell in your body. In particular, omega-6 fatty acids are required for proper cell integrity and healthy nervous and immune system function. And they're a major contributor to skin health.

Proper development of your mammary glands, placenta, and uterus are dependent on sufficient levels of healthy fats in your body. Your breasts and uterus change rapidly and the placenta develops during your first trimester, so be sure to include lots of good fats, such as the omega-6 fatty acids found in tahini.

Take That Steak Away!

Food aversions can be a major problem during pregnancy, to the point that many a pregnant woman has had to tell her partner to take that steak he's eating and go outside. Pregnancy heightens a woman's sense of smell, likely an evolutionary trait to help you stay alert to protect your offspring from dangers. But this heightened sense of smell can cause trouble getting certain foods in, especially meat. One woman described her first-trimester food woes as a crash course on eating like a vegetarian. If you're experiencing meat aversion, finding nonmeat sources of protein may be really helpful. Tahini contains 5 g of protein in just 2 tablespoons. Seeds, nuts, and beans are also great sources of protein. Try tahini, almond butter, and other nut butters if your stomach isn't happy with your efforts to get sufficient protein into your diet.

Jonny's Tasty Tips

Hummus and baba ghanouj are two Middle Eastern spreads that are both delicious and nutritious. And not surprisingly, both contain tahini! Baba ghanouj is made with mashed roasted eggplant, tahini, lemon juice, garlic, and salt. The best baba ghanouj is made with fire-roasted or grilled eggplant, which gives it a delicious smoky flavor. If you don't feel like roasting your own eggplant, you can find baba ghanouj wherever hummus is sold. And these days, that's pretty much everywhere!

You can buy hummus ready to eat in a number of variations, including with cracked black pepper or sweet red bell pepper. But it's also easy to make your own hummus at home. Drain a can of chickpeas (garbanzos) and cream them in a blender or food processor (add a little vegetable stock if they're too dry). Add tahini, garlic, lime juice, and a little cracked black pepper, and you're good to go! The texture will get thicker and the flavors will blend better if you let your homemade hummus chill in the fridge for an hour or more before eating. Like so many other foods in this chapter, you can enjoy hummus or baba ghanouj spread on whole-wheat pita wedges or as dips with carrot sticks, bell pepper strips, celery stalks, broccoli florets, or your favorite veggies.

Tilapia

IS IT SAFE TO EAT FISH DURING PREGNANCY?
What about all the concerns about mercury?
It's time to debunk the myths behind fish
consumption and mercury risk. Experts
from the University of British Columbia
reported at a conference in Toronto, Ontario, in
2007 that the benefits of eating fish during pregnancy
outweigh any risks.

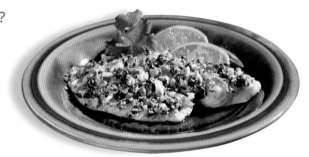

TILAPIA AT A GLANCE

Serving Size: 100 g	Calcium: 1%
Calories: 128	Vitamin A: 0%
Saturated Fat: 1 g	Vitamin C: 0%
Protein: 26 g	Iron: 4%
Fiber: 0 g	

Tilapia is known as a "safe" fish, since it's not high
in mercury. Admittedly, it's not the healthiest fish for
pregnancy (fatty fish like salmon and tuna are better
choices). But tilapia has one big thing in its favor: It's
very bland and lacks the characteristic "fishy" smell
that may be offensive, or even unbearable, if you're
having first-trimester issues with food aversions or
morning sickness.

Super Selenium
Tilapia is an excellent source of selenium, with over
50 mcg in a 100-g serving—that's close to your entire
daily needs in a few bites of fish. Selenium works with

BITING BACK AGAINST BAD GENETICS

Researchers from the Manchester Metropolitan
University reported in 2007 that eating certain nutrients during pregnancy may help
reduce the expression of some harmful genes
in babies. (*Expression* means that the gene's
potential, in this case to create harmful effects,
is allowed to emerge.) When the researchers
reviewed the information available, they found
that mothers who consume adequate levels of
B vitamins, choline, and methionine may reduce
the expression of potentially harmful genes
in their fetuses. More research is needed, but
once again, a diet rich in healthy foods like
tilapia may play a role in helping your baby's
healthiest genes prevail.

Jonny's Tasty Tips

Tilapia may be bland, but it doesn't have to be boring! Here are some great ways to boost this flaky white fish's flavor while keeping it healthy. Try topping tilapia fillets with sliced leeks and fresh parsley and baking them in olive oil and lemon juice. Grill the fillets and top them with fresh mango salsa and a slice of lime. Poach tilapia fillets in olive oil and white wine (the alcohol content evaporates during cooking). Bake tilapia fillets in olive oil and lemon juice and then serve topped with a creamy sauce of plain yogurt and fresh dill weed.

vitamin E, the most important fat-soluble vitamin in your body. It preserves the elasticity of your skin, a great benefit as your breasts and belly start to grow. Plus, selenium stimulates an increase in antibody response, which can help you respond faster to germs like the common cold or the flu.

Bland, Boring, but Nutritious

There's more nutrition hiding in this seemingly boring fish. Tilapia is a source of protein, the B vitamin niacin, vitamin B12, and choline. Protein is key to a healthy pregnancy and good energy levels during your first trimester. B vitamins are also great sources of energy, plus they play a key role in your baby's development. There are close to 5 mg of niacin and 2 mcg of vitamin B12 in a serving of tilapia, which is over a quarter of your daily needs of these energizing nutrients. In a serving of tilapia, there are 42 g of choline, a nutrient required for the healthy development of your baby's brain and nervous system.

MERCURY AND THE MEDIA

A well-publicized January 2001 federal advisory recommended that pregnant women limit consumption of certain fish because of concerns about mercury contamination. Recent studies have suggested that prenatal exposure to mercury among populations with high fish consumption may cause developmental delays in the baby. (Populations with high fish consumption, by the way, would be the Japanese and Scandinavians, for example. Pregnant women in North America do not eat very much fish.)

When researchers looked into the fallout from this report, they found that pregnant women decreased their consumption of dark-meat fish, canned tuna, and white-meat fish. This resulted in a reduction in total fish consumption of approximately 1.4 servings per month. This is of grave concern, because the consumption of the healthy fats in fish offers benefits to the fetus such as reduced risk of preterm delivery and enhanced infant cognition. These benefits could outweigh any harm from mercury exposure.

Experts overwhelmingly recommend eating fish. The American Heart Association has suggested that adults should consume fish at least twice weekly to promote cardiovascular health. Nutrition experts have advised that pregnant women consume sufficient levels of good fats (essential fatty acids, or EFAs) equivalent to approximately three oil-rich fish meals per week.

So shop smart when you buy fish, and don't eat ridiculous amounts of fish (or anything else). You can even choose to buy organic or wild fish, which have been touted as "cleaner" choices—an option we both recommend.

Watermelon

WATERMELON IS MORE THAN A SUMMER TREAT to be enjoyed at the park or at the neighborhood barbecue. This fruit is packed with B vitamins, lycopene, vitamins C and A, as well as water and fiber, making it a great food for any diet and a pleasing food for women suffering from various first-trimester symptoms like food aversions, thirst, and morning sickness.

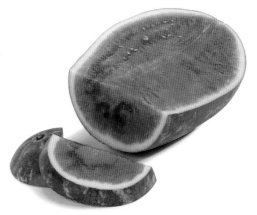

WATERMELON AT A GLANCE

Serving Size: 1 cup (154 g)	Calcium: 1%
Calories: 46	Vitamin A: 16%
Saturated Fat: 0 g	Vitamin C: 20%
Protein: 1 g	Iron: 2%
Fiber: 1 g	

FAST FACT

Most of the time, the watermelon you'll find in stores is red- or pink-fleshed. But watermelons can also have yellow, orange, or even white flesh.

A Healthy Slice

A slice of watermelon contains fewer than 50 calories—about the same as a stick of licorice. Yet unlike watermelon, a stick of licorice offers you or your baby no benefits. Watermelon is rich in some of nature's most effective antioxidants, including vitamins A and C. A cup of watermelon contains more than 400 IU of vitamin A and 12 mg of vitamin C. These antioxidants are fat- and water-soluble, respectively, which means that together, they can neutralize free radicals—unstable compounds that damage cells—in every part of your body and your baby's body. Red or pink watermelon is also a source of lycopene, another potent antioxidant. Concentrated amounts of lycopene are found in tomatoes, but watermelon offers a hefty dose of this antioxidant as well.

Bring on the Bs

Watermelon provides about 1 percent of your dietary needs of vitamin B1 (thiamin) and 3 percent of vitamin B6 (pyridoxine). These B vitamins are necessary for energy production. Your body requires energy to help support the changes in your uterus and breasts and to keep up with increased hormone production during your first trimester. Plus, vitamin B6 is an ally in the fight against morning sickness.

Thirst Quencher

Did you know that a watermelon is 92 percent water by weight? Besides the many nutrients it provides that support your health, watermelon hydrates too. A common symptom experienced by women in their first trimester is thirst. This may be due to the increase in blood volume in your body or the sheer increase in your need for nutrients as your body moves into over-drive to get your little baby developed in a mere nine months. Try watermelon cold as a great food to quench your thirst in hot weather.

Jonny's Tasty Tips

A cold, juicy slice of watermelon needs no embellishment in my book! But that doesn't mean you can't go to town if you want to dress it up. Sprinkle lime juice over that slice for a sweet-tart treat. Or cube your watermelon (or reach for the melon baller) and make a fresh fruit salad with cantaloupe, blueberries, and strawberries. Eat with a squeeze of lime juice or a little dressing made of orange juice and olive oil.

Here's a trick if you need a break from those endless glasses of water. Take a melon baller, make watermelon balls, and then pack them in a plastic container and keep them nearby. You can toss some in your mouth any time you're feeling thirsty or just need a little pick-me-up. Don't forget to choose seedless watermelon to make preparation super-fast and easy. Watermelon is also a great substitute for tomatoes in salad. Add some feta and basil and enjoy.

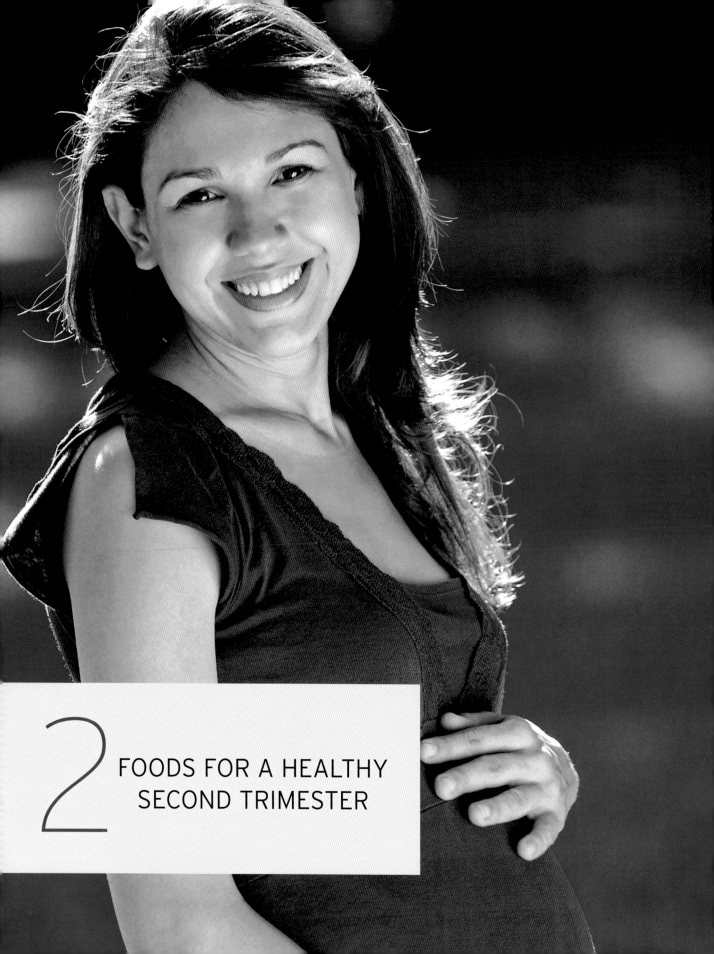

2 FOODS FOR A HEALTHY
SECOND TRIMESTER

YOU'VE MANAGED TO SURVIVE THE FIRST trimester. Now it's time to enjoy your pregnancy! The nausea will mostly have passed, and your baby is still too small to cause you much discomfort. Plus, many women find a renewed feeling of energy in their second trimester.

There's more to your second trimester than just feeling better. That beautiful pregnancy glow will appear this trimester, and your little bump will attract many loving smiles and excitement from friends and family. It's very exciting when your belly starts to grow, and this is usually the time to announce your pregnancy to the whole world, including your coworkers. It's an exciting time! Many women consider the second trimester to be the best months of pregnancy.

In the meantime, your baby is still growing at an amazing rate. In fact, if the rate of growth your baby will experience over the next few months were to continue without change, your baby would be thirteen feet tall by the time he or she was a month old! Obviously, this kind of growth needs the right kinds of fuel. So let's take a look at the nutrients you and your baby need during your second trimester and the best foods to find them in.

BIG AND BIGGER

Your "baby belly" will definitely start showing in this trimester, but your rate of growth is nothing compared to your baby's. Sure, you may have to consign the skinny jeans and slinky tops to the closet for a while, but it's all worth it. These outward changes you're experiencing (growing belly and enlarged breasts) are a great reminder of how much you and your baby are changing—and how important eating lots of the right nutrients is to helping you both keep up.

FAST FACT

The second trimester is officially from week 13 to week 27 of pregnancy, but most people think of it as the fourth to sixth months of pregnancy.

You'll need to eat the right foods in your second trimester to keep your energy levels up and your baby growing strong and healthy. Let's take a closer look at the changes that are occurring in your second trimester of pregnancy and what foods are the best choices during this period.

DEALING WITH COMPLAINTS

Once you've passed the first trimester, the types of complaints you may experience are different. You may not be having morning sickness, but backaches, breast tenderness, leg cramps, acne, gas, heartburn, constipation, low energy, and a few other discomforts can arise over the next few months. Massage therapy and regular exercise can help relieve some of the aches and pains in your back and legs.

Eating a healthy diet abundant in fiber-rich foods will help alleviate some of the gas, heartburn, bloating, and/or constipation some women experience. Acne can be brought on by your high hormone levels—the same thing that caused it in your teenage years. Regular cleansing of your skin and eating foods that support healthy skin can help fight acne. Look for them in chapter 4, beginning on page 173.

NUTRITIONAL NEEDS FOR THE SECOND TRIMESTER

Because every woman's body is different, it's important to work closely with your obstetrician or midwife to develop a nutritional program that's ideal for you. Factors from your health, age, and weight to your activity level, heredity, and the amount of stress you're experiencing combine to create unique nutritional needs. And since each pregnancy is different, your nutritional needs may be too. This chart will give you nutritional guidelines for a healthy second trimester. You'll read about these nutrients in detail later in the chapter.

Key Vitamins

Vitamin A: 2,700 IU daily

Folate: 800 mcg daily

Vitamin B12: 2.2 mcg daily

Vitamin C: 85 mg daily

Vitamin D: 400 IU daily

Key Minerals

Calcium: 1,000 mg daily

Iron: 27 mg daily

Sodium: 2,400 mg daily

Zinc: 15 mg daily

Other Key Nutritional Needs

Calories: 300 extra calories a day

Protein: a minimum of 60 g daily

Fiber: 25 to 30 g daily

Fluids: eight to twelve 8-oz glasses of liquid daily

WHAT'S HAPPENING?

Did you know all of your baby's major organs have formed by the 15th week of pregnancy? Some organs, such as the heart, lungs, and kidneys, will continue to develop this trimester. Your baby's eyebrows and fingernails will form now, and his or her reddish, wrinkled skin will soon be covered with fine hair. By the end of this trimester, your baby will have grown to between 11 and 14 inches long and about 2 to 2 1/2 pounds. He or she will be able to swallow and hear. You may also notice periods of activity and quiet as he or she moves, kicks, sleeps, and wakes.

And what's happening with your body? Your breasts will be getting larger. That's because of two things: First, stimulated by estrogen and progesterone (the two main hormones in the female body), the milk-producing glands inside your breasts get larger. Second, fat will accumulate in your breasts, which may result in as much as one pound of extra breast tissue, or up to two additional cup sizes. You may also notice that your pants are getting a little tighter around the waist. Your growing belly is stretching to make room for your uterus, which is becoming heavier and larger to make room for the baby.

At times, your uterus may even contract in an attempt to build strength for the big job ahead. These contracts are called Braxton-Hicks contractions and are perfectly normal. However, if the contractions become painful or regular, consult your obstetrician or midwife to make sure they're not signs of preterm labor.

The increase in size of your uterus can also lead to more pressure on the veins that return blood from your legs to your heart. Leg cramps, especially at night, may occur, but luckily stretching and walking can help. And don't forget about the effects on your intestinal tract. Your stomach and small and large intestines get sort of pushed out of the way, which can lead to heartburn and constipation. Luckily, eating lots of healthy foods, particularly those rich in fiber, can help combat these problems and keep your digestive tract moving despite its increasingly cramped environment. Check out our "Top Foods for the Second Trimester" beginning on page 83 for some great high-fiber choices like chickpeas and hemp seeds.

More Blood

As blood circulation increases, you'll notice a few other symptoms. An obvious one is that healthy glow to your skin. The "pregnancy glow" is beautiful, and we hope you enjoy it. So many people say that pregnant women are beautiful, and this may in part be due to the increase in blood flow to your skin. Eating foods that are rich in skin-healthy ingredients like coconut oil, cherries, and avocados can help keep your skin looking radiant into your later months.

The increase in blood flow can lead to a few less lovely side effects as well. Certain areas of your skin may also become darker, such as the skin around your nipples. The increase in circulation also moves more blood through your nasal passage and gums. This may cause the lining of your nose and airway to swell, leading to congestion, snoring, and/or nosebleeds. For your gums, you may have minor bleeding when you brush or floss your teeth. Eating foods rich in nutrients that support healthy tissues may help your gums. For example, foods that are rich in vitamin C can help your tissues build collagen to maintain structure and strength. While enjoying that slice of orange or handful of strawberries to get your vitamin C, why not grab a few spoonfuls of yogurt? The good bacteria it contains makes yogurt a mouth-healthy choice.

SIGNS AND SYMPTOMS: THE SECOND TRIMESTER

Don't panic if your body, symptoms, cravings, and needs change during your second trimester. It's perfectly normal! But be sure to share any changes with your obstetrician or midwife. Look for these signs:

- You need to eat more nutritious foods to support your baby's growth. (Don't cheat on your healthy diet now! Keep eating the healthy foods in this book.)

- You may want to eat more and/or have cravings. Eat smart for you and your baby.

- Nosebleeds and/or gum problems can occur with your increased blood volume (focus on getting more iron and water if you suffer from these).

- Skin can become blotchy and darker. Nourish with good oils and fruits and vegetables.

- Your body may increase its fat stores (there is nothing you can do about it).

- You may develop backaches, cramps, swollen legs and ankles, and/or varicose veins.

- You may experience heartburn and/or constipation, so eat smaller meals, drink lots of water, avoid fatty and spicy foods, and eat more high-fiber foods.

- Your breasts and belly will get bigger.

With more blood, your blood vessels will dilate, which can lead to some dizziness. If you experience dizziness, try to avoid prolonged standing and rise slowly after lying or sitting down to help combat it. Eating healthy foods like avocados and watercress that contain plenty of iron, sodium, potassium, and protein will ensure your blood has what it needs to stay healthy.

Can't Keep Up

Experiencing a shortness of breath during pregnancy is common. It is caused by the increasing demands on your lungs. In fact, your lungs are processing up to 40 percent more air now than they did before your pregnancy. This allows your blood to carry more oxygen to your placenta and thus to your baby. Eating energizing foods can help. Green leafy foods like spinach, kale, and nori contain iron needed to carry oxygen, and antioxidant-rich seeds and fruits like hemp seeds and cherries can help prevent damage caused by free radicals.

Infections

A thin, white vaginal discharge is common during pregnancy. This acidic discharge works to prevent the growth of harmful bacteria and yeasts in the vaginal tract. Besides yeast infections, pregnant women can experience bladder and kidney infections. That's because hormonal changes and your growing uterus can slow the flow of urine, which normally keeps bacteria out of these organs. To help prevent infections in your urinary tract, stay hydrated by drinking safe herbal teas like peppermint and chamomile, chocolate milk, and water.

Probiotics are also a good option for battling bacterial and yeast infections. Probiotics are the good microbes that keep the lining of your mouth, intestines, urinary tract, and vagina healthy and free of overgrowths of bad bacteria and yeasts. Probiotics are found naturally in fermented foods like yogurt and kefir, and they're available in capsule and powder form from most health food stores. Remember to refrigerate them!

Research suggests that the use of probiotics by pregnant women has a number of healthy benefits and is considered safe. However, as with all supplements, pregnant women should discuss the use of probiotics with their obstetrician or midwife.

Top Foods for The Second Trimester

Now that you're not fighting morning sickness, you can really enjoy eating in your second trimester. So dig in! There are many healthy foods to enjoy during this trimester, including sweet berries, savory vegetables, nutty grains, satisfying nuts, mouthwatering meats, and more. Salads, fruits, nuts, seeds, whole-grain breads, crackers, pasta, and low-fat meats are always a good choice during your second trimester. Try to eat a diet that has variety, balance, and moderation to make sure that you're getting sufficient amounts of all nutrients and energy sources in your diet.

Obviously, you can still enjoy all the first-trimester foods we recommended in chapter 1. But certain nutrients are of particular benefit to you and your baby during the second trimester. So we've compiled a list of delicious, healthy foods especially for your second-trimester diet.

HERE ARE THE 20 HEALTHIEST FOODS FOR THE SECOND TRIMESTER:

- AVOCADO
- BASIL
- CARROTS
- CHIA SEEDS
- CHAMOMILE
- CHERRIES
- CHICKPEAS
- CHOCOLATE MILK
- COCONUT OIL
- FIGS
- HEMP SEEDS
- KALE
- NORI
- ROMAINE LETTUCE
- SCALLIONS
- TOFU
- TURMERIC
- TUNA
- TURKEY
- WATERCRESS

Let's look at each of these second-trimester favorites and see what makes them so great. And please, don't be afraid to try them! Even if you're not used to cooking with coconut oil, adding chia or hemp seeds to your food, or seasoning it with turmeric, "Jonny's Tasty Tips" will give you some wonderful ways to enjoy them.

Avocado

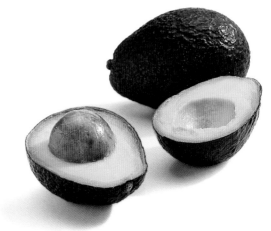

"RICH AND LUXURIOUS" IS A STRANGE WAY TO describe most fruits, but avocados are one of the most decadent fruits on earth and one of the healthiest, too. Avocados are packed with vitamins, antioxidants, minerals, fiber, and healthy fats to help you and your baby enjoy a healthy pregnancy.

AVACADO AT A GLANCE

Serving Size: 1 cup (150 g)	Calcium: 2%
Calories: 240	Vitamin A: 8%
Saturated Fat: 3 g	Vitamin C: 25%
Protein: 3 g	Iron: 5%
Fiber: 10 g	

Note: The nutritional facts data provided in this book are approximations based on the nutrient value of the foods and a pregnant woman's RDA.

Too Fattening?

Fat! That's what usually comes to mind when people think of avocados. This fruit has definitely gotten a bad rap, thanks to the popularity of low-fat and anti-fat diets. But it is important to not let the fat content of any food cause you to immediately dismiss it. Remember that not all fats are created equal. We're not talking about french fries here. The fat in avocados is mostly healthy fat, and you *need* that fat. That's right: You need to be eating fat! As of week 17, your baby starts to accumulate fat under his skin. This fat will provide energy and help keep your baby warm after birth, plus it will give him or her those cute baby cheeks we all love to kiss.

How much fat is in an avocado? In 1 cup, there are 22 g of fat. But wait—before you flip the page and write off avocados, consider that a cup of avocado contains only 3 g of saturated fat, and it's saturated fat that you actually need to help build cell structures like membranes. As your baby grows, he is creating millions of new cells, and each one consists of a series of membranes, each of which is made of fat. Most of the fat in an avocado is monounsaturated fat, the kind found in plants (about 15 g in 1 cup of avocado). These healthy fats are important to provide your body with adequate energy, for cell membrane health, and for many other functions. And that growing belly of yours will love that your avocado contains 3 g of polyunsaturated fat in the form of omega-6 fatty acids. These good fats are important for your skin's health—and with all that stretching and growing going on, you'll be glad to have these fats helping your skin stay pliable.

A Nutritional Powerhouse

There is much more to that avocado than fat. In each cup of avocado, there are also 16 g of fiber to help balance out your diet. Plus, there are 205 mcg of folate, which is almost a third of a pregnant woman's daily needs. Even though your baby's neural tube has closed

EAT FAT, ABSORB MORE NUTRIENTS

Eating fat is important because it helps your body absorb more nutrients. Certain nutrients like vitamin A and E can't be absorbed unless there's fat in your digestive system. In a study from Iowa State University, people who ate a salad with fat-free dressing didn't absorb any carotenoids (a type of vitamin A), whereas those who ate a salad with a reduced-fat or full-fat dressing had substantially greater absorption of these important compounds. Avocados have nutrient-absorption-supporting fats and over 200 IU of vitamin A in just 1 cup. Vitamin A is a key antioxidant in your body and in your baby's body. Plus, vitamin A plays a role in regulating growth—something that is happening very quickly in your second trimester as your belly continues to expand. So don't skip the dressing on your salad or better yet add some avocado to your salad and let the fat help your body get more nutrients from your food.

well before your second trimester, folate is still very important for your baby's proper development. And a cup of avocado has 22 mg of choline, a nutrient needed for your baby's healthy nerve and brain development.

The good news about avocados isn't over yet. Your cup of avocado has more than half of your daily needs of vitamin K and a third of your daily needs of vitamin B6. Plus, it's a good source of vitamin C, niacin, and riboflavin, as well as a source of thiamin and every important mineral in your diet: copper, magnesium, manganese, sodium, potassium, selenium, calcium, phosphorus, and iron. Wow!

Jonny's Tasty Tips

There are so many easy ways to get this nutritious, luxurious fruit into your diet. The easiest of all is to simply cut up some avocado and add it to your salad. It's particularly delicious with red grapefruit and thinly sliced red onion over baby spinach—and that's a recipe for a nutritional powerhouse of a salad. Or, for a great snack, mash up some avocado and add some garlic and a splash of lemon for a great dip for whole-grain tortillas or crudites. I've even been known to eat a whole avocado as a mini-meal right out of the skin!

FAST FACT

You may think of avocados as vegetables—the main ingredient in guacamole or sliced on salads—since they're not sweet like an apple or peach. But technically, they're considered fruits.

Basil

BASIL IS EVERYBODY'S FAVORITE HERB.
It's not just a delicious and indispensable ingredient in Italian dishes and homemade salad dressings. It's packed with nutrients for you and your growing baby.

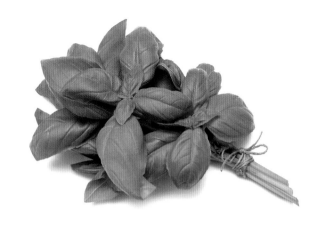

BASIL AT A GLANCE

Serving Size: 1 ounce (28 g or about 10 Tbsp fresh basil)	**Calcium:** 5%
Calories: 6	**Vitamin A:** 30%
Saturated Fat: 0 g	**Vitamin C:** 8%
Protein: 0 g	**Iron:** 5%
Fiber: 0 g	

FAST FACT

Anemia can show up during your second trimester if you're not getting enough iron.

Pregnancy Superfood

Basil contains every major nutrient you need during your pregnancy. This anise-flavored herb is packed with iron, calcium, and folate, nutrients most women of child-bearing age don't consume enough of. Iron is vital for keeping your energy levels up, and anemia caused by low iron levels can appear in your second trimester (remember, your body's making all that new blood), so it's especially important to get plenty of iron now.

We all know how important it is to consume a calcium-rich diet for strong bones and teeth, but it's even more essential during pregnancy. Your baby has 300 bones to build and grow! That requires a *lot* of calcium. Luckily, that fresh and flavorful basil pesto on your whole-wheat pasta contains 50 mg of calcium to help your baby's bones grow.

Folate, a B vitamin best known for its ability to prevent neural-tube defects, is vital for many processes in your growing baby, including cell growth and division. Basil is also a great source of folate, offering about 20 mcg per ounce. Basil really is a superfood for your pregnancy.

Fresh Is Best

Fresh basil is also a good source of protein, vitamin E (alpha-tocopherol), riboflavin, and niacin, and a it's very good source of dietary fiber, vitamin A, vitamin C, vitamin K, vitamin B6, magnesium, phosphorus, potassium, zinc, copper, and manganese. Whenever possible, choose fresh basil, since it contains more of these nutrients than dried basil. Luckily, most markets now offer fresh basil year-round.

BYE-BYE, BACTERIA

Basil contains many volatile oils (estragole, linalool, cineole, eugenol, sabinene, myrcene, and limonene), and that's a good thing. Not only do they contribute to its spicy, complex flavor, but laboratory studies have shown that the volatile oils in basil can restrict the growth of numerous bad bacteria, including *Listeria monocytogenes, Staphylococcus aureus, Escherichia coli, Yersinia enterocolitica,* and *Pseudomonas aeruginosa.* It's great to know that this tasty herb goes to battle for you against these nasty bugs.

Herbs for Health

Basil leaves also contain flavonoids. Flavonoids are health-protective plant compounds. They act as antioxidants, helping keep your body free of damage caused by free radicals and freeing up your energy for baby-making tasks. Herbs and spices used in traditional Mediterranean cooking, like basil, oregano, and thyme, even when used in small quantities, significantly contribute to flavonoid intake in your diet, particularly if you eat them often. So feel good about adding basil and other flavor-enhancing herbs to your dishes. It's a healthy choice.

Is It Safe?

A quick search on the Internet about the safety of basil during pregnancy will bring up a number of conflicting Web pages. It is important to note that, in this book, we are talking about fresh basil used as a culinary ingredient. We are *not* talking about holy basil or using basil in medicinal amounts. In both

Jonny's Tasty Tips

Want to get more basil bang for your buck? Enjoy the fresh, spicy leaves in a caprese salad. It's best with flavorful, ripe tomatoes (I like heirloom tomatoes for a real blast of flavor), fresh mozzarella or bocconcini (the white kind sold in balls), and fruity extra-virgin olive oil. And it's not only yummy, it's super-easy to put together and rich enough to make a satisfying lunch all by itself. Here's what you do: Line your salad plate with buttery lettuce leaves (like Boston or Bibb lettuce). Then create a circle of alternating half-slices of tomato, mozzarella, and basil leaves, fanning them on top of each other. (If you want, you can put a whole slice of tomato over the hole in the center of the circle, top it with a slice of mozzarella, and lay a big, beautiful basil leaf on top.) Drizzle olive oil (and balsamic vinegar if you like) over the salad, add a sprinkling of salt (you need that iodine), and enjoy!

cases, there is some concern as to its safety during pregnancy. Culinary basil has been a major ingredient in Italian cooking for centuries without cause for concern, and using it to enhance the flavors of your meals is also considered safe. In fact, to eat enough basil to be anywhere close to levels of concern for your pregnancy, you'd have to slather *every* meal with pesto! So grab a handful of basil leaves and enjoy their refreshing, mouthwatering flavor in your meals.

Carrots

CARROTS AREN'T JUST BUNNY FOOD. AND they're not all orange, either—carrots also come in white, yellow, red, and even purple varieties. Carrots are packed with good nutrients like vitamin A, vitamin C, fiber, and vitamin K, making this portable vegetable a healthy and easy addition to your pregnancy diet. So listen to your mom and eat your carrots!

CARROTS AT A GLANCE

Serving Size: 1 cup (128 g)

Calories: 52

Saturated Fat: 0 g

Protein: 1 g

Fiber: 4 g

Calcium: 4%

Vitamin A: 700%

Vitamin C: 13%

Iron: 2%

FAST FACT

Omega-6 fatty acids help keep your belly's skin soft and supple as it stretches.

Better Sight Day and Night

Eating carrots is good for your eyes because carrots are rich in beta-carotene, an orange-colored nutrient that is converted to vitamin A in the body. A lack of vitamin A can cause poor vision, particularly night vision, and eating more carrots or other vegetables that are rich in vitamin A can help maintain or restore your eyesight. In 1 cup of raw carrots, you'll find roughly 700 percent (20,000 IU) of your recommended Daily Value of vitamin A! When you're pregnant, this is doubly important, especially now, since during your second trimester your baby's eyes are developing.

Too Much of a Good Thing?

Even if you love carrots, it's important not to go carrot-crazy. Eating a heaping helping of carrots every few hours may not be good for you or your baby. For one thing, eating too many carrots can cause your skin to turn orange, a condition called hypercarotenemia. Luckily, your risk of getting hypercarotenemia is low since you'd have to eat at least 20 mg of beta-carotene per day (that's about three 8-inch carrots). We all know people who love eating carrot sticks, but even they would have a hard time eating that many carrots in a day!

You may also be worried because you've heard (correctly) that vitamin A can lead to toxic symptoms—including birth defects—if consumed at high dosages. This is because vitamin A is a fat-soluble vitamin that can accumulate in your tissues. But it's important to remember that there are two different types of vitamin A: retinol and beta-carotene. Retinol is found in animal foods. Carrots and other plant sources of vitamin A offer you beta-carotene. Beta-carotene is converted in the body to retinol, the form the body can use. But this conversion isn't highly efficient. In other words, eating a lot of carrots will not lead to toxic levels of vitamin A. Feel free to dig into that pile of carrots—it's healthy for you, and safe. Some supplements contain high amounts of vitamin A. Most multivitamins, including prenatal vitamins, contain less than 5,000 IU of retinol, which is well below your daily upper levels of 10,000 IU.

So combining a healthy diet that contains foods like carrots that are rich in vitamin A with a prenatal vitamin is not a cause for concern. But while it's on your mind, it's not a bad idea to check the label on your vitamin supplement and make sure it contains no more than 5,000 IU of vitamin A. And this is another good reason not to take "extra" vitamins on your own. If you're concerned that you might not be getting enough of a particular vitamin or mineral, discuss it with your obstetrician.

Jonny's Tasty Tips

One really great thing about carrots is that they're so easy to eat. Think of Bugs Bunny: no fuss, no muss. Buy organic carrots and you don't even have to peel them! Raw, chopped, or diced carrots make a good snack. Take your salad from boring to bright with the simple addition of grated carrots. Cooked carrots make a colorful side dish on their own, and they're a great addition to hearty winter dishes like stews, soups, and pot roast. They're versatile enough to add to recipes ranging from mixed roasted root veggies to vegetable curry.

What about baby carrots? These mini-carrots aren't any better for you and your baby than the full-size version, but they sure are fun and convenient to eat. Baby carrots are a fast food pregnant women should fall in love with. You can buy baby carrots in single-serving bags, so they're easy to take along as a healthy snack to help keep you going during your busy day. Dip them in yogurt, hummus, or low-fat ranch dressing for an extra dose of flavor and nutrition.

Hey, that may be the first time you've heard the words *ranch dressing* and *nutrition* used together, but there's sound science behind the link: The carotenoids and vitamin A in carrots are more bioavailable when you eat your carrots with a little fat. One more great thing about carrots: Because they're root vegetables, they store well. You can buy a week's worth (or more) and not have to worry about them going bad before you get to them, as long as you keep them in the veggie crisper until you're ready to use them. How convenient!

Chia Seeds

EVER HEARD OF CHIA SEEDS? IF THEY'RE A NEW food to you, you're not alone. This relatively unknown seed is popular in South America, and it's gaining popularity in North America as a health food. Chia seeds contain lots of healthy nutrients for you and your baby, including amino acids and fiber. But chia seeds' real claim to fame is their omega-3 fatty acid content.

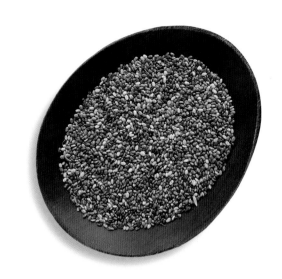

CHIA SEEDS AT A GLANCE

Serving Size: 1 ounce (28 g)	Calcium: 18%
Calories: 137	Vitamin A: 0%
Saturated Fat: 1 g	Vitamin C: 0%
Protein: 4 g	Iron: 0%
Fiber: 11 g	

FAST FACT

Around week 15, your baby's skin is forming, and shortly afterward, your baby starts to make facial expressions, such as squinting and frowning.

The Alpha of Omega

The omega-3 fatty acid content is even higher in chia seeds than in the previous king of omega-3 seeds, flaxseeds. Chia seeds contain about 5,000 mg of omega-3 fatty acids per ounce. Flaxseeds contain about half of that amount per ounce. (Don't toss your flaxseeds, though: They also have high lignan content. Lignans are fats known for their ability to help battle conditions caused by hormone imbalances, like PMS and menopausal symptoms such as hot flashes, and for promoting breast and prostate health.)

Mega Fatty Benefits

What's so great about omega-3s? Omega-3 fatty acids are essential, which means that your body needs them for health but can't produce them; you have to consume them. The type of omega-3 fatty acid found in plant seeds, like chia seeds, is alpha-linolenic acid (ALA). ALA is a healthy fat that plays an important role in your body. A diet rich in healthy fats like ALA and low in bad fats (trans fats, fried foods) results in healthier cells in your body, which means your brain, nerves, skin, and other organs can work better. (That's right—your skin is considered an organ.)

True confession: The most important types of omega-3 fatty acids are eicosapentaenoic acid (EPA) and docosahexaenoic acid (DHA), found naturally in fish. Unfortunately, the conversion of ALA into EPA and DHA in your body is a highly inefficient process, so fish is a far better source of these nutrients. Read the Tuna entry on page 118 for more EPA and DHAs. But ALA offers its own benefits, and as we're about to see, it's only part of the chia seed story.

More than Fat

Important as they are to good health, there is much more to chia seeds than some good fats. One ounce of chia seeds contains 11 g of fiber, 4 g of protein, and 9 g of fat (most of which is good fat). That tells us that chia seeds are a well-balanced source of energizing nutrients. Plus, these little seeds also contain about a third of your daily recommended intake of phosphorus and about 25 percent of your needs of manganese, two minerals needed for proper development of your baby's skeletal system. An ounce of chia seeds also contains about 180 mg calcium, another crucial mineral for bone development.

Jonny's Tasty Tips

You may remember sprouting chia seeds on those infamous clay figurines known as "chia pets" in the 1980s. You can even still find chia pets for sale, but please, don't try eating the seeds in those packages! Instead, look for chia seeds in your local health food store. You don't even have to sprout them: Just add them to a smoothie or sprinkle them on top of cereal or yogurt for a fast, easy nutrition boost.

Chamomile

CHAMOMILE IS A POPULAR HERB TEA, SINCE drinking it can calm and relax you. And staying calm and relaxed during pregnancy is definitely a goal! But as with all foods, moderation is key when you're pregnant. When used orally and in amounts

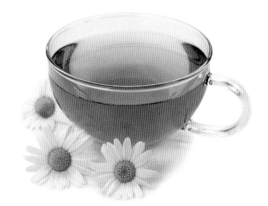

commonly found in foods, chamomile (specifically, German chamomile) has "generally recognized as safe" (GRAS) status in the United States. A cup of chamomile tea would qualify as an "amount commonly found in foods." So feel free to unwind with a soothing, steamy cup of chamomile tea. For other great teas you can enjoy during pregnancy, see chapter 5, beginning on page 210.

CHAMOMILE AT A GLANCE

Serving Size: 1 cup (8 fl oz)	Calcium: 0%
Calories: 0	Vitamin A: 1%
Saturated Fat: 0 g	Vitamin C: 0%
Protein: 0 g	Iron: 1%
Fiber: 0 g	

There are nutritional benefits to enjoying a cup of chamomile tea. It's mostly water, and you need to drink plenty of water during pregnancy, especially if you live in a hot or humid climate or are exercising. There are also some vitamins and minerals in a cup of chamomile tea, making it a healthy choice. One cup of chamomile tea contains vitamin A, iron, manganese, copper, zinc, and magnesium.

A Mine of Minerals

A cup of chamomile tea does more than calm you down. Each cup contains 0.2 mg of iron, about 1 percent of your daily needs. Iron is helpful in promoting a feeling of energy during pregnancy because it is part of hemoglobin, the compound in your blood that carries oxygen to your tissues to help them feel energized. Your cup of chamomile tea also has copper, which helps iron absorption, improving your ability to get iron into your body. There's about 1 percent of your daily needs of potassium, magnesium, manganese, copper, and zinc in a cup of chamomile tea. This is a trivial amount of the major minerals potassium and magnesium, but it's a great way to get more of the trace minerals zinc, copper, and manganese into your diet. Zinc and manganese are involved in hundreds of enzyme reactions in your body, keeping it going. Zinc is also required for the development and growth of your fetus, the transport of vitamin A, and wound healing.

Nighty-Night, Sleep Tight

Chamomile can be helpful as a sleep aid for mothers-to-be. Sleep may not be a problem in your second trimester, but as your body continues to grow and change, your belly may start to cause some discomfort at night. If insomnia is starting to be a problem for you, chamomile tea can calm you so you can relax into sleep. Many sleepy-time teas use a combination of peppermint and chamomile as a relaxing blend to soothe the digestive tract and promote a feeling of restfulness. If you enjoy the flavor of peppermint, look for one of these in the herb tea section of your grocery or health food store.

Kick the Caffeine Habit

If you need a nice cup of something hot and lemon-laced hot water isn't doing it for you, reaching for some soothing herb tea instead of coffee or caffeinated tea is a smart choice. Check out chapter 5, beginning on page 210, for a more detailed rundown on herbal teas and which ones are safe choices during pregnancy.

In the January 2008 issue of the *American Journal of Obstetrics and Gynecology*, a study noted the potential harm of caffeine to an unborn child. The study found that consuming more than 200 mg of caffeine daily—that's 10 ounces of coffee (about one and a half cups) or 25 ounces of tea (about 3 cups)—may double the risk of miscarriage. The lead author suggested that pregnant women should try to give up caffeine for the first three or four months of pregnancy.

Why the fuss? It is known that caffeine crosses the placenta to the developing fetus, but just how this contributes to miscarriage remains unclear. Experts from the Motherisk Program at Toronto's Hospital for Sick Children, a group that is considered an authority on pregnancy, suggests moderating caffeine consumption during pregnancy. Moderation would mean drinking only two to three cups of coffee a day. Note

Jonny's Tasty Tips

I love the pure, unsweetened flavors of herb teas, so I drink mine straight. But if that's not your, uh, cup of tea, you don't need to load up on sugar or honey to enjoy herb teas. Start small—see if a half-teaspoon of honey, well stirred, makes enough of a difference. Or add a little fruit juice, choosing a flavor that will complement your herb tea. (Orange juice and chamomile tea are a nice pairing.)

Don't forget that herb teas are delicious iced, too! Add a sprig of mint and a slice of lemon or lime and then sit back and say "Aaaaahhh..."

that a cup means six to eight ounces—not a big mug or a "grande"! Switching to decaf coffee and tea can help lower your caffeine intake levels, but remember that decaf is *not* caffeine-free! See the chart "Caffeine Content of Commonly Consumed Foods" on page 221 for a rundown on the caffeine content of various drinks. And beware of foods that contain caffeine, since they add to your total daily caffeine intake. Coffee (espresso, cappuccino, latte), black tea, green tea, white tea, chocolate, hot chocolate (cocoa), soft drinks (including diet sodas), and popular energy drinks all contain caffeine. Some medications can also contain caffeine. It can really add up.

★ Cherries

HAVING TROUBLE SLEEPING? SOME PREGNANT women will suffer from insomnia during their pregnancy even if they've never had any issues with it before. It is not known why this happens. It could be the hormonal changes in your body or the physical changes that are making your normal sleeping position uncomfortable. Even thinking about having a baby may be keeping you up! Sleep medications may not be safe during pregnancy, but there's one delicious fruit that's safe and may help you sleep: cherries.

CHERRIES AT A GLANCE

Serving Size: 1 cup (138 g)	Calcium: 2%
Calories: 87	Vitamin A: 2%
Saturated Fat: 0 g	Vitamin C: 16%
Protein: 1 g	Iron: 3%
Fiber: 3 g	

FAST FACT

You're not the only one who needs oxygen now. Your baby's lungs are developing during the second and third trimester.

Melatonin Madness

Cherries contain a compound called melatonin, an antioxidant hormone. Scientists have found that tart cherries contain more of this powerful antioxidant than your body normally produces. An 8-ounce serving of tart cherry juice generally contains 473.47 nanograms of natural melatonin. If you prefer sweet cherries, they also contain some melatonin, just less than tart cherries. Melatonin is produced by the pineal gland in the brain. It helps the body know when it's time to sleep and when it's time to wake up, explaining why some people claim they simply can't "sleep in" on weekends. Melatonin is released at night or in the dark, letting your body know that it's time to sleep. Eating cherries can improve your body's levels of melatonin and may help you sleep better.

That's not all melatonin's good for. It also stimulates cell growth that can help your skin, which is growing and stretching around your breasts and belly. Plus, melatonin may help protect your skin by preventing damage like stretch marks and wrinkles. Eating some cherries may make you a healthy, younger-looking mom. Now that sure sounds sweet!

Powerful C

Cherries are also a good source of vitamin C, with about 10 mg per cup. Vitamin C is a friend to your immune system, keeping it strong and helping you fend off infections like the common cold. This vitamin also helps strengthen blood vessels, which during your pregnancy are working hard to ensure that enough blood is getting to the placenta and eventually to your baby.

Getting More Iron

Even better, vitamin C plays a role in iron absorption. This key mineral helps your bloodstream carry oxygen around your body and to your baby. If you've been feeling winded, you may find some relief with more iron in your diet. If you're still feeling lethargic, despite moving past the fatigue associated with the first trimester, you may want to get your blood iron levels checked by your obstetrician to make sure you aren't anemic. (When you're anemic, you don't have enough iron in your bloodstream.) Vitamin C helps you make the most of every bit of iron you consume or take.

C for Collagen

Vitamin C also plays a role in the production of collagen, the main strength compound in your skin. Collagen is like the scaffolding of your skin. You may have heard collagen mentioned in commercials for high-end facial care cosmetics. Collagen plays a part in your skin's ability to stretch and rebound after stretching. When collagen levels drop in your skin, it looks bumpy, wrinkled, and old. Your skin is stretching during your second trimester and will stretch even more in your third trimester. As your uterus grows and breasts enlarge, you'll be glad to have vitamin C in your diet helping your skin produce collagen to keep your skin strong, resilient, and beautiful.

Jonny's Tasty Tips

Fresh cherries are most available—and most affordable!—in the summer. If you're pregnant then, indulge! But buy organic cherries, please, for your sake and your baby's. The Environmental Working Group lists conventionally grown cherries on its 2003 list of twelve foods most contaminated with pesticides. And remember, the redder the cherries, the better they are for you.

Luckily, frozen cherries have a nutritional value fairly close to fresh cherries', and they're available year-round. So buy a bag and keep it in your freezer for adding to smoothies or yogurt. Or try my own favorite dessert—organic red cherries straight from the freezer and topped with some milk or yogurt. The milk or yogurt semifreezes on the cherries, and when I stir it up, it creates my healthy alternative to Cherry Garcia ice cream. It's my secret weapon against The Attack of the Ice Cream Craving. Now it can be yours, too!

Cherry juice is another good choice. Look for organic, 100 percent pure cherry juice that is not from concentrate, since concentrated juice loses most of its water-soluble nutrients during processing.

I know we said that sour cherries were even better for you than sweet, but that isn't an excuse for pigging out on sugar-drenched, calorie-laden cherry pie or dried cherries! Instead, think of ways to use sour cherries where their tartness is an advantage: baked with chicken, duck, or pork roast; in a salad with orange segments and almonds; or in a delicious Indian rice dish. Or try sneaking some into brown rice pudding or bread pudding for a luscious comfort food.

★ Chickpeas

ALSO KNOWN AS GARBANZO BEANS, CHICKPEAS ARE one of the best foods you can eat during your pregnancy. These tasty beans are full of nutrients to help you and your baby enjoy a healthy pregnancy. Plus, they're easy to add to many dishes, including salads, pasta, chili, and soups. Oh, and did we mention hummus?

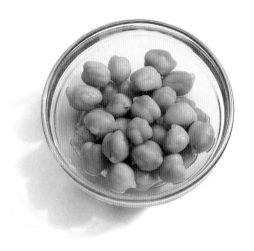

CHICKPEAS AT A GLANCE

Serving Size: 1 cup (164 g)	Calcium: 8%
Calories: 269	Vitamin A: 1%
Saturated Fat: 0 g	Vitamin C: 4%
Protein: 15 g	Iron: 26%
Fiber: 12 g	

Eating for Two

You can expect to gain about 25 to 40 pounds over your pregnancy, with about 4 pounds coming on monthly in your second trimester. This is caused by your baby's rapid growth during these months. To help ensure that the weight you are gaining is the right kind for your baby, fill your plate with healthy foods like chickpeas, instead of fried, fatty, or processed foods.

Heart-Healthy Chickpeas

Population studies have found a positive effect from eating legumes like chickpeas—low rates of cardiovascular disease and obesity. In one study, food intake patterns were compared to the risk of death from coronary heart disease in more than 16,000 middle-aged men in the United States, Finland, the Netherlands, Italy, former Yugoslavia, Greece, and Japan for 25 years. They found that, typically, each population ate a different diet: higher consumption of dairy products in Northern Europe; higher consumption of meat in the United States; higher consumption of vegetables, legumes, fish, and wine in Southern Europe; and higher consumption of cereals, soy products, and fish in Japan.

When researchers analyzed this data in relation to the risk of death from heart disease, they found that legumes were associated with a whopping 82 percent reduction in risk. Chickpeas and other legumes are a healthy choice for your heart (which is working hard to pump a lot of extra blood these days) and your waistline, so be sure to seek these foods out during your pregnancy and afterward too!

Chock-Full of Goodness

Chickpeas are packed with lots of nutrients. In a cup of chickpeas your body gets 12 g of dietary fiber, 15 g of protein (that's about a quarter of your daily needs), more than half of your daily needs of vitamin B6, and about a quarter of your daily needs of iron. Plus, your cup of chickpeas contains some choline needed for nerve and brain development. There's even some pantothenic acid in chickpeas, a B vitamin needed for the formation of some fats. Fats are especially important to your baby now, because he or she is laying down that important layer of fat under the skin during the second trimester.

Mega Manganese

A whopping 65 percent of your daily needs of manganese (about 1.5 mg) can be found in just a cup of chickpeas. Manganese is vital to the health of your rapidly growing baby. This important mineral is an enzyme activator—in other words, it helps turn on certain enzymes that make certain processes occur. Manganese also helps in skeletal development, and your baby is going to need all the help he can get with 300 bones to build! Plus, that cup of chickpeas contains 75 mg of calcium, another bone-building nutrient.

Forgotten Minerals

Selenium, zinc, and copper are minor minerals that we tend to forget about in our nutrient discussions. Chickpeas are rich in all three: 6 mcg selenium (8 percent RDA), 2.5 mcg zinc (13 percent RDA), and 0.6 mg copper (28 percent RDA). They're natural antioxidants, so they play a key role in keeping you and your baby safe from damage caused by free radicals, damaging compounds that form in your body. Antioxidants are known to help prevent disease and aging and may also play a role in a healthy pregnancy. Researchers from the University of North Carolina reported in 2004 that antioxidants may be able to help prevent malformations in babies exposed to alcohol during pregnancy.

LEGUMES FOR LIFE

The Food Habits in Later Life Study examined the eating habits of people over the age of 70 in four different countries: Japan, Sweden, Australia, and Greece. Beans and other legumes, including chickpeas, emerged as the food most linked to longer life. In fact, legumes were the only food consistently and significantly linked to survival across all populations.

Jonny's Tasty Tips

To keep from having to cook them practically forever, you need to soak dried chickpeas for at least 12 and up to 24 hours. Then they'll get soft if you boil them for half an hour. But if you use canned chickpeas, you don't need to cook them at all. Just open a can and rinse them well before adding them to a salad, stew, or curry or using them to make baked or barbecued beans.

Chickpeas are used in many kinds of dishes around the world, including Middle Eastern falafel patties. But you probably know them best in that delicious dip, hummus. Hummus is easy to make in a food processor, or pick up a tub (or several) and a package of whole-wheat pita bread next time you're at the store. It's a great dip for carrot sticks, pepper strips, and other raw veggies, too.

Here's another delicious, easy way to cook chickpeas that I picked up from noted natural-foods expert Rebecca Wood: Simmer them till tender with garlic and toasted cumin seeds for a taste sensation. No matter how you eat them, chickpeas are a super addition to your pregnancy diet.

Chocolate Milk

GOT MILK? HOW ABOUT CHOCOLATE MILK? SURE, go ahead and reach for a glass of chocolate milk during pregnancy—it's healthier than most people think. Chocolate milk is simply low-fat milk with added cocoa powder and some sugar. And milk is packed with tons of healthy nutrients your body needs during your second trimester. Plus, cocoa is high in antioxidants and has become well known as a healthy addition to any diet. If you're not a plain-milk drinker, chocolate milk is the way to go. Even if you love milk, it will provide some delicious variety to your diet. Enjoy!

CHOCOLATE MILK AT A GLANCE

Serving Size: 1 cup (250 ml)	Calcium: 29%
Calories: 157	Vitamin A: 10%
Saturated Fat: 2 g	Vitamin C: 4%
Protein: 8 g	Iron: 3%
Fiber: 1 g	

Low Fat, High Protein

Every healthy diet recommends eating foods that are low in fat and high in protein. Chocolate milk is both of these. Most chocolate milk is low in fat, since it's usually made from 1 percent milk. And just one cup of chocolate milk contains 8 g of protein. You can feel good about getting that chocolate milk mustache.

Exercise Is Important

Exercise and a healthy diet are two equal components of a healthy pregnancy. A pregnant woman needs to be active every day. To know how much you should do, consult your obstetrician or midwife. In general, do what feels good and listen to your body. Don't try to start a challenging new exercise routine or train for a marathon—just be active. Take a walk, hit the local pool for a few casual laps, or hop on a stationary bike. Make sure your heart rate stays below 80 percent of your max. Exercise is good for you, your baby, and your partner too! And guess what? Chocolate milk may be a helpful companion to your workout routine.

Chocolate milk is being touted as the next great postworkout drink. Researchers in the Department of Kinesiology at Indiana University reported in 2006 that chocolate milk may be a good recovery aid post-exercise. In the study, nine male athletes were asked to perform a tiring bout of exercise. Then they consumed either a glass of chocolate milk, a carbohydrate replacement drink, or a fluid replacement drink. A few hours later, they were asked to exercise again until they reached exhaustion. Each athlete repeated this process three times—once with each kind of drink. The researchers found that the athletes were able to go between 49 and 54 percent longer on the second stint of exercise after they had drunk the chocolate milk. So chocolate milk could be a good choice for helping your tired body recover. (However, this study was small and was supported in part by the Dairy and Nutrition Council. More research will be needed before this study will be deemed conclusive.)

Staying Hydrated

Many beverages, including coffee, tea, and sodas, are not hydrating. In other words, they don't offer your body all of the water they contain. But chocolate milk hydrates your body and quenches your thirst, since milk is 90 percent water. Mind you, water is still the healthiest drink option during pregnancy, but for both hydration and a protein boost, you can't beat milk.

Consider the Caffeine

Remember, when you're pregnant, you should consider the caffeine content of everything you eat or drink. Researchers are suggesting that pregnant women should not consume more than 200 mg of caffeine per day (about 1.5 cups of coffee). The caffeine in chocolate bars, sodas, and chocolate milk all add up, so don't overlook them when you're calculating your daily caffeine intake. The good news: There are only about 8 mg of caffeine in a glass of chocolate milk.

Jonny's Tasty Tips

Plain chocolate milk is good. But there's an easy way to make it great: Fill a blender halfway with ice, add chocolate milk, and blend. Instant healthy milkshake! And that extra water helps you stay hydrated. For a creamy treat that's good for you and your bones, toss a banana into the blender with the ice and chocolate milk. (This is a great trick with plain milk, too.)

FAST FACT

Around week 13, your baby first can move in a jerky fashion, flexing the arms and kicking the legs. He or she may even be able to put a thumb in his or her mouth.

A Bone-Healthy Choice

Offering close to 300 mg of calcium per cup, milk is a bone-healthy choice for you and your baby. With hundreds of bones to grow and rapid growth occurring during the second trimester, your baby's calcium needs are at an all-time high, and since he or she gets that calcium from you, so are yours. Be sure to get plenty of calcium into your diet by eating green leafy vegetables, nuts, grains, and dairy products like chocolate milk. Plus, chocolate milk is rich in other nutrients needed for healthy bone growth, such as phosphorus, magnesium, and vitamin D.

Coconut Oil

COCONUT OIL IS ONE OF THE MOST MISUNDER-
stood foods. It's solid at room temperature and
it contains saturated fat, two of the signs people
use to tell bad fats from good fats (good fats are
liquid at room temperature—think of olive oil—
while bad fats are solid). But not all saturated fats are
alike, and coconut oil breaks all the rules. It's a great fat to
include in your diet. Jonny's personal favorite is Barlean's Extra Virgin Organic
Coconut Oil, and it's available at health food stores everywhere. Jonny even cooks
eggs and vegetables in it!

COCONUT OIL AT A GLANCE

Serving Size: 1 Tbsp (15 ml)	Calcium: 0%
Calories: 130	Vitamin A: 0%
Saturated Fat: 13 g	Vitamin C: 0%
Protein: 0 g	Iron: 0%
Fiber: 0 g	

FAST FACTS

Coconut oil is a safe food choice. The United
States has given coconut oil GRAS (generally
recognized as safe) status, and medical data-
bases list coconut oil use in oral and appropriate amounts in pregnant and lactating women
as safe. In other words, if you use coconut oil
in your cooking in moderate amounts, it is considered a safe food to eat.

A Great Cooking Oil

Around the world, coconut oil is used for a wide variety
of health purposes, including promoting weight loss,
improving skin conditions, and even as a hair moistur-
izer. (Try it on your hair. It's a safe and natural condi-
tioner.)

But it's coconut oil's cooking characteristics that
make it such a healthy food choice during pregnancy.
Coconut oil has a high smoke point (it can be heated
to very high temperatures before it is destroyed or

altered), making it a great choice for sautés and other high-heat cooking methods. Try using a spoonful of coconut oil instead of another oil or butter in your next high-heat culinary adventure.

Don't Fear Fat

Fat in your diet helps you absorb fat-soluble vitamins (vitamins A, E, D, and K). It also helps you absorb valuable plant carotenoids (like beta-carotene) and lycopene, which are found in fruits and vegetables. So don't skip the fat; just choose the healthiest kinds, like the fats found in foods such as nuts, seeds, and fish. (Believe it or not, a coconut is really a sort of giant seed, though technically, it's a drupe—a one-seeded fruit.)

Breast Milk Component

Because it's high in saturated fat, coconut oil was once considered a bad fat. But one type of saturated fat in coconut oil, called lauric acid, is a health hero. Lauric acid is also naturally found in breast milk. Scientists think that the lauric acid in breast milk helps prevent infants from viral and bacterial infection. Because of this, researchers are working on discovering if these helpful benefits also apply to adults if they consume lauric acid in foods like coconut oil.

Coconut oil contains antimicrobial fats that help support a healthy immune system. And if that weren't enough, the main type of saturated fat in coconuts (and coconut oil) is MCT (medium-chain triglycerides), which the body tends to use for energy rather than for fat storage. Jonny included coconut oil in his best-selling book *The 150 Healthiest Foods on Earth* and even gave it a star: Along with a growing number of experts, he considers virgin coconut oil a true superfood.

So cook with coconut oil! Researchers from the Oregon Health Sciences University found that when lactating women consumed coconut oil, their breast milk contained higher amounts of antimicrobial lauric acid within 6 hours.

Jonny's Tasty Tips

Make sure you choose the right kind of coconut oil when you're shopping for this amazing superfood. Some of the original bad press on coconut oil came from studies in which they used a hydrogenated, inferior product (loaded with trans fats) that behaves very differently in the body from the real thing. When buying coconut oil, go for the best: virgin or extra-virgin coconut oil. (Jonny recommends Barlean's Extra Virgin Coconut Oil.) It's never hydrogenated or partially hydrogenated, and it's processed without high heat and chemicals.

DON'T LET IT SMOKE!

When choosing your cooking oil, bear in mind that certain oils hold up to heat better than others. When oil starts to smoke, it means that the oil has changed in structure and is no longer healthy for you. So pick the right oil for the job. Olive oil is best used at room temperature or only in cooking at low temperatures. Canola oil can handle medium heat, and coconut oil is the best choice for medium-high to high-temperature cooking.

Figs

WOW! THERE'S A WHOPPING 5 g OF FIBER
in just 1 cup of figs. These dried fruits should
no longer be an exotic treat reserved for
Christmas fruit assortments. Figs should be
a part of your healthy diet. Figs are packed
with fiber, calcium, iron, and other nutrients that
make it a top choice for pregnant women.

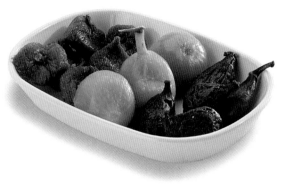

FIGS AT A GLANCE

Serving Size: 1 cup (about 8 figs)	Calcium: 6%
Calories: 133	Vitamin A: 2%
Saturated Fat: 0 g	Vitamin C: 4%
Protein: 1 g	Iron: 3%
Fiber: 5 g	

FAST FACT

Dried figs contain more calcium, potassium,
and iron than other dried fruits like raisins and
dried cranberries, making them a better choice
for athletes, pregnant women, and anyone who
needs high-nutrient foods.

Sweet Treat

Figs are definitely sweet. They contain more than four
times more sugar than fiber. Plus, they can stick to
your teeth, which can lead to poor oral health. So be
sure to brush after eating this tasty treat! But the high
sugar content doesn't mean you should pass up this
sweet food. Figs are a great nondairy source of calcium, containing about one-quarter of your daily needs
in just 1 cup. And while your teeth may not appreciate
the sugar, they will appreciate the potassium, phosphorus, and magnesium in figs. These tooth-supporting
nutrients aren't just great for your own mouth, they
are essential to the 28, plus 4 wisdom teeth, forming
below the gums in your growing baby's mouth.

Pump Up

Iron deficiency can cause anemia in pregnant women,
thanks to increases in mom's blood volume and growing
demands by the baby for iron to produce the millions
of red blood cells. Figs are a good source of iron, with
stewed figs offering you about 3 mg (about 10 percent
of your daily recommended intake) in 1 cup. Plus, this
many figs will offer your body 23 mcg of vitamin K,
a vitamin needed for proper blood clotting and bone
formation.

Jonny's Tasty Tips

You may never have even eaten a whole dried fig. But I'll bet you've eaten plenty of dried figs in the form of fig cookies. Sure, these cookies contain the calcium, iron, vitamins, and fiber of figs, but they also contain added sugar and fat. If you *must* have a cookie, fig cookies are one of the better choices, but eating real figs is the healthiest choice of all. Don't like the seedy texture of dried figs? Try some fresh figs, now increasingly available in groceries. They're considered one of the greatest of all delicacies in India and the Middle East.

Here's another cool way to use figs that I learned from Louisiana State University nutritionist Catrinel Stanciu: Puree them and then use the puree as a sweetener or fat substitute in recipes. You can make fig puree by combining 8 ounces of figs with ¼ to ⅓ cup of water in a blender.

Need More Reasons?

Not that you need other reasons to add figs to your next gourmet appetizer plate alongside other pregnancy-healthy foods like hard cheeses and whole-grain crackers but here are three: Figs are also a healthy choice due to their low-fat content and lack of sodium and cholesterol.

JUNK FOOD MAKES WEAK BABIES

It may seem like a no-brainer that avoiding junk foods (foods high in sugar, salt, and fat) is a good idea to promote proper growth and development of your baby, giving him or her the best start at a healthy life. But since junk foods are so addictive, you may need every reason you can find to keep your hand out of the chip bag or candy jar.

Here's one you may not have heard about: Researchers from England reported in the *European Journal of Nutrition* in 2008 that they found evidence suggesting that a diet high in junk food during pregnancy and lactation may reduce the muscle in the offspring. They found in a rat model that offspring of mothers eating a junk-food diet had weaker muscle strength and were less capable of exercising as they aged, thus increasing their risk of becoming obese.

Hemp

THERE IS A LOT OF CONFUSION ABOUT HEMP, since most people think of it as the source of marijuana. Yes, there is a compound in hemp leaves called delta-9-tetrahydrocannabinol (THC) that can be used for its psychoactive properties. But there's a lot more to hemp than marijuana.

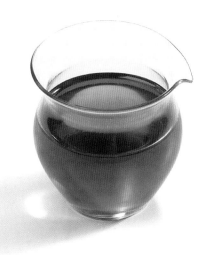

HEMP OIL AT A GLANCE

Serving Size: 1 cup (240 ml)	Calcium: 0%
Calories: 160	Vitamin A: 0%
Saturated Fat: 0.7 g	Vitamin C: 0%
Protein: 11 g	Iron: 20%
Fiber: 1 g	

Most hemp isn't smoked. Hemp plants have been used for years as a food source, and hemp fibers are used to make paper and clothing. (At one time, it was the major source of rope.) The strains of hemp plant used for food have been naturally selected to produce very little THC, causing it to lose any psychoactive properties. Hemp foods are packed with fiber, protein, and healthy fats, making hemp one of the healthiest food choices for your second trimester.

Good Fats

Hemp is one of nature's perfect sources of good fats. Hemp-seed oil contains omega-6 fatty acids (primarily gamma-linolenic acid, which is the best form of this fat for your health) and omega-3 fatty acids (primarily alpha-linolenic acid) in a ratio of about 3:1. That is close to the 4:1 ratio of these two fats recommended by the World Health Organization for an ideal diet.

Vegan Protein

If you're a vegan, it can be hard to find easy and tasty ways to add appropriate sources of protein to your diet. And as you know, it's ultra-important to get plenty of protein when you're pregnant. Luckily, hemp is a well-balanced source of ten essential amino acids. In particular, hemp is a good source of arginine (123 mg/g protein) and histidine (27 mg/g protein). These two amino acids are important for growth during childhood. In addition, hemp contains the sulfur-containing amino acids methionine (23 mg/g protein) and cysteine (16 mg/g protein), which are needed for proper enzyme formation in your body and for your growing baby.

Constipation Relief

During pregnancy, fiber may just become your new best friend. It's because fiber could provide the relief you've been looking for if your body has a hard time with bowel movements. It's common and understandable: Your baby grows, reducing the space your intestines have to work with, and elevated levels of the relaxing hormone (progesterone) slows the speed of your intestinal transit, leading to constipation. Hemp seeds are a great source of fiber.

There are 4 grams of fiber in each serving (about 5 tablespoons) of hemp seeds. That is a lot of fiber. You need about 25 to 30 grams of fiber a day. A few scoops of hemp in your yogurt can get you a long way toward a healthier digestive system. Be sure to increase your water intake as well, as water helps push things through your digestive system to help keep you regular. Stop having to hate the toilet! Eat lots of fiber during pregnancy to avoid constipation, and a diet high in fiber can even help you avoid developing hemorrhoids, too.

Shelled hemp seeds are the form of hemp you are most likely to find at your local market or health food store. In addition to fiber, hemp seeds are also a great source of protein and healthy fats (18.5 g protein, 4 g fiber, and 20g polyunsaturated fats per 5 tablespoons).

Jonny's Tasty Tips

Shelled hemp seeds are the form of hemp you're most likely to find at your local market or health food store. Hemp seeds are a great source of protein, fiber, and healthy fats (11 g of protein, 1 g of fiber, and 8 g of polyunsaturated fats per cup). And I can tell you that they're delicious! Add them to your cereal, shake, or yogurt, or sprinkle them on any dish. I even love eating them straight from the bag.

Hemp-seed butter is another tasty way to enjoy the nutritional benefits of this plant. And it's worth seeking out hemp-seed oil (aka hemp oil), too. Use this delicious, nutty-flavored oil on salads and cooked vegetables, or mix it half-and-half with softened organic butter for a terrific-tasting "essential fatty acid butter." Don't cook with hemp-seed oil, though! Store it in the fridge and use it quickly so it stays fresh.

Kale

KALE IS ANOTHER GREEN LEAFY VEGETABLE THAT'S ideal for your pregnancy diet. Even government health agencies, such as Health Canada, are recommending that all adults consume at least one green leafy vegetable a day. Whether it's kale, spinach, collards, turnip or beet greens, or mustard greens, be good to your body and add some green to your routine!

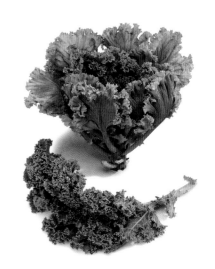

KALE AT A GLANCE

Serving Size: 1 cup (67 g)	Calcium: 7%
Calories: 33	Vitamin A: 200%
Saturated Fat: 0 g	Vitamin C: 125%
Protein: 2 g	Iron: 5%
Fiber: 1 g	

Sulfur for Safety

Kale and other *Brassica*-family vegetables like Brussels sprouts, cabbage, and broccoli have gained recent widespread attention due to the health-promoting sulfur-containing phytonutrient sulforaphane. When kale is chopped or chewed, sulforaphane is formed. It triggers your liver to produce enzymes that detoxify (neutralize) cancer-causing chemicals. In fact, research studies have found that sulforaphane can inhibit breast cancers caused by chemicals and can even tell colon cancer cells to commit suicide. Since cancer's the last thing you want to worry about when you're pregnant, make this tasty precaution a part of your weekly diet.

Protect the Ovaries

If you're having a girl, during your second trimester her ovaries are already producing the millions of eggs that will be formed by birth and will last for the duration of her reproductive years and enable her to have children of her own. Ovaries are amazing organs. They are even responsible for producing the majority of estrogen in your body from cholesterol. So when researchers discovered that foods like kale may prevent ovarian cancer, this healthy food became even more essential as one of the top foods for a healthy pregnancy and for your daughter to eat for years to come.

The Nurses' Health Study surveyed more than 60,000 women and found that women whose diet provided the most kaempferol (a flavonoid found in the highest amounts in kale, blueberries, onions, leeks, and broccoli) had a 40 percent reduced risk of ovarian cancer.

MYTH BUSTERS!

A common myth is that women can suffer losses in their cognitive ability during and after pregnancy. Mental performance normally declines with age, but having a baby has nothing to do with it! If you're worried about declining memory, get in the habit of eating more greens now. According to the Chicago Health and Aging Project, eating three servings of leafy green, yellow, and cruciferous vegetables like kale each day could slow mental decline by 40 percent.

Super Protector

Kale is also rich in manganese (0.5 mcg, more than 20 percent of your daily needs). Manganese is a critical component of an important antioxidant enzyme called superoxide dismutase (SOD). SOD is found exclusively inside your cells' mitochondria (the energy factories), where it provides protection against damage from the free radicals produced during energy production.

Jonny's Tasty Tips

Recently kale has become one of my favorite foods. I eat it about five times a week! My favorite way to use kale comes from the Sherman Oaks Whole Foods deli manager. He mixes raw kale leaves with pine nuts and cranberries and then softens the whole mixture by tossing it in olive oil. It's amazing!

Tender kale greens are perfect for adding body to any salad. I like to mix them with strong-flavored ingredients like tamari-roasted almonds or red pepper flakes. If you've never tried kale raw, add some to your next salad. You may find that even if cooked kale has always left you cold, you'll become addicted to the delicious, mild flavor and great body of raw kale.

Then again, maybe you love cooked kale. Like many other green leafy vegetables, it's so easy to prepare. Just wash it well and steam it to make a beautiful and nutritious bed for your main dish. Or add it to pasta or casseroles and let it wilt down for a fun flash of green on your plate. Serve it as a side dish with a splash of balsamic vinegar. Or sneak it into soups, stews, chilis, or even stir-fries for an extra dose of delicious nutrition.

Nori

NORI IS A KIND OF SEAWEED. BUT PLEASE don't head out to the local beach and dredge up some greens for tonight's salad! Buy your nori sheets at your local market or health food store instead.

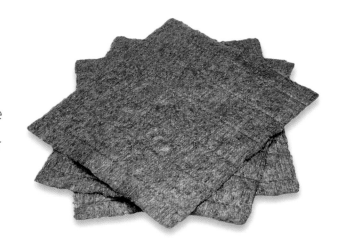

NORI AT A GLANCE

Serving Size: 1 sheet (2.5 g)	**Calcium:** 0%
Calories: 13	**Vitamin A:** 10%
Saturated Fat: 0 g	**Vitamin C:** 13%
Protein: 1 g	**Iron:** 0%
Fiber: 1 g	

Nori sheets are typically used to make sushi. Sushi itself is not recommended for pregnant women since there are real concerns that eating raw fish increases the risk for bacterial poisoning or parasite infection. However, not all sushi contains raw fish. Making vegetarian sushi at home is not only fun, but it's a delicious and nutritious meal.

Nori has many of the nutritional benefits of other dark green vegetables. It's packed with nutrients and contains over 270 IU of vitamin A in just one sheet. During your second trimester, your baby's eyes and skin are developing, and vitamin A is necessary for both to develop normally.

KELP SUPPLEMENTS: SAFETY FIRST!

Make sure you're choosing nori, the sheets of edible seaweed you use in sushi, soup, and stir-fries, *not* the concentrated kelp (also a form of seaweed) found in supplements. The most common kelp supplements contain the plant species *Fucus vesiculosus* and *Ascophyllum nodosum*, more commonly called bladderwrack or Atlantic kelp. These supplements are commonly used for their high iodine content. Pregnant or lactating women shouldn't use these supplements, since they can contain very high amounts of iodine and heavy metals. Speak with your obstetrician or midwife before taking kelp or related supplements.

Dense Nutrition

Nori is amazingly nutrient-rich. Besides vitamin A, nori is a very good source of riboflavin, vitamin B6, vitamin B12, and magnesium, offering over 100 percent of your daily needs of each. Plus, it is a great source of iron. As a pregnant woman, your needs for iron will increase in your later weeks of pregnancy as your baby pulls on your iron stores to help build up his or her own blood supply before birth.

From A to Zinc

Nori is also a good source of zinc (0.3 mg per $\frac{1}{3}$ cup). According to researchers from the University of California, zinc deficiency during pregnancy may affect a baby's lung development, leading to improper formation of air sacs and the lining of the lungs.

Having low levels of zinc in your body will lower your ability to absorb vitamin A, perhaps explaining why vitamin A deficiencies are one of the most common nutritional deficiencies around the world. This is a huge concern for pregnant women because low zinc levels could lead to low circulating vitamin A levels in the mother, reducing the transport of vitamin A to the fetus and into breast milk.

Jonny's Tasty Tips

Keeping things simple but flavorful is one of my goals, and when you're pregnant, it's bound to be one of yours, too. I'd suggest buying your vegetarian sushi from a local sushi bar and making these Nori Rice Balls at home. I found the recipe on a Web site called Nori Recipes (www.norirecipes.com), and you can find plenty of other great nori recipes if you check out this site.

To make Nori Rice Balls, cook 1 cup of quick brown rice in 1 $\frac{1}{2}$ cups water with $\frac{1}{4}$ teaspoon salt. Cook the rice over medium heat until the rice is tender and the water is absorbed. Allow rice to cool to room temperature. Meanwhile, cut half a carrot into half-inch matchsticks and steam lightly. Place several spoonfuls of rice into the center of each of 8 nori sheets, add several carrot matchsticks, and top with a dollop of umeboshi paste. Roll each filled sheet into a ball. Serve with a sauce made from soy sauce and grated ginger.

Romaine Lettuce

GO GREEN! THE DARKER YOUR LETTUCE, THE better it is for you. Romaine lettuce is becoming a more popular choice among North Americans as the benefits of dark green vegetables are becoming a common dinner table topic. That cup of romaine lettuce you've served on your salad plate contains about 2,000 IU of vitamin A, 12 mg of vitamin C, and more than half of your daily needs of vitamin K, as well as about 70 mcg of folate and 0.5 mg of iron.

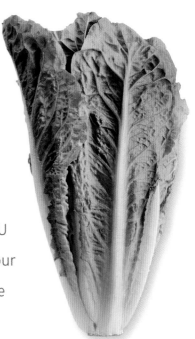

ROMAINE LETTUCE AT A GLANCE

Serving Size: 1 cup (47 g)	Calcium: 2%
Calories: 8	Vitamin A: 75%
Saturated Fat: 0 g	Vitamin C: 17%
Protein: 1 g	Iron: 3%
Fiber: 1 g	

FAST FACT

Iceberg lettuce is a nutritional weakling. Romaine lettuce is much better. Here's the rule: The darker the green, the more nutritional value it has.

Dark leafy greens are a great choice for both you and your baby. And don't forget that the higher the nutrient content in your food, the better your body's defense against disease.

Baby Nutrients

Your baby needs all of the vitamins and minerals in your diet as much as you do. But some nutrients get the lion's share of attention during pregnancy because pregnant women tend to have lower intake levels of nutrients such as folate and iron. Folate is a key nutrient required for red blood cell formation, neural-tube formation, and cell division. Iron is also needed for red blood cell formation, and it promotes proper growth. Romaine lettuce and other dark leafy green vegetables are good sources of both these nutrients.

Iron-Folate Interactions

Many nutrients in your diet interact with each other, enhancing or reducing absorption. Folate and iron are both essential during pregnancy. But some sources of folate will prevent iron absorption. Folate in milk will interact with iron, reducing your ability to absorb the iron. This may be why some newer prenatal vitamins are split into two dosages: one containing iron and nutrients that don't interact with it and the other containing folate and its complementary nutrients.

Keep this "divide and conquer" mentality in mind when you're eating. When choosing foods to serve at each meal, divide your dairy products from your meats and dark leafy greens. For example, skip that glass of milk over dinner so the iron in your meat and vegetables has a chance to be fully absorbed. You can still get plenty of calcium in your diet by enjoying dairy, nuts, and other sources of calcium at breakfast, in snacks, and at lunch.

More Than Fiber and Water

Lettuce is sometimes considered a nutritional lightweight. But it's high in fiber and water, both essential to a healthy pregnancy. And hiding in those leaves is much more. Romaine lettuce is a great source of vitamin A, vitamin C, vitamin K, thiamin, potassium, and manganese. And it's also a good source of calcium, magnesium, phosphorus, copper, vitamin B6, and riboflavin. So forget that "rabbit food" stuff and eat your salad!

Jonny's Tasty Tips

Thank heavens for Caesar and Greek salads! They're responsible for taking romaine lettuce from obscurity to stardom in the American salad bowl. First we ate romaine in these salads for its delightful crunch. Then we learned about its great nutritional value. Now we can feel even better about filling our salad bowls!

Caesar salad combines romaine lettuce with another pregnancy superfood, anchovies. I like to skip the croutons and heavy dressing and add plenty of anchovies, sunflower or pumpkin seeds (pepitas), and some shredded Parmesan or Asiago cheese and then dress the salad with a blend of extra-virgin olive oil and hemp-seed oil and some balsamic vinegar. Bliss!

Greek salad gives you another healthy, delicious salad variation. I like to top a big bowl of romaine lettuce with ripe tomatoes (lots of lycopene), diced red and orange bell peppers, fresh oregano and thyme, sliced scallions (green onions), chopped cukes, kalamata olives, and yummy feta cheese. (I've been known to sneak some anchovies in here, too.) Then I add some fruity organic extra-virgin olive oil, some lemon juice, and dig in.

Romaine is not just for salads, either. Those crunchy leaves are ideal for sandwiches. They hold their own with any kind of filling, whether you're making a turkey club, an egg or chicken salad sandwich, a pita filled with hummus and tomatoes, or a classic BLT.

Scallions

SCALLIONS—OFTEN KNOWN SIMPLY AS green onions —may be small, but they're nutritionally mighty. These green onions are mild, crunchy, and a great addition to many dishes. Just a few tablespoons of scallions provide essential nutrients to support the healthy growth of your baby and your body during your second trimester, making them a great food to include in your diet.

SCALLIONS AT A GLANCE

Serving Size: 1 cup (100 g)	Calcium: 7%
Calories: 32	Vitamin A: 18%
Saturated Fat: 0 g	Vitamin C: 28%
Protein: 2 g	Iron: 8%
Fiber: 3 g	

Onion Power!

Scallions contain almost four times the vitamin C and up to 5,000 times the vitamin A (as beta-carotene) that is found in red, white, or yellow onions. If there is so much beta-carotene in these onions, why are they green? The carotenes are masked by the green chlorophyll pigments in the mature part (upper section) of the onion.

FAST FACT

Your baby's taste buds develop around week 22 of pregnancy. Research hasn't revealed many food flavors that a baby can perceive in the womb, but garlic is one of them. Maybe eating a variety of healthy foods during this stage of pregnancy, including some spicy ones like garlic and scallions, can help keep your child from becoming a picky eater! Who knows if it works, but we agree it's definitely worth a shot!

Antioxidant Oomph

Cornell University researchers found that pungent onion varieties like scallions have the highest antioxidant activity. Having lots of antioxidants in your diet is more than a great way to fight off the common cold, help you fight wrinkles, or even inhibit cancer growth. Antioxidants also play a major role in a healthy pregnancy.

Studies have found that nitric oxide, a soluble gas, is one cause of oxidative stress (a process that causes damage to cells and structures in the body), which can affect both placental function and fetal growth. Luckily, having lots of antioxidants in your bloodstream from eating a diet filled with antioxidant-rich foods like onions could reduce oxidative stress in an expectant mother, promoting health for her placenta and fetus.

Grab a Bunch

On your next visit to the market, be sure to grab a bunch or two of scallions. They're a very good source of vitamin A, vitamin B6, and manganese, and a good source of vitamin C, folate, and potassium. These crunchy onions make a spicy, colorful topping for dips, baked potatoes, and salads. And, like all onions, they taste delicious when paired with garlic.

Jonny's Tasty Tips

I love the bold spicy flavor of scallions, so I go through several bunches a week. I load them on salads and in stir-fries and omelets. I heap them on refried beans, chili, potatoes, and soups. I even eat them whole (minus the roots, of course), using them like any other crunchy raw vegetable to scoop up hummus or a yogurt-herb or cheese dip.

Another favorite way to eat these delicious green onions may surprise you, but if you try it, you'll probably find it addictive, too. Have you heard how the French eat their breakfast radishes, sliced on a piece of buttered baguette with a sprinkle of salt? Does this sound weird? You may not consider that breakfast food, but for lunch or an afternoon snack it's amazing. But what's really amazing is when you use a healthy chunk of artisanal multigrain bread instead of a baguette, spread on organic butter, and top it with sliced radishes and scallions. Want to up the nutritional ante? Add some shaved Parmesan on top of the butter before you put on the veggies.

Worried about onion breath? Forget the breath mints and try this tip from India, where strongly flavored food is the norm: After you eat oniony food, chew a spoonful of fennel seeds. They're naturally sweet, they're great for your breath, and best of all they soothe the stomach and aid digestion.

Tofu

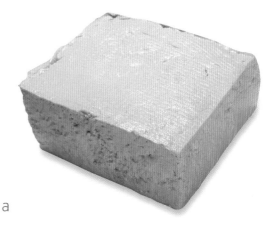

SOFT, SPONGY, BLAND, AND A LITTLE frightening (or at least boring) to some people, tofu (aka bean curd) has gotten a bad rap in North America because it's often badly prepared. (Or just cut into cubes and thrown on a salad bar as if to say "I dare you to eat it!") But when it's well prepared—think Thai curry or Chinese bean curd home style—tofu is delicious. So give it another chance. It is so easy to work with, and it's a fast way to add protein into your busy day. Even that initially bland flavor can be a plus, since you can add tofu to almost anything you're making without changing the flavor of the dish.

TOFU AT A GLANCE	
Serving Size: 1 slice (84 g of firm tofu)	**Calcium:** 8%
Calories: 55	**Vitamin A:** 0%
Saturated Fat: 0 g	**Vitamin C:** 0%
Protein: 7 g	**Iron:** 5%
Fiber: 0 g	

Nutritionally, tofu is more than a protein powerhouse. It's also a good source of essential minerals: calcium, iron, magnesium, phosphorus, copper, and selenium. Tofu is definitely one of the best foods for pregnancy.

The Power of Protein

We've said it and said it, but we can't emphasize enough the importance of protein during pregnancy. Protein is necessary for growth and development, two

processes working overtime during these nine months. The hormones needed to develop your breasts sufficiently to produce enough milk for your baby are made from protein. Enzymes and antibodies (messengers of the immune system) are also made from protein. Plus, protein is an important source of heat and energy—two things both your baby and your body need. One serving of tofu (about 80 g, or one-quarter of a typical block of tofu) contains about 7 g of protein and very little saturated fat.

Not Getting Enough Protein?

Vegetarians and vegans need to be especially careful that they're getting plenty of protein during pregnancy, and tofu can be a godsend. It will keep you and your baby healthy, but it can also guard your baby from obesity later in life. Say what?

Researchers from the University of Nottingham in the United Kingdom reported in the *British Journal of Nutrition* that restricting nutrient consumption during pregnancy can lead to adult obesity in the offspring. When a rat model was used to see how a mother's intake of protein would affect the offspring's obesity later in life, the researchers found that low-protein diets eaten by mothers during pregnancy promote changes in the babies' systems. These changes are involved in control of appetite and perception of palatability (taste). The babies of mothers who ate a low-protein diet had a preference for high-fat foods. Eating right during pregnancy is not just important for your health, it may help your child develop healthy eating behaviors too.

Lactose-Friendly

Tofu is also a good source of calcium. For those moms-to-be who are lactose intolerant, consider tofu as another nondairy alternative source of calcium. One serving of firm tofu prepared with calcium sulfate provides over 160 mg of calcium, about a sixth of your daily needs.

WHAT IS TOFU, ANYWAY?

Tofu originated in China, where it has long been a part of the Chinese diet. (Though if you go to a Chinese restaurant, you'll see tofu listed on menus as bean curd. *Tofu* is the Japanese word for this food.) Tofu is made from soymilk, which in turn is produced from yellow soybeans.

Tofu has very little taste, but it absorbs the flavors of anything it's cooked with or marinated in. There are two main kinds of tofu: silken or soft tofu and firm or extra-firm tofu. Silken tofu is often used in "yogurt," tofu "ice cream," "cheesecakes," and other nondairy desserts and in dips and spreads. Firm and extra-firm tofu are used in savory dishes like curries and stir-fries. Now you can even buy extra-firm tofu precut into cubes, as well as pressed tofu that's flavored with herbs, barbecue, and many other flavorings. How convenient!

Jonny's Tasty Tips

When cooking with firm or extra-firm tofu, you should drain, rinse, and press it dry between some paper towels first. Some recipes may even ask for you to freeze and thaw your tofu before using it, removing even more moisture for a firmer, chewier, more meatlike texture. (Or you can save yourself the trouble and buy the flavored pressed tofu at your local grocery or health food store instead.) I like to take the middle road, buying the pre-cubed extra-firm tofu when I can find it and simply buying a block of extra-firm tofu and cubing it myself when I can't.

Before you start using tofu at home, you should taste it prepared well. On your next visit to a Thai, Chinese, Vietnamese, Japanese, or Indian restaurant, order your dish with tofu instead of chicken or beef, and let an expert chef introduce your taste buds to this highly nutritious source of protein. But watch out: Some delicious and deadly appetizers and even main courses use fried tofu as the main ingredient. Here you are trying to avoid french fries, fried chicken, doughnuts, chicken-fried steak, and all those other bad-fat, bad-for-you foods. Don't replace them with fried tofu! There are plenty of healthy tofu-based choices to try instead.

Tumeric

TURMERIC IS BEST KNOWN AS A MAJOR INGREDIENT in curry powder. This bright yellow-orange powder is sometimes called the "wonder spice." But it's no wonder why when you read the review of 300 papers done by researchers at the University College of London. Research has linked turmeric to low risk of heart disease, cancer, diabetes, Parkinson's disease, and cataracts. There is ample evidence that the consumption of turmeric both prevents and treats disease.

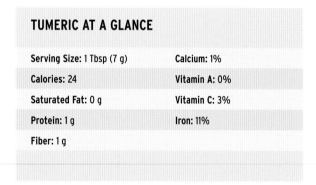

TUMERIC AT A GLANCE

Serving Size: 1 Tbsp (7 g)	Calcium: 1%
Calories: 24	Vitamin A: 0%
Saturated Fat: 0 g	Vitamin C: 3%
Protein: 1 g	Iron: 11%
Fiber: 1 g	

FAST FACT

Amazingly, your baby begins to hear as early as week 18 and may even be startled by loud noises. In a few weeks, he or she can pick up your voice in conversations. Make sure your baby's hearing develops normally by including plenty of manganese-rich foods like turmeric in your diet.

Used regularly in the foods you eat every day, turmeric is a great food to include in your nutritious pregnancy diet. (Jonny gave turmeric a star in his best-selling book, *The 150 Healthiest Foods on Earth*. He uses it on everything from scrambled eggs to vegetables!)

Working Together

One tablespoon of turmeric contains about 3 mg of iron. Plus, turmeric is a source of vitamin C (about 2 mg per tablespoon). This combination of nutrients is ideal because vitamin C helps iron be absorbed into your body via your digestive tract.

Mineral Impact

Manganese is an enzyme activator, and it helps your body use fat and carbohydrates to keep you energized. Manganese is even more important for your baby: In your growing baby, manganese plays a role in normal skeletal development and is involved in sex-hormone production. Insufficient intake of manganese during pregnancy could increase the risk that your baby will suffer from blindness and/or deafness.

Luckily, including spices like turmeric in your diet can easily help you get lots of manganese in your diet. Almost one-quarter of your daily recommended intake of manganese can be found in 2 tablespoons of turmeric.

Curious about Curcumin?

Curcumin is one of the healthiest nutrients in turmeric. It works as an antioxidant, anti-inflammatory, antiviral, and antifungal in your body. Its anti-inflammatory actions may be its most impressive characteristic now that studies have shown that inflammation may be responsible for so much harm in the body. Curcumin can help your body stay healthy from head to heart to toe.

Curcumin has another amazing health benefit: Studies have found that curcumin can bind with heavy metals such as cadmium and lead, which are harmful to you and your growing baby. By binding these heavy metals so they're not free to damage your body, curcumin reduces their toxicity. This explains why curcumin has been found to be protective of the brain and makes it a great nutrient to include in a healthy pregnancy to help reduce the risk heavy metals pose to you and your baby.

It's Everywhere!

The most common use for turmeric is in making curry. But it's also used in many foods as a coloring agent because of its great yellow color. You'll find curcumin in foods like mustard, margarine, processed cheese, cakes, soft drinks, and sweets. But that's not an invitation to indulge in junk food! Just because your slice of cake may contain curcumin, remember that you really should get this powerful nutrient from turmeric used to spice healthy dishes like delicious vegetable curry.

Jonny's Tasty Tips

If there were ever a contest for a spice that deserved a whole book written about it, turmeric would be the clear winner. It's pretty much my favorite spice, not only for its encyclopedia list of health benefits but also for its incredible taste. Turmeric is a staple in India: It's the spice that gives Indian food its distinctive flavor. It's an important part of curry sauce, but that's only the beginning. I use it on just about everything, but my latest discovery is how great it tastes on scrambled eggs and veggie omelets.

FAST FACT

Curcumin is the active compound in turmeric. It gives it that characteristic yellow color. UCLA researchers and Department of Veteran Affairs concluded that curcumin may be a powerful weapon against Alzheimer's.

Tuna

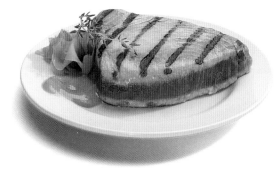

A NUMBER OF STUDIES HAVE FOUND THAT eating high amounts of fish during later stages of pregnancy and lactation (3 to 4 servings per week) has many healthy benefits. Tuna is one of the easiest fish to add into your busy lifestyle. Pack a can of tuna in your lunch bag and toss it on top of your salad for a great dose of protein (42 g of high-quality protein for under 200 calories!), good fats, and other nutrients. Or enjoy a meaty tuna steak as an upscale dinner option.

TUNA AT A GLANCE

Serving Size: 1 can (165 g)	Calcium: 2%
Calories: 190	Vitamin A: 2%
Saturated Fat: 0 g	Vitamin C: 0%
Protein: 42 g	Iron: 12%
Fiber: 0 g	

Bone-Healthy

Japanese women have lower rates of osteoporosis, even though they generally don't consume high amounts of calcium. Why? Fish, especially high fat fish like salmon and tuna, is rich in vitamin D. Japanese women have high intakes of vitamin D because they eat fish frequently (about 4 or 5 times more per week than American women). High vitamin D intake is believed by many researchers to protect against osteoporosis, and the latest research shows it's also protective against heart disease and against some cancers.

Essential Fats

The fats found in fish are essential, which means your body cannot make them, and if you don't eat them, you and your growing baby will be deficient. DHA is required in high levels in the brain and retina as a physiologically essential nutrient to provide for optimal neuronal functioning (learning ability and mental development) and visual acuity in young and old alike. There are more than 300 mg of DHA in a can of water-packed tuna!

Eat More Fish *Now*

Usually the importance of essential fatty acids is discussed around the third trimester because the majority of these fats are absorbed during this later period of pregnancy. But it's important to include sufficient amounts of EPA and DHA in your diet earlier in pregnancy to ensure that if your baby is born prematurely, he or she has had the opportunity to get as much of these good fats as possible. In addition, 70 percent of your baby's brain cell development takes place in the womb. The fetal liver is not mature enough to metabolize shorter-chain fatty acids like alpha-linolenic acid (ALA), found in plant oils like flax, into the long-chain omega-3s eicosapentaenoic acid (EPA) and DHA until 16 weeks after birth.

Jonny's Tasty Tips

Water-packed or oil-packed? That might be your first question when buying canned tuna. But believe it or not, there's no easy answer. Oil-packed tuna is more likely to retain those essential omega-3 fatty acids, but if you drain the oil, they'll go right down the drain along with it. Instead, use that oil on your salad instead of salad oil and save your omega-3s! Water-packed tuna has less omega-3s, but you won't lose them if you drain off the water. My pick? I recommend you seek out the small specialty companies like Vital Choice (reachable through a link on Jonny's Web site, www.jonnybowden.com) that produce a better-quality product, like gourmet or premium canned Pacific tuna, and enjoy the flavor and the extra omega-3s.

In other words, your dietary choices will play a major role in whether your baby gets enough of these essential fatty acids. It's time to add more fish into your diet. And if you need more motivation, research studies have found that women who are deficient in DHA are more likely to have preterm deliveries or low-birth-weight babies, and these women are also more likely to develop behavioral or mood disorders, including postpartum depression.

Eat the Right Fats

The typical North American diet of pregnant women includes high levels of omega-6 fatty acids found in corn and soybean oils (about 8,000 mg a day), high levels of ALA omega-3 fatty acids found in flax and canola oils (about 1,300 mg a day), but low levels of DHA (80 mg a day) and EPA (35 mg a day on average). This low intake in North American women is a drastic contrast to the amount consumed by Japanese women.

PREGNANT WOMEN: EAT MORE FISH!

You may be leery of eating fish while you're pregnant because you've heard the reports of mercury and other heavy metal contamination. The main concern is that methyl-mercury, the contaminant found in certain fish, can increase the risk of impaired brain development in the infant. And who wants to risk that?

But here's the scoop: The Food and Drug Administration recommends that pregnant women avoid eating shark, swordfish, king mackerel, and golden snapper. Otherwise, eating fish isn't just safe, it's vital to a healthy pregnancy and a healthy, well-developed brain in your baby.

Top researchers recommend that pregnant women eat fish. The benefits of sufficient docosahexaenoic acid (DHA) levels in pregnant women far outweigh any potential risks of eating fish. DHA is the primary fat required for proper brain cell development and functioning. Having enough DHA in your diet has been linked to lower depression level and babies with higher IQs and advanced learning abilities. And DHA, found predominantly in fish and seafood, isn't consumed nearly often enough: just once every 10 days during pregnancy. Eating fish like tuna 3 or 4 times a week will give your baby the best chance of developing a great brain, not to mention a strong liver and other organs.

Turkey

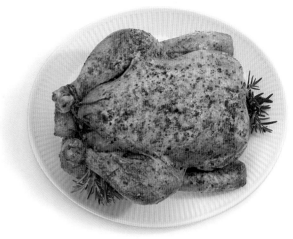

ACCORDING TO THE NATIONAL TURKEY Federation, the average American eats an estimated 17 pounds of turkey each year. (We know, you're still reeling from the idea that there actually *is* a National Turkey Foundation!) But here's the thing—when you're pregnant, you should *definitely* be gobbling up some turkey. Turkey is a great source of protein that is low in fat and packed with healthy nutrients for you and your developing baby. Just one 4-ounce serving provides about 60 percent of your daily recommended protein intake.

TURKEY AT A GLANCE

Serving Size: 1 cup (140 g white meat)	Calcium: 2%
Calories: 220	Vitamin A: 0%
Saturated Fat: 1 g	Vitamin C: 0%
Protein: 42 g	Iron: 8%
Fiber: 0 g	

A Radical Bird

Turkey is high in cysteine and selenium, nutrients that are important during pregnancy because they're potent antioxidants. Both nutrients also support healthy levels of one of the body's most powerful antioxidants, glutathione peroxidase. Glutathione peroxidase neutralizes free radicals that form from exposure to harmful chemicals in the environment (including ultraviolet radiation from sunlight, detergents, cosmetics, cigarette smoke, and pesticides on food).

SAY NO TO LUNCH MEAT

Don't buy your turkey at the deli counter. Many deli meats contain added fat and sodium. Plus, there are concerns that pregnant women and the elderly should avoid lunch meats because they have a higher risk than other foods of being contaminated with harmful bacteria like Listeria. For a healthier and safer sandwich, prepare a turkey breast at home and slice it into your own deli-style cold cuts.

Free radicals can damage any part of your body. But they're most dangerous when they attack your blood vessels or mitochondria. Blood supply to your baby is vital, and your mitochondria are responsible for making energy, something you're in serious need of as your baby grows and increases the amount of extra weight you're having to lug around all day. In just 4 ounces of roasted turkey breast, you'll find 45 percent of your daily recommended value of selenium.

The Feel-Good Food

Turkey's not just about nutrients. It's rich in trypto-phan, which is converted in the body to serotonin. And as you've probably heard, serotonin boosts your mood and reduces sugar cravings. Since you may not always feel so well when you're pregnant, be it from discomfort or raging hormones, it's great to know that a safe, effective mood booster is only a sandwich away!

Jonny's Tasty Tips

Thanksgiving and Christmas may be peak times for turkey consumption, but don't wait for the holidays to take advantage of its wonderful taste and nutritional offerings. Sliced turkey is a perfect sandwich meat, and cooked, cubed turkey is a great substitute for beef in stews and chili. In place of chicken, make a turkey pot pie or turkey salad. In fact, turkey's a great substitute for chicken anytime. (But please, skip the deep-fried turkey!) Buy turkey breast so you don't have to cook the whole bird every time. Turkey is a healthy way to add more protein into your diet and to keep your energy levels high as your pregnancy progresses.

Watercress

CRISP, PEPPERY WATERCRESS IS A GREAT addition to any salad. And it's packed with nutrients to support your changing body and growing baby. Watercress is a good source of protein, folate, copper, magnesium, manganese, potassium, vitamin K, and phosphorus. And that's not all!

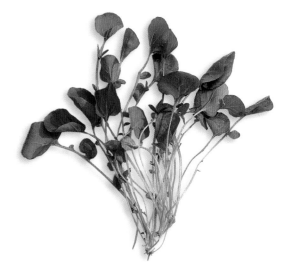

WATERCRESS AT A GLANCE

Serving Size: 1 cup (34 g)	Calcium: 3%
Calories: 4	Vitamin A: 37%
Saturated Fat: 0 g	Vitamin C: 20%
Protein: 1 g	Iron: 0%
Fiber: 0 g	

FAST FACT

Most miscarriages are caused by unspecific causes. There is usually nothing you can do to prevent a miscarriage.

Antioxidants to the Rescue

During pregnancy, a woman's body is going through a lot of changes and stress, and as a result, her levels of oxidative stress increase. Oxidative stress is the scientific way to explain how many damaging free radicals (reactive oxygen species) are in your body, causing damage to cells and organs. Luckily, antioxidants like vitamin C, vitamin E, and vitamin A, found in many healthy foods like watercress, can battle back against these free radicals, neutralizing them so they can't cause damage.

Eye It Up

Lutein and zeaxanthin are more key nutrients in watercress. These nutrients are found in high levels in the lens and retina of the eye, and since your baby's eyes are developing quickly now, they're especially important. Plus, watercress is a source of vitamin A (about 500 IU per half-cup), which is needed for healthy night vision.

Get Your Bs

This nutrient-rich green leafy vegetable is also a good source of a number of B vitamins. B vitamins are most famous for their role in energy production, helping you feel good. Watercress is especially rich in the B vitamins pantothenic acid and riboflavin (about 0.1 mg per cup). Pantothenic acid helps the body form certain fats, but more important, it helps improve your cells' ability to resist stress, which your body will certainly experience during pregnancy and particularly during labor.

Riboflavin plays a role in the formation of cell blood cells and antibodies (messengers of the immune system). Low intake levels of riboflavin are associated with eye problems in infants and may be associated with prematurity or stillbirth. Luckily, riboflavin is present in many healthy foods, including watercress. You'll also find some vitamin B6 in watercress, which can help maintain your sodium/phosphorus balance, helping you stay properly hydrated.

Jonny's Tasty Tips

Grab some watercress at your next visit to the market and enjoy its fresh, crisp fragrance and peppery flavor in your next salad, omelet, or stir-fry. It's great as a topping on chili, black bean soup, and refried beans, too. You may find that, like me, you enjoy the flavor so much that you'll want to make it a stand-alone salad topped with a squeeze of lemon and a dribble of organic extra-virgin olive oil. And if you're a fan of tomato and cottage cheese salad, add some beautiful green watercress and see how much better it tastes. Ditto for tuna and egg salad sandwiches. It's great to know that you're boosting flavor and nutrition at the same time!

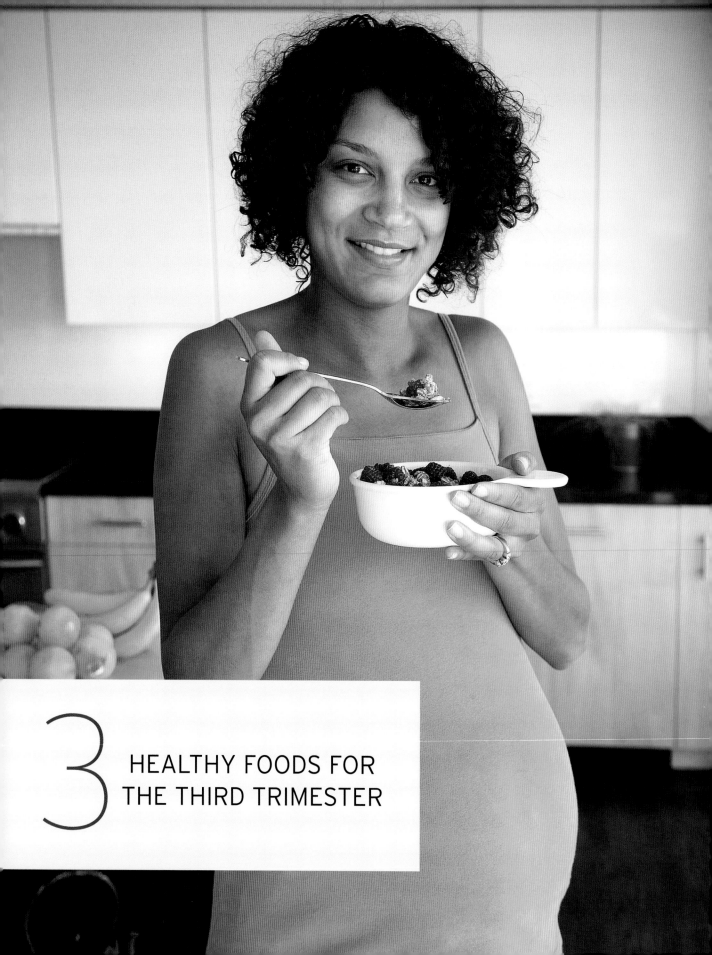

3

HEALTHY FOODS FOR THE THIRD TRIMESTER

STARTING TO FEEL LIKE YOU'RE GOING TO BE pregnant forever? The third trimester is the last stage of pregnancy, and with it comes a very large belly. Sorry about that. Your widening midsection will change the way you move, bend, and feel. But it's not all bad news. On the plus side, you'll get to enjoy baby hiccups and somersaults, both of which can make you feel excited about your soon-to-be-born baby.

From week 28 until labor, you'll be in your third trimester. And with this final stage of pregnancy comes a whole new range of changes in your body and a whole new range of nutrient needs.

In this chapter, we'll discuss what's happening during this home stretch and which foods are best to support your needs.

NEW TRIMESTER, NEW COMPLAINTS

Because you and your baby are heading to the finish line, you'll be experiencing a lot of body changes. As your baby's muscle and fat tissue is developing, you'll experience steady weight gain. And because the baby's growing fast and taking up more and more room, your internal organs are going to be squeezed to make space, which may result in digestive discomfort, heartburn, increased urination, and back pain. Are you having fun yet?

Let's quickly discuss the not-so-pretty side of the third trimester and address some common complaints. Keep in mind that not all women will experience these symptoms. Every pregnancy is different! You may be one of the lucky ones.

Puffy Mommy

Swelling of your feet and ankles may become an issue in your third trimester. Your growing uterus and baby are putting pressure on the veins that return blood from your legs to your heart. To reduce swelling, try cold compresses on the affected areas, lying down, or using a footrest. If you avoid standing for too long, it will not only help with swelling but with back pain, too.

NUTRITIONAL NEEDS FOR THE THIRD TRIMESTER

Because every woman's body is different, it's important to work closely with your obstetrician to develop a nutritional program that's ideal for you. Factors including your health, age, and weight to your activity level, heredity, and the amount of stress you're experiencing combine to create unique nutritional needs. This chart will give you nutritional guidelines for a healthy third trimester. You'll read about these nutrients in detail later in the chapter.

Key Vitamins

Vitamin A: 2,700 IU daily

Folate: 800 mcg daily

Vitamin B12: 2.2 mcg daily

Vitamin C: 85 mg daily

Vitamin D: 400 IU daily

Key Minerals

Calcium: 1,000 mg daily

Iron: 27 mg daily

Sodium: 2,400 mg daily

Zinc: 15 mg daily

Other Key Nutritional Needs

Calories: 450 extra calories a day (only if needed)

Protein: a minimum of 60 g daily

Fiber: 25 to 30 g daily

Fluids: Eight to twelve 8-ounce glasses of liquid daily

Watching your fluid intake, as well as your potassium and sodium intake, can help battle back against swelling. When it comes to watching your fluid intake, you need to make sure you're getting enough water. I know this may seem like a contradiction, but drinking lots of water and other "good liquids" like pure juice can help your body maintain a proper water balance, which doesn't include swelling.

As for sodium (salt), eating foods in their natural state instead of eating them in packaged or processed forms can help you control your intake of this fluid-retaining mineral. And don't forget potassium—it helps you keep the extra sodium in your body from building up and causing swelling. There's lots of potassium in bananas and other fruits and vegetables. Reaching for lots of water and natural foods like fresh vegetables, fruits, seeds, and grains is a great way to help your body maintain a healthy fluid level.

Burning Up

The walk from the car to the office building may also seem like a harder feat as your pregnancy progresses and your uterus expands. In your last trimester, your uterus has expanded to the point that it now sits just below your diaphragm muscles—the ones that help expand your lungs when you breathe. This pressure in the upper part of your abdomen can also push your stomach out of its normal position and cause heartburn. To help keep stomach acid in your stomach where it belongs and not in your throat, eat small meals and drink plenty of fluids. Avoiding spicy and fatty foods may help, too. And eating high-fiber foods like black beans and celery can also help you battle heartburn.

The Big Stretch

Your skin may also be experiencing some changes you're not going to enjoy, such as spider veins or varicose veins, caused by your increased blood volume. Stretch marks—pink, reddish streaks along your abdomen, upper arms, breasts, and/or thighs—may show up now. Stretching around your breasts is due to continued breast growth in preparation for breast-feeding. In your third trimester, you may have up to an additional one to three pounds of breast tissue! But eating enough protein can help your body repair any stretching muscles and skin. The same is true for many fruits, which are packed with skin-healthy nutrients to keep you looking your most beautiful.

Can't Get Comfortable

Your baby's size and position may make it hard for you to get comfortable. To compensate for the discomfort, get plenty of rest. Wear comfortable clothes. (You can resume being a fashion diva *after* the pregnancy!) Use lots of pillows to help make you comfortable at night. Many women find that sleeping on their left side is the most comfortable position. And remember that your diet plays a major role in how you feel, so eat right to help keep you feeling your best.

Weight Gain

By your 28th week of pregnancy, your baby will weigh about 2.5 pounds (1.1 kg). This is amazing when you consider that over the last 11 weeks your baby has increased his or her weight 10 times. And in just the last month, your baby has *doubled* him or her weight! By the end of the third trimester, the average baby birth weight is about 7.5 pounds (3.4 kg). Your baby is starting to put on weight and so are you (about 3 to 4 pounds each month). Some women will find their weight gain slow in the last weeks of pregnancy.

Depending on your prepregnancy weight, you can expect to put on a total of 25 to 40 pounds during your pregnancy (underweight women should gain more weight, and overweight women may gain less). But here's the good news: If you've been eating healthy foods like the ones we recommend throughout your pregnancy and making sure you have plenty of colorful foods on your plate, sufficient protein, and whole grains, your weight gain is likely to be within your body's appropriate range.

If you're worried about your weight gain, talk to your obstetrician or midwife. And if you've indulged in the occasional chunk of chocolate or sweet or salty treat, don't worry: "Everything in moderation" is the rule for every healthy diet. And the occasional treat counts as moderation!

COUNTING DOWN

If you're eight months and counting, you may feel as though you're in a holding pattern, waiting for your baby to make its entrance into this world. However, there's a lot going on inside of you. That pain under your ribs is thanks to the cramped conditions in your belly. Your uterus is less roomy now than in previous months, when your baby was able to amuse him or herself with somersaults. Now your baby is doing some stretching, and once he or she settles into the head-down position (the position that 97 percent of babies assume before labor), he or she'll be stretching by pushing his feet under your ribs.

More Side Effects

One thing you'll notice is a lot of movement going on, and it's not you who's doing the moving. Hiccups and other baby movements are common in your third trimester. You can also experience sudden movements, such as when your baby tries to get his or her thumb back in his or her mouth, which is a habit that starts before birth. And as your baby descends into your pelvis toward the final days of your pregnancy (this may occur as early as a few weeks ahead of time), his or her head begins pressing against your perineum (the area between your anus and your vagina), which may make walking and even sitting uncomfortable.

Abdominal cramping, groin pain, and/or a persistent backache can all be attributed to the new, lower position your baby has assumed. It increases pressure on your pelvis and rectum. You may start to think that

GETTING BIGGER

The other day, over a glass of lemon water, a friend of mine described her experiences during her third trimester of pregnancy. Her growing belly was the biggest attraction of her pregnancy. She loved being able to see on the outside all of the changes happening on the inside.

However, there came a point where she believed that it was going to be simply impossible for her belly to grow any bigger. Yet upon waking the next morning, there it would be—an even bigger belly than before. The amazing ability of your uterus to grow from the size of a small piece of fruit, such as a lime, to the size of a large watermelon in a mere nine months means that your organs have to move over, and your skin has to stretch.

Luckily, eating certain foods can arm your body with nutrients it needs to help support these changes. Nutrients like fiber, water, vitamin C, vitamin E, silica, and good fats can help get your intestines and your skin through these months of stretching and squeezing. Check out the top foods for the third trimester, beginning on page 130, for some fast, delicious relief.

WHAT IF I'M *LOSING* WEIGHT?

Some women may actually lose weight (a pound or two) in their last month of pregnancy, despite their baby's increasing weight. This is nothing to be concerned about. The total amount of amniotic fluid in your body is decreasing, a change triggered by hormonal fluctuations occurring late in pregnancy. This weight loss may also be caused by the decreased space around your stomach. With little room to expand, you may find you're not able to eat as much as you used to. If you're worried about your inability to eat enough, be sure to focus on the foods in this book—foods that are rich in nutrients, protein, good carbohydrates, and good fats that will keep you and your baby going.

FAST FACT

During the third trimester, your baby's eyes and brain are developing more, along with his taste buds. It's true: Your baby can taste foods like garlic even before he's born.

your baby is using your bladder as a squeeze toy: The feeling that you have to urinate every hour is common and is unfortunately just part of the program.

YOU STILL NEED TO EAT

Of course, we're most concerned about your third-trimester eating habits. You may find in this later stage of pregnancy that your large uterus is not just cramping your bladder but your intestines and stomach too. Eating lots of healthy foods that are rich in fiber like fruits, vegetables, nuts, and seeds will help keep your intestinal tract moving despite its confined conditions.

Your stomach also has less room to expand, which may cause you to feel full even after just a few bites of food. Trying to eat smaller, more frequent meals may help. This may make it harder to keep track of which nutrients you're taking in, so be sure that each mini-meal offers you as many healthy nutrients as possible.

Eat More Fish

Research has shown that women who eat fish during their last trimester of pregnancy have babies with healthier weights. The *Journal of Epidemiology and Community Health* reported in 2004 that in a study of over 11,580 women, those who ate more fish at 32 weeks of pregnancy had lower rates of restricted growth in their babies, where the baby is not able to grow in the womb to a healthy size and weight. (Restricted fetal growth normally occurs in one in ten pregnancies.)

The researchers found that on average the women ate almost 33 g of fish or the equivalent of about a third of a small can of tuna a day, which gave them 0.15 g of omega-3 fatty acids. They concluded that the more fish the women ate, the lower the rates of restricted fetal growth. So eating fish regularly in late pregnancy may help your baby grow.

PREECLAMPSIA

One last issue we need to discuss before we dive into the top foods for your third trimester is the issue of preeclampsia (or, in Canada and Europe, pre-eclampsia). Preeclampsia is a disorder that occurs only during pregnancy (typically after 20 weeks of gestation) and the postpartum period. It affects both the mother and her unborn baby.

Preeclampsia is a rapidly progressive condition characterized by high blood pressure and protein in the urine. Swelling, sudden weight gain, headaches, and changes in vision are potential symptoms. Besides high blood pressure, preeclampsia can cause damage to your kidneys and reduced blood flow to the placenta, which can complicate your pregnancy.

Obviously, preeclampsia is a very serious condition, and if you experience signs of it, you need to contact your obstetrician immediately. Globally, preeclampsia and other hypertensive disorders of pregnancy are a leading cause of maternal and infant illness and death. The good news is that it's uncommon, only affecting about 5 to 8 percent of all pregnancies.

Researchers are trying to determine the cause of preeclampsia. Meanwhile, prevention remains the key to avoiding this condition. Different drugs and supplements, such as evening primrose oil and fish oil, and healthy eating habits, including getting enough protein, calcium, and magnesium, are excellent precautions. We're about to tell you more about them as we get into the top foods for the third trimester.

GET ENOUGH GOOD FATS

One of the most important nutrients to consider during your last trimester of pregnancy is an omega-3 fatty acid with the unwieldy name of docosahexaenoic acid (DHA for short). Don't worry—you'll never have to spell it—but it's important that you know about it. During the last trimester of pregnancy, your baby's brain—which is about 60 percent fat by weight—is developing really fast. And the majority of the fat in your baby's brain is that very same omega-3 fatty acid: DHA.

Eating sufficient amounts of DHA, found most abundantly in fish, is important to you and your baby. (Now you know why your grandmother correctly called fish "brain food." It is!). DHA supports proper brain development. In fact, eating enough DHA during the third trimester has been linked to impressive cognitive abilities in toddlers. Maybe your baby won't be the next Einstein, but it's smart on your part to give him or her the best brain you can! See the section on fish oil beginning on page 147 for more on the benefits of getting plenty of DHA.

Top Foods for The Third Trimester

Finally it's time to dig your teeth into the healthiest foods for your third trimester. These foods are rich in nutrients needed for your body's third-trimester growth and changes, as well as for your baby's unique developmental needs during these last few months. Remember that all of the foods in this book, including the ones in the lists of healthiest foods for your first and second trimesters, are healthy choices for moms every day. Keep enjoying them, but make sure you add these to your diet, too.

HERE ARE THE 21 HEALTHIEST FOODS FOR THE THIRD TRIMESTER:

- BLACK BEANS
- CELERY
- COHO SALMON
- CRANBERRIES
- CRIMINI MUSHROOMS
- EGGS
- EGGPLANT
- EVENING PRIMROSE OIL

- FISH OIL
- GARLIC
- GREEN PEAS
- HERRING
- MOLASSES
- NUTS
- PAPAYA
- PARSLEY

- PEPPERMINT
- RED RASPBERRY LEAF TEA
- RHUBARB
- SESAME SEEDS
- SWISS CHEESE

Let's look at each of these healthy third-trimester foods and see what makes them tops on our list. By now, you're used to us telling you to break with routine and try these fabulous foods, even if you've never eaten herring or sipped a cup of red raspberry leaf tea or taken evening primrose or fish oil supplements before. "Jonny's Tasty Tips" will give you some great ways to enjoy them.

Black Beans

A FAVORITE IN MEXICAN DISHES, BLACK BEANS (also known as turtle or black turtle beans) are a tasty and nutritious addition to your pregnancy diet. The *Journal of Agriculture and Food Chemistry* reported that black beans are as rich in antioxidant compounds called anthocyanins as grapes and cranberries, two fruits that are antioxidant stars. Try adding black beans into your diet—they're packed with nutrients that you and your baby need.

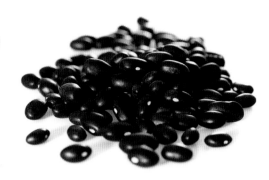

BLACK BEANS AT A GLANCE

Serving Size: 1 cup (172 g)	Calcium: 5%
Calories: 227	Vitamin A: 0%
Saturated Fat: 0 g	Vitamin C: 0%
Protein: 15 g	Iron: 18%
Fiber: 15 g	

Note: The nutritional facts data provided in this book are approximations based on the food's nutrient value and a pregnant woman's RDA.

Black beans are also a good source of manganese, iron, thiamin, phosphorus, and magnesium. So toss some into your next chili or salad for a fun twist packed with great nutrients to keep you and your baby feeling great.

Beans and Berries

When we think of antioxidants, we tend to think of berries, but beans are also antioxidant rich, with black beans at the top of the list. University of Guelph researchers tested the antioxidant activity of plant compounds called flavonoids from the skin of 12 common bean varieties. Black beans came out on top, followed by red, brown, yellow, and white beans. In general, darker-colored beans had higher levels of flavonoids and higher antioxidant activity.

Good Things in Small Packages

Black beans have always been appealing, because of their great flavor, vibrant dark color, and cute, tiny size. But they offer more than good looks and taste: These beans are packed with nutrients. In just one cup of black beans, there are an astounding 15 g of fiber, more than half of your daily needs. Plus, there's tons of folate (over 250 mcg per cup).

Molybdenum Detox

Black beans are an excellent source of the trace mineral molybdenum. This is definitely one of the lesser-known minerals, but its role in the body is nothing to ignore. Molybdenum is an integral component of the enzyme sulfite oxidase, which is responsible for detoxifying sulfites. Sulfites are a type of preservative commonly added to prepared foods like delicatessen salads and salad bars and even to dried fruit. In a cup of black beans, you'll get a whopping 160 percent of your daily

Jonny's Tasty Tips

You may have seen black bean salsas selling for big bucks in gourmet stores and catalogs. But it's so easy to make your own, there's no excuse for spending the money. Take a can of black beans, a package of frozen corn, and a jar of salsa that's the heat you like it. I love adding minced fresh cilantro and a finely chopped fresh sweet onion to the mix, too. Stir them all together and enjoy this incredibly tasty dip!

Another all-time favorite is black bean soup. Yum!!! It adds a ton of flavorful nutrients to a basic can or two of black beans. The way I make it is fast and easy, too. I sauté chopped sweet onion and minced garlic in olive oil with whole cumin seed, black mustard seed, and plenty of dried Greek oregano. Then I add diced green pepper and diced paste tomatoes, splash in a little fresh-squeezed lemon juice and a dollop of hot sauce, and toss in a couple of cans of black beans. When it's bubbling, I mash the beans with a potato masher to make the soup thick and rich. After stirring well, I serve up this luscious soup with a dollop of plain yogurt and some minced cilantro on top. You can pour it in a bowl over a scoop of brown rice for a complete protein meal. And don't forget, leftovers make the ideal dip for chips or veggie sticks!

needs of molybdenum. And since it's almost impossible to avoid sulfites, you really need that molybdenum to make food safe!

Feelin' Good

A cup of black beans also has about 180 mg of that famous feel-good compound tryptophan. Tryptophan is an essential amino acid (you have to eat it because your body can't make it). In your body, tryptophan is used to make niacin (a B vitamin) and serotonin (a feel-good hormone that is thought to stabilize mood and promote sleep). With your baby kicking and squeezing your insides, sleep can be hard to come by right now, so eat your beans before bedtime!

Meat Equivalent

These smoky-flavored beans are a good source of protein. If you eat them with a whole grain, such as whole wheat pasta or brown rice, or corn, it provides a protein comparable to that of meat or dairy foods (called a complete protein source) without the high calories or saturated fat found in these foods.

Celery

CRISP AND DELICIOUS, CELERY IS MORE THAN A HEALTHY

snack: Consider it your new skin-beautifying food during your pregnancy. Celery is rich in silica, a mineral that is important to the tone and firmness of your skin. With all the stretching and expanding going on during this final trimester of pregnancy, your skin needs all the support it can get. In fact, silica can help your skin hold water, keeping it hydrated and healthy while it gets pulled to its fullest extent.

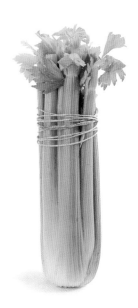

CELERY AT A GLANCE

Serving Size: 1 cup (100 g)	**Calcium:** 4%
Calories: 16	**Vitamin A:** 8%
Saturated Fat: 0 g	**Vitamin C:** 4%
Protein: 1 g	**Iron:** 4%
Fiber: 2 g	

Silica for Your Skin

Even though silica is the second most abundant element on earth, people commonly suffer from a silica deficiency and have weak, saggy skin as a result. During pregnancy, your skin is stretched to its limits, and then after birth, the skin contracts back toward its normal position. Now, don't get any illusions that after labor, your belly goes flat and the skin around your stomach is perfect—it took you nine months to get that big, and it's certainly going to take a few months to get your body back to normal. Patience and a healthy diet can help you regain that prepregnancy shape. Eating foods like celery that contain skin-healthy nutrients can help your skin rebound quickly.

You Need More

If you're an older mom, it's especially important to make sure you're getting enough silica. Experts have not yet come up with a recommended daily intake of silica, since it's not considered an essential nutrient, but estimates suggest that women could benefit from about 40 mg a day. This is the amount in studies that have been associated with increased bone-mineral density. Men and premenopausal women who have higher dietary intake of silica seem to have higher bone mineral density, which could reduce the risk of osteoporosis. You need more silica as you age, because as you get older, you become less able to absorb silica; your stomach acids weaken, making it difficult for your body to digest this mineral properly. For these reasons, you need to eat plenty of celery and other skin-healthy foods during pregnancy and lactation to help your skin survive this ordeal.

Jonny's Tasty Tips

I love to eat celery with a spoonful of peanut or almond butter on it as a filling snack. Or vary your routine by dipping a stalk in hummus or plain yogurt, with or without shredded cheese mixed in. It's so easy to pack some celery sticks and carry them with you or chop up a stalk or two and throw it on a salad or into soups, stews, or pot roast.

But here's my favorite way to enjoy celery: juiced. Surprised? Toss a few cut-up stalks into the blender with a cut-up pear and a couple of inches of peeled ginger-root and then strain and serve over ice for a spicy, refreshing pick-me-up. (Actually, if you don't mind it pulpy, you don't even have to strain!) Better yet, if you have a juicer, just juice the celery, pear, and gingerroot. I think you'll love it as much as I do!

One word of warning: The Environmental Working Group put celery on its 2003 list of twelve foods most contaminated with pesticides. For your sake and your baby's, buy organic celery to be safe.

There's More?

Celery is just fiber and water, right? Think again. Besides being rich in silica, celery is a source of many nutrients, including potassium and sodium, the most important minerals for controlling fluid balance in your body. Celery was used traditionally as a diuretic and can help you get rid of excess fluid, such as the puffiness that can build up under your eyes and in your feet during pregnancy. And celery is a source of another potent antioxidant, vitamin C, that can help you and your baby fight off damage caused by free radicals.

C for Collagen

Celery is a source of vitamin C, another nutrient known to give you natural skin support. Vitamin C is needed for specialized cells in your skin called fibroblasts to make collagen. Collagen is like the scaffolding of your skin—it keeps it strong and gives it structure. You'll need it during your third trimester as the skin around your breasts and belly is being stretched. This extra stress on the skin may cause your collagen to break down. Keep your skin strong with the help of vitamin C-rich foods like celery and help your skin rebound faster from its out-of-shape condition. Celery is an excellent source of vitamin C—one cup of celery provides roughly 5 percent of your recommended daily needs.

Grab a Glass

Celery has a very high water content, which helps hydrate your body, your baby, and your skin. You may not feel as thirsty as you did during your first trimester, but your need for water is ramping up now. And as you begin breast-feeding, you'll need more and more water. Foods rich in water like celery are a great way to help you get more water into your diet.

⭐ Coho Salmon

SALMON IS ONE OF THE HEALTHIEST FOODS YOU can eat during pregnancy. Wild salmon is considered the healthiest type of salmon, and one of the tastiest is Coho salmon. Rich in omega-3 fatty acids, protein, and vitamins, salmon is a perfect food to include in your diet during your third trimester.

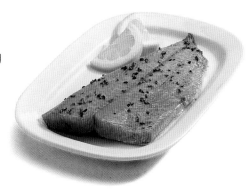

COHO SALMON AT A GLANCE

Serving Size: ½ fillet (175 g)	Calcium: 8%
Calories: 250	Vitamin A: 4%
Saturated Fat: 2 g	Vitamin C: 4%
Protein: 42 g	Iron: 5%
Fiber: 0 g	

Fats for Life

Omega-3s are essential for all age groups and stages of life. To ensure that you're getting enough of these essential fatty acids, eat a fatty type of fish such as salmon at least twice a week (a portion is about the size of a deck of cards) and snack on nuts and seeds to get other valuable essential fatty acids. Essential fatty acids (EFAs) are required for good health and are especially crucial during pregnancy. In particular, the fats docosahexaenoic acid (DHA), eicosapentaenoic acid (EPA), and arachidonic acid (AA) are absolutely critical for the development of your baby's nervous system, brain, and retinas.

Salmon for Smart Kids

Once scientists realized that the good fats in fish are so important to brain and eye development, they started to look at whether an expectant mother's diet could affect her child's mental abilities later in life. Today, thanks to researchers around the world, we know that eating fish during your pregnancy can in fact make your baby smarter. There is evidence from published clinical trials that pregnant women whose diets had higher amounts of the good fat DHA from eating fish (researchers estimated these women consumed 4 servings of various types of fish each week) or by taking supplements (about 1,100 mg DHA and 800 mg EPA daily) gave birth to babies with higher cognitive development scores. These children grew up to have higher IQ scores and better mental processing scores by the age of 4.

So give your kid a head start and send him or her to the front of the class by adding fish rich in DHA, like Coho salmon, to your diet this trimester. A half-fillet serving of coho salmon includes 1,250 mg of DHA and 850 mg of EPA, almost the same amount taken in daily supplements by the women in the study cited above!

Jonny's Tasty Tips

Wondering where you can get wild Alaskan salmon? Worried about mercury contamination? One company I'm particularly fond of that harvests toxin-free salmon from pristine Alaskan waters and ships it—and other "clean" fish—direct to your door is Vital Choice. You can find them on my website, www.jonnybowden.com, in the shopping section under "Healthy Foods."

Sleep Tight

A few weeks after you give birth, you'll be begging for a good night's sleep as the endless midnight cries from your new baby ring in your ears. But there's something you can do right now to give your baby—and you!—more restful nights. Researchers have found that women who eat lots of DHA during pregnancy give birth to babies with improved sleep patterns. So to help your little one sleep better, add some fish to your diet today.

How Much Is Safe?

A recent Canadian study indicated that the consumption of two to three servings weekly of fatty fish (fish that contain a high amount of good fats), like wild salmon or rainbow trout, provides a daily average DHA intake of at least 300 mg/day during pregnancy without containing amounts of mercury, polychlorinated biphenyls (PCBs), dioxins, or furans anywhere near as high as the "tolerable" levels set by the World Health Organization.

Women in the study cited in "Salmon for Smart Kids" ate four servings of fish per week, which would also not contain dangerous levels of mercury, PCBs, or other contaminants of concern. DHA-enriched ingredients like fish oil supplements and other omega-3-enhanced foods are free from environmental contaminants, making them a good option for expectant mothers to consider as additional sources of DHA.

It's very important to note that the study we just cited was done in Canada, and fish from different locations may have different levels of mercury and toxins. We strongly prefer wild salmon over farmed salmon. A 2003 study showed that farmed salmon from U.S. grocery stores were likely the most PCB-contaminated protein source in the U.S. food supply. If possible, get wild salmon.

Fresh Is Best

At the local market, you can find fresh, frozen, smoked, and canned salmon. Always pick fresh fish. Frozen fish may not have as delicious a flavor and could have added preservatives or other unwanted ingredients, so be sure to read your labels carefully. Smoked fish is not recommended for pregnant women (see page 229 in chapter 5 for more on this). Canned fish can contain added sodium, fat, and other unwanted additives. As with most foods, with salmon go fresh—fresh is always best.

Cranberries

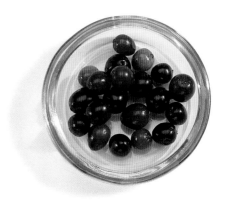

PUCKER UP TO A GLASS OF CRANBERRY JUICE
and kiss your bad bacteria goodbye. Cranberries
are not only a great source of vitamin C and other
antioxidants, they also have a unique ability to keep
your body free from bad bacteria that can cause
problems such as urinary tract infections, a common problem for pregnant women.

CRANBERRIES AT A GLANCE

Serving Size: 1 cup (110 g)	Calcium: 1%
Calories: 51	Vitamin A: 0%
Saturated Fat: 0 g	Vitamin C: 22%
Protein: 0 g	Iron: 2%
Fiber: 5 g	

Gotta Pee?

One of the symptoms of your growing uterus is a lack
of space in your gut. And one organ that really feels
the squeeze is your bladder. The effect on your bladder
is minor—it just doesn't have the same room it used to
in order to expand and hold more urine, making your
potty breaks more frequent. In fact, for some women,
the added pressure on their bladder can mean that
they have to run for the bathroom every hour, and that
can get old fast.

It can also lead to urinary tract infections. Here's
why: Because you're urinating more frequently and in
smaller amounts, there's a lack of gushing urine, which
blasts out bad bacteria that might be trying to infect
your urinary tract and bladder. If bad bacteria are
allowed to grab hold of the lining of your urinary tract
or bladder, they will start to grow and could develop
into a urinary tract infection. Luckily, cranberries can
help you fight back. Cranberries are great protec-
tors of your urinary tract. Scientists have found that
cranberries can prevent bacteria from binding to your
bladder lining, which is why they can prevent urinary
tract infections. They can do this because they contain proanthocyanidins, a powerful phytonutrient that
inhibits bacteria's ability to attach to the lining of your
urinary tract.

Heartburn Culprit

One common cause of heartburn is a form of
bacteria called *H. pylori*. These nasty bacteria live in
your stomach where, under certain circumstances,
they can grow, cause damage to your stomach lining,
and even lead to ulcers. Cranberries can prevent bacteria from adhering or attaching to your stomach lining
the same way they prevent bacteria from attaching
to the lining of your bladder and can help fight back
against *H. pylori*. Here's some good news: During pregnancy, your heartburn is usually from the upward pressure on your stomach from your growing uterus and
not from this bacteria. But better safe than sorry!

Jonny's Tasty Tips

Love your dried cranberries (a.k.a. Craisins)? Better bear in mind that you're taking in a lot of extra calories, as in 370 per cup compared to 51 per cup for raw cranberries. Instead, enjoy cranberries' flavor and health benefits the way I do: in smoothies. I add the raw berries to my smoothies and sweeten them up with xylitol, a healthy natural sweetener. You can find it at health food stores and some local grocery stores too.

Don't forget that cranberries don't *have* to be sweet to taste good! True, you wouldn't want to munch on a handful of raw cranberries. But you can toss them in dressing for baked chicken or turkey or in a rice dish and enjoy them as a savory, colorful addition to your meal. Cranberries really shine in wild rice dishes. They're also good in dal (Indian lentil stews) and stewed fruit soups. Challenge yourself to think of new ways to use cranberries!

Sweet Tarts

These tart berries are full of great nutrients like vitamin C. A cup of raw cranberries contains about one-quarter of your daily needs of vitamin C. But you're not likely to eat a cup of raw cranberries unless you really love tart things that make your mouth pucker!

You're more likely to drink your cranberries as cranberry juice. This is still a great source of vitamin C, but you do lose the fiber found in the berries (5 g per cup). If you do drink cranberry juice, be sure to look for pure cranberry juice, not a cranberry cocktail. Let's face it, cocktails are just sugar and water: Don't buy them. Pure (not from concentrate) cranberry juice is your best choice. If you find it too sour, mix it with some orange or grape juice to sweeten it up a little.

As for the traditional canned cranberry sauce that accompanies the family turkey dinner, it lost most of its vitamin C and fiber content when it was manufactured, and has a lot of added sugar. A better option is to simply boil fresh cranberries in a bit of water and then add a pinch of sugar or honey to sweeten to taste.

Crimini Mushrooms

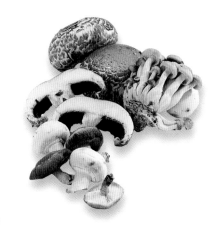

MUSHROOMS CONTAIN MANY NUTRIENTS THAT
are hard to find in other foods, such as selenium
and B vitamins. With the help of this potent antioxidant and these energizing vitamins, your body will
be armed and ready to take on this third trimester
of pregnancy. But why crimini mushrooms specifically?
Not all mushrooms are equally nutritious. Criminis (sometimes sold as "creamies")
are also a good source of folate, another important nutrient for pregnancy. Plus, they
offer you a vegetarian source of protein.

CRIMINI MUSHROOMS AT A GLANCE

Serving Size: 1 cup (87 g)   Calcium: 2%

Calories: 23   Vitamin A: 0%

Saturated Fat: 0 g   Vitamin C: 0%

Protein: 2 g   Iron: 2%

Fiber: 1 g

A Cup of Selenium

When it comes to selenium content, the crimini mushroom gets top billing since it contains more of this mineral than its white button or portabella counterparts.
Compared to other known food sources of selenium,
however, all three of these mushrooms are at the head
of the class. Only turkey is a better choice, as the High-
Selenium Foods chart shows.

High-Selenium Foods

Food	Quantity	Daily Value of Selenium
Turkey, light meat	3 oz.	45 percent
Crimini mushrooms	5 medium	31 percent
White button mushrooms	5 medium	22 percent
Portabella mushrooms	1 medium	21 percent
Eggs, whole	1 medium	20 percent
Brown rice	½ cup	15 percent

Jonny's Tasty Tips

Don't stop at crimini mushrooms! There are many other mushrooms you should try. Shiitake, oyster, king oyster, reishi, and maitake mushrooms also deliver healthy nutrients. They are larger and have more distinct flavors. Portabella mushrooms are another tasty choice—their large, flat shape and steak-like flavor make them a hit with vegetarians and meat-eaters alike.

Ditch the White Stuff

If there's one thing we'd like to make sure you take home, it's the message that white mushrooms are a waste of time! The white button mushroom is the most popular variety of mushroom consumed in the United States, but with a few exceptions like selenium, they aren't very high in nutrients compared to their mushroom cousins like criminis. Ditch those white mushrooms and reach for healthier mushrooms, like crimini mushrooms (they are most similar in taste and shape to a traditional white button mushroom). The coffee-colored crimini mushrooms have a richer flavor and more nutrients than their white button cousins.

New Antioxidant

Mushrooms contain the powerful antioxidant L-ergothioneine, which was once thought to be available only in chicken liver and wheat germ. According to researchers at the Pennsylvania State Mushroom Research Laboratory, mushrooms contain significant levels of this antioxidant, which acts as a scavenger of strong oxidants. Oxidants, also called free radicals, are unstable molecules that cause damage to parts of your body. You can prevent them from causing damage by consuming lots of antioxidants. Better yet, the presence of selenium in mushrooms enhances this antioxidant's activity.

PLACENTAL ABRUPTION

Premature separation of the placenta from the wall of the uterus, a condition called placental abruption, can occur in rare cases. (Estimates from the National Library of Medicine are about one in every 150 pregnancies have some small degree of separation, with only one in every 750 resulting in fetal death.) The cause of placental abruption is unknown. Certain conditions may increase its chance of occurrence, including physical injury to the mother (such as a car accident), a short umbilical cord, hypertension, or nutritional deficiency.

Your baby relies entirely on circulation from the placenta. If the placenta separates, your baby cannot receive blood from the umbilical cord, which is attached to the placenta. Vaginal bleeding, tenderness of the uterus, fetal distress, or even contractions are potential symptoms of placental abruption. Studies indicate that folic acid deficiency can play a role in causing placental abruption. Crimini and most other mushrooms are a good source of folate (about 15 mcg per cup).

Eggs

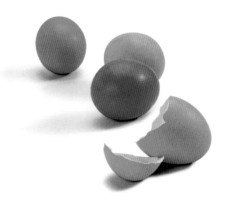

DO YOU LOVE EGGS, BUT AVOID THEM OUT OF fear of high cholesterol? Then you'll share my "eggcitement" over the latest egg research. We all know that eggs are full of cholesterol. In fact, there are more than 200 mg of cholesterol in an egg; most of which is concentrated in the yolk.

Our egg phobia is based on the belief that eating cholesterol will elevate our blood cholesterol levels. But it turns out that this is simply wrong.

EGGS AT A GLANCE

Serving Size: 1 cup (99 g)

Calories: 211

Saturated Fat: 4 g

Protein: 17 g

Fiber: 0 g

Calcium: 7%

Vitamin A: 14%

Vitamin C: 0%

Iron: 8%

The Real Deal on Cholesterol

For years, we've been told that people on low-cholesterol diets should avoid eggs. This is because the high cholesterol level in egg yolks was thought to elevate blood cholesterol. However, it is well known that dietary cholesterol intake has a very insignificant effect on your blood cholesterol levels. There are other factors, such as the rest of your diet (including fiber, antioxidants, and good fat intake).

Cholesterol isn't the villain it's been made out to be, either. Cholesterol is produced in the liver by the enzyme called HMG-CoA. Our bodies require lots of cholesterol, which is an important component of cell membranes and hormones, including estrogen and testosterone. The liver produces about 1,000 mg of cholesterol each day, while the typical diet contributes only a few hundred milligrams. Thus, dietary cholesterol plays only a small part in our overall cholesterol levels.

Cracking the Cholesterol Myth

According to research published in the *Journal of Nutrition* in 2006, eating eggs does not elevate your blood cholesterol. A randomized crossover-design study was conducted on 33 men and women over the age of 60. They were asked to eat one egg every day for five weeks. When the researchers looked at the blood concentrations of total cholesterol, there was no difference between egg consumption and no egg consumption. In addition, the researchers found similar results in the subjects' bad cholesterol (LDL), good cholesterol (HDL), and triglyceride levels.

Jonny's Tasty Tips

I can't say enough good things about eggs. They're nature's most perfect food. But how you cook them matters. That's because the less you scramble or expose the yolk to oxygen, the less the yolk gets oxidized and the better the egg is for you. Poaching and boiling are both better ways to go.

I'd rather see you eat scrambled eggs than not eat eggs at all. But instead, why not go for an omelet, frittata, or *huevos rancheros* and up the veggie content? And skip the fried eggs, please. No reason to turn a good food bad!

You Need Cholesterol

Since you're not likely to be reading this book if you're over 60, you may be wondering what that study has to do with you. But we all need cholesterol, and as a pregnant woman, your needs for cholesterol are even higher. Every cell in your body contains cholesterol—it's part of the basic structure of every cell membrane. To make a baby, your body will produce millions of new cells, and cholesterol is needed for every one. It's a relief to know that you can eat superfoods like eggs without worrying about clogging your arteries. And don't forget that egg yolks are one of the best sources of choline (see page 63), an important nutrient for the brain!

Help with the Load

Eggs are an excellent source of protein, containing all the essential amino acids. During your third trimester, your muscles need all of the support they can get from your diet. Protein in your diet will help your muscles keep up with the extra weight they are asked to carry around all day from your growing belly. In fact, the demands on your muscles during your third trimester are about the same as if you were to carry a 25-pound plate strapped to your waist all day—it's a serious workout. Help your muscles rebuild and stay strong with the help of good-quality protein sources like eggs.

Eyeing Up Some Eggs

Eggs are also a great source of other nutrients, including the antioxidant lutein. There's about 1 mg of lutein in a regular egg, with some specialty eggs containing up to 6 mg. Lutein is a nutrient involved in eye health. Your baby's eyes are still developing, and they'll appreciate all the nutritional help you can offer by eating healthy foods like eggs.

Eggplant

A HEALTHY DIET IS A RAINBOW ON YOUR PLATE.

Every day, you should be able to think back about what you've eaten and see a rainbow of colors. Each color of food offers you a different set of nutrients. And one of the most commonly missed colors is purple. Blueberries, plums, grapes, and eggplant are all purple foods, packed with healthy nutrients for you and your baby.

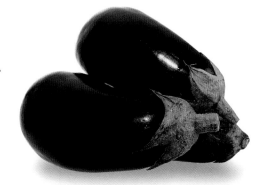

EGGPLANT AT A GLANCE

Serving Size: 1 cup (99 g)	**Calcium:** 1%
Calories: 35	**Vitamin A:** 1%
Saturated Fat: 0 g	**Vitamin C:** 2%
Protein: 1 g	**Iron:** 1%
Fiber: 2 g	

Eggplant gets a lot of press about being a healthy food choice, but surprisingly, it's not particularly high in any single vitamin or mineral. Eggplant's claim to nutritional fame is that it's very filling, low in calories, and virtually fat-free. And it contributes a meaty texture to dishes (think eggplant parmigiana), making eggplant popular in vegetarian dishes. One cup of cooked eggplant offers just 35 calories and 2.5 g of fiber.

Nutrients for You

That doesn't mean that eggplant is nutrient free by any means. Eggplant contains about 4 percent of your daily value of vitamin K, thiamin, vitamin B6, and manganese. But it isn't the standard nutrients in eggplant that makes it so healthy for you. It's the compounds that make the skin of an eggplant purple. These are powerful antioxidants, nutrients we need in high amounts in our body to fight off disease and keep our cells (and your baby's cells) healthy and working optimally.

When researchers at the United States Department of Agriculture investigated the antioxidant levels of eggplant, they found chlorogenic acid, a great antioxidant with immune benefits, and 13 other phenolic acids (antioxidants) present at varying levels. Purple really is powerful!

Jonny's Tasty Tips

While available year-round, eggplants are at their peak in August and September in North America. Choose smaller, immature eggplants. Larger, puffy ones may have hard seeds and have a bitter flavor. Choose eggplants that are firm, smooth skinned, and heavy for their size. Avoid any eggplant with soft or brown spots. If you enjoy Asian cuisine and/or stir-fries, look for the sausage-shaped Asian eggplants instead of the heavy teardrop shapes we associate with Italian cuisine.

I discovered my favorite way to eat eggplant at an amazing little Japanese restaurant in Studio City. They serve cooked eggplant in a miso-ginger sauce that just knocks my socks off. I can easily make a meal out of an entire eggplant prepared this way, and since the eggplant itself is only 132 calories, all you have to do is use the sauce judiciously and you've got a great dish. Add a couple of eggs for protein—I know it's unconventional, but it's great!—and you have a terrific and complete meal with very moderate calories.

Here are other delicious options: Try eggplant sliced and grilled with a sprinkle of olive oil. Or enjoy that super-healthy, addictive eggplant spread, baba ghanouj, which combines grilled eggplant in a puree with olive oil and garlic. If you're making a big salad for the family and you can manage to include one whole eggplant, grilled and sliced up, you'll be giving them great tastes and a variety of nutrients in every bowl. And let's not forget ratatouille, the French specialty that combines eggplant, tomatoes, zucchini, herbs, olive oil, and garlic in an irresistible dish that's good hot or cold, over brown rice, in an omelet, or even as a sandwich filling.

FAST FACT

Eggplants may not look much like potatoes, tomatoes, or peppers, but they're all in the same family, the nightshade or solanum family. And like tomatoes and peppers, eggplants are technically fruits. But that's no big deal: So are many plants commonly eaten as vegetables. Unlike *fruit*, *vegetable* is a word applied to anything eaten as a savory (not sweet) dish, from shoots like asparagus to tubers like potatoes, roots like carrots and radishes, leaves like lettuce and spinach, bulbs like onions and garlic, or even flower buds like artichokes. What's in a name?

Brain Protector

There is one more compound in the skin of eggplant that makes it a great candidate for our list of healthiest foods for your third trimester: nasunin. Nasunin is an anthocyanin with potent antioxidant and free-radical-scavenging abilities. Researchers have found that nasunin is particularly helpful at protecting the fat in the membranes of brain cells. Cell membranes are almost entirely composed of lipids (fats) and are responsible for letting nutrients in to the cell and wastes out as well as receiving and sending messages. Your baby's brain is developing rapidly and in complex ways during its last few months, making eggplant a great addition to your next ratatouille, curry, or stir-fry.

Evening Primrose Oil

IT'S CERTAINLY NOT YOUR COMMON COOKING OIL, but evening primrose oil (EPO) should be a part of every pregnant woman's pantry. EPO is one of the best sources of the essential fatty acid gamma-linolenic acid (GLA). GLA is essential, which means your body can't make it; you need to ingest it to have it in your body. It plays a major role in your health. In fact, thanks to dozens of research studies, we know today that GLA is beneficial to your joints, heart, and skin.

EVENING PRIMROSE OIL AT A GLANCE

Serving Size: 1 g	Calcium: 0%
Calories: 9	Vitamin A: 0%
Saturated Fat: 0 g	Vitamin C: 0%
Protein: 0 g	Iron: 0%
Fiber: 0 g	

Regulators

EPO contains linoleic acid (LA) as well as GLA. Under ideal conditions, the body uses LA to produce GLA. In turn, GLA is used to produce beneficial hormone-like compounds called prostaglandins. Prostaglandins affect the function of virtually every system in the body. These molecules are used in the regulation of inflammation, pain, blood pressure, fluid balance, and blood clotting. Prostaglandins also affect hormone production and function. Many of these body functions need to be perfectly balanced to have a healthy pregnancy, making GLA an important player in your health.

Not Getting Enough

The key to understanding the need for getting oils rich in GLA is that many of us can't convert LA to GLA efficiently. Dietary deficiencies, disease conditions, aging, and eating poorly (as many of us do, consuming sugar, processed oils, trans fatty acids, heated oils, and alcohol) all slow down the enzyme that converts LA to GLA. In fact, virtually all North Americans are deficient in GLA.

Supplementing your diet with EPO can enrich your body's GLA supply and restore the production of beneficial prostaglandins derived from GLA. Research completed over the last 20 years has confirmed that supplementation with evening primrose oil has beneficial effects on numerous diseases and conditions, ranging from pregnancy, premenstrual syndrome, and menopause to fibrocystic breast pain, eczema, rheumatoid arthritis, diabetes, heart disease, osteoporosis, and ulcerative colitis.

Jonny's Tasty Tips

Keep EPO refrigerated and buy a small enough bottle so you can use it quickly. If you don't take it in capsule form, mix it in your salad dressing right before you eat your salad or stir it into hummus before making a pita sandwich (I like whole-wheat pita with hummus, sliced tomato, and romaine lettuce or arugula) or veggie dip.

EPO and Preeclampsia

EPO, containing GLA, has been hailed as an effective treatment against pregnancy-induced high blood pressure, known as preeclampsia.

A study published in 1992 looked at the effects of EPO and fish oil compared to magnesium oxide and a placebo in preventing preeclampsia during pregnancy. The group of pregnant women given the mixture of evening primrose and fish oil had a significantly lower incidence of swelling compared to the women receiving magnesium oxide or a placebo. In addition, the women receiving the mixture of evening primrose and fish oil had a lower rate of preeclampsia than the public average, suggesting that these oils have a preventive effect. See page 129 for more on preeclampsia.

Check with Your Obstetrician

We recommend that you discuss evening primrose oil with your obstetrician or midwife before taking it. There are medical resources that list concerns about the proof of evening primrose's safety for pregnant women, despite the wide use of EPO by midwives. Traditionally, midwives have used EPO to hasten cervical ripening in an effort to shorten labor and decrease the incidence of pregnancies going past due dates. New research supports the use of this oil during pregnancy, and thus we've added it to our list of healthiest foods for your third trimester. But dosages should be kept to low amounts (avoid taking large supplemental amounts) and should be used with the supervision of your obstetrician. Using EPO in small amounts in salad dressings or in a smoothie are great ways to help get some GLA in your diet. As for the safety of taking EPO during pregnancy, despite the old studies, new research has found it safe. Researchers from the University of Munich reported in a 2008 issue of the *British Journal of Nutrition* that healthy women supplementing with fish oil and EPO experienced healthy increases in their blood levels of good fats (such as GLA and DHA). The researchers also commented that the use of fish oil and EPO during pregnancy appears safe and well tolerated. The safety of using EPO during lactation (breast-feeding) is also well supported.

Fish Oil

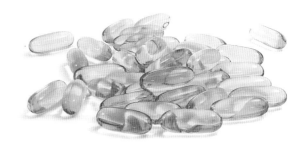

IF THERE WAS ONE PIECE OF ADVICE WE'D love for every woman to know, it's the value of including fish in your diet during and after pregnancy. Countless health associations are recommending that women consume about three to four servings of fish per week. And the best fish are those that are high in good fats, like salmon, sardines, and anchovies, to list a few. However, for some women, the idea of eating fish is disgusting. For whatever reason, fish simply doesn't appeal. But no worries. Even if you're one of these gals, we've got an answer: fish oil supplements.

FISH OIL AT A GLANCE

Serving Size: 1 Tbsp (14 g)	Calcium: 0%
Calories: 41	Vitamin A: 0%
Saturated Fat: 1 g	Vitamin C: 0%
Protein: 0 g	Iron: 0%
Fiber: 0 g	

Supplementing with fish oil is a solution all but vegetarian women can consider. In fact, many women will supplement with fish oil and still eat fish in their diet a few times a week, since fish is a good source of protein and is lower in bad stuff (like hormones and antibiotics) than red meat. Plus, fish oil supplements are easy to add into your diet, require no prep time, and are portable. You're already taking a prenatal multivitamin and mineral, so it's easy to put a bottle of fish oil supplements beside your prenatal so you'll remember to take it too. You'll find that this is one of the easiest changes you can make to your diet.

If the idea of fish oil supplements still bothers you, some new products have come to market that may interest you. There are new liquid products that taste great, including flavors like lemon pudding and strawberry cream. There's not the slightest fishy taste in some and it's so good that kids will eat it (as long as you don't tell them it's fish oil).

Start Now

Getting fish oil into your diet is a healthy choice since it's an easy way to get fabulous amounts of essential fatty acids into your diet. Plus, a diet that includes fish oils has been associated with many other health benefits, including lower risks of heart disease. Start eating fish or taking fish oil today if you aren't already. It's never too late. Even starting from the 30th week of pregnancy, studies have shown women can have positive effects on their baby by adding fish to their diet.

Jonny's Tasty Tips

Here's a true confession: I don't know what I'd do without my juicer. I start *every* single day–and I mean every day, 365 days a year–with a glass of homemade juice. And here's a secret: I add 2 tablespoons of omega-3-rich fish oil to my freshly made juice. The omega-3 fat in the fish oil makes the carotenoids in the vegetables and fruits more available to my body. And guess what? Nobody in my family can taste the fish oil, just the delicious juice.

Women at their 30th week of pregnancy who consumed 2.7 g of fish daily until labor had longer gestations (by 4 days) and higher birth weights (107 g heavier) compared to the control group of women, who received olive oil.

Experts on fish oil have concluded that consuming as little as 150 mg of fish oil a day is known to increase birth weights, which is important because low birth weight (below 7 pounds) is associated with less healthy babies. Supplementing your diet with 150 mg of fish oil daily during your pregnancy may also be helpful in reducing the risk of preterm delivery and appears to be associated with longer gestations (i.e., full-term, which is healthier than premature birth).

How Much?

Based on current research, it appears that pregnant women should be consuming an average of at least 1 g of fish oil per day (up to 4 to 6 g is considered perfectly safe). In your last trimester, one of the most important aspects of your fish-oil supplement is the amount of docosahexaenoic acid (DHA) it contains. You want to consume about 300 mg of DHA each day. So make sure your supplement measures up!

Tough Choices

There are so many different fish-oil supplements on the market, you may find it hard to find the right one for you. First, look for a brand with a good quality record. If you don't know which brands are better than others, visit a good health food store in your community and speak with a qualified person at the store; they can help you choose a good brand. Next, make sure your fish-oil supplement has a guarantee that it is mercury- and PCB-free. Most fish-oil supplements in North America meet this standard today.

Your next choice is more personal. You'll need to decide what kind of supplement is best for you and your lifestyle. Let's face it: If you won't take the supplement, there's no point in buying it. Fish-oil supplements come in capsules of various sizes, some easier to swallow than others. The smaller the capsule, the less oil in each, and the more capsules you'll have to take each day.

You can also buy fish oils as liquids, in more flavors than you can imagine. Some are delicious flavors like lemon meringue or orange. Other fish oils are just plain, which we'd suggest you hide in a smoothie. Otherwise, a spoonful of this medicine may be hard to swallow!

That Fishy Burp-Up

If you find you're burping up the fish oil from your supplement, here are a few tricks that help. First, take your fish oil with food: the more food, the better. Second, try a fish-oil capsule with an enteric coat. Enteric-coated capsules dissolve in the small intestine rather than the stomach. This means the fish oil is never actually in your stomach, so you won't have to taste it if you burp. Plus, research in the *New England Journal of Medicine* in 1996 showed that enteric-coated capsules are actually three times better absorbed. So you get more nutrients per capsule, and you never have to taste or smell fishy!

Finally, try putting your fish oil capsules in the freezer. This works really well to eliminate any fishy burps!

★ Garlic

AS YOUR BODY REACHES ITS FINAL MONTHS OF pregnancy, the toll on your cardiovascular system is more taxing. You've probably already noticed this. It's amazing how exhausted you can feel only after walking around a few aisles in the grocery store. You've got a lot of extra weight and blood to pump around your body these days. You could probably use some heart-healthy garlic.

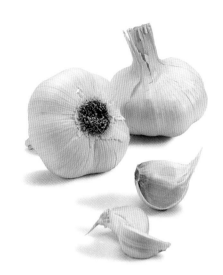

GARLIC AT A GLANCE

Serving Size: 3 cloves	Calcium: 2%
Calories: 13	Vitamin A: 0%
Saturated Fat: 0 g	Vitamin C: 4%
Protein: 1 g	Iron: 1%
Fiber: 0 g	

Happy Hearts

For years, researchers have been working with garlic because it has amazing heart-healthy benefits. Studies have confirmed that garlic can reduce many factors that lead to heart disease, including atherosclerosis (hardening of the arteries). In fact, a study in Preventive Medicine reported that garlic even prevents calcification, a process that leads to plaque formation on your blood vessels. Researchers around the world have discovered that garlic can help lower bad cholesterol, total cholesterol, and triglycerides, which is good for your heart.

Garlic also helps prevent your blood from clotting. (Think of clotting as leading to a problem much like a fender-bender on the highway can cause a backup. In this case, a clot can back up blood in your blood vessels.) Garlic has been shown to help lower risk factors of heart disease and improve blood pressure. Plus, garlic is a great antioxidant.

The Italians, who love garlic, are considered to have one of the healthiest diets on earth. Maybe garlic is their secret ingredient!

More Garlic Goodness

Garlic contains some conventional nutrients, too. In fact, in just 3 cloves of garlic you'll find 8% of your daily value of manganese, 6% of vitamin B6, and 4% of vitamin C. Garlic also has decent amounts of selenium, phosphorus, and calcium. All of these nutrients support a healthy body, healthy bones, and a healthy baby. As you can see, garlic is one of the healthiest foods for your third trimester of pregnancy.

Jonny's Tasty Tips

Garlic: In tomato sauce, ratatouille, hummus, baba ghanouj, stir-fries, roasted, and used a thousand different ways—it's delicious. But is garlic good for health? The fresher the garlic the better it is. Garlic experts advise crushing a little raw garlic and combining it with the cooked food shortly before serving. (Eating it raw isn't recommended because it can be irritating to the stomach—not what you need right now!) Microwaving appears to destroy the healthful compounds in garlic completely—sorry.

Garlic and Preeclampsia

Since garlic offers so many heart-healthy benefits, including the ability to help lower blood pressure, inhibit platelet aggregation, and reduce oxidative stress, it's possible that it may have a role in preventing preeclampsia and its complications. Researchers from Tarbiat Modarres University in Iran reported that when a group of women were given a garlic supplement during pregnancy, they had lower blood pressure. However, studies have yet to determine how much garlic is best and if or how much it reduces preeclampsia and its related problems during pregnancy. (See page 127 for more on this dangerous condition.)

For You and Your Baby

For many years, people have used garlic as a way to fight off the common cold. You may be one of them. But did you ever think that garlic could help your immune system in your placenta? According to a paper in *Placenta* in 2005, garlic may have an immunomodulatory effect (i.e., it helps regulate the immune response) on the placentas of both normal and eclamptic women. In other words, a healthy immune system for you and your placenta may be just a few cloves of garlic away.

Strep B Prevention

Group B strep is the most common cause of sepsis (blood infection) and meningitis (infection of the fluid and lining around the brain) in newborns. Group B strep is a frequent cause of newborn pneumonia, and it's more common than other, more well-known newborn problems such as rubella, congenital syphilis, and spina bifida. In 2002, the Centers for Disease Control wrote new protocols that called for the pregnant women in the United States to have a rectal/vaginal culture for strep B at 36 weeks. According to *Midwifery Today with International Midwife* 2004, garlic kills strep B and can prevent it in newborns. Speak with your obstetrician for more information.

Green Peas

IN JUST ONE CUP OF FROZEN PEAS (BECAUSE, let's be honest, for most of the year, that's the easiest way to buy these green peas), you'll find tons of nutrients. Sure, you can head to the local market for a few weeks each spring and find some fresh peas and shuck them, but for most of the year, the frozen bag of peas in your grocery's freezer section is the best option.

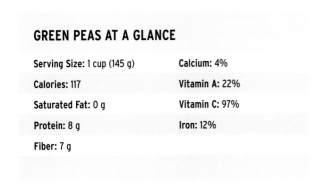

GREEN PEAS AT A GLANCE

Serving Size: 1 cup (145 g)	Calcium: 4%
Calories: 117	Vitamin A: 22%
Saturated Fat: 0 g	Vitamin C: 97%
Protein: 8 g	Iron: 12%
Fiber: 7 g	

Frozen peas are made from fresh peas in their prime. Freezing vegetables like peas causes very little change to their nutritional value, making frozen peas a healthy and easy way to add more vegetables to your diet. Peas are a primo source of vitamin A, vitamin C, vitamin K, thiamin, and manganese. Per cup, you're also offering yourself and your baby a good source of protein, niacin, folate, iron, and phosphorus.

The Green Nutritional Giant

Peas are small, but they sure are good for you. Let's take a closer look at some of the nutrients in peas and how they help you during your last trimester. Vitamin A is needed for your baby's developing eyes and skin that are getting ready in the last trimester for their debut in the outside world—and your cup of frozen peas contains more than a quarter of the daily value.

Vitamin C strengthens blood vessels, keeping them healthy and strong. During labor, you'll ask your body to perform an amazing feat that will require energy and stretching and will put at lot of stress on your body, particularly your blood vessels. Vitamin C in foods like peas can help keep your blood vessels healthy, and you'll need them to build strength (collagen) in your skin after all that stretching. A cup of green peas offers your body almost the entire daily value of this nutrient.

Thiamin, also known as vitamin B1, stimulates growth and good muscle tone. You'll need all the muscle tone you can get when you're asked to bear down and deliver that baby. A cup of green peas contains 0.4 mg of thiamin.

Sugar Makes Fat Babies

Midwives have a saying for newly expectant moms: "Sugar makes fat babies." In other words, healthy eating is not just a good idea for controlling your weight

Jonny's Tasty Tips

When I was a kid, green peas were my favorite vegetable. I couldn't get enough of them! I still love them, but I've learned to love other forms of green peas like edible-podded snow and snap peas, too. I'll eat peas fresh, frozen, dried, popped straight from the pod into my mouth—any way but canned. Ugh! That dull green canned-pea color signals a lack of chlorophyll and nutrients, and the mushy taste would turn anybody off peas. So skip the canned peas and enjoy the natural sweetness and goodness of fresh or frozen peas in rice dishes, salads, pasta sauces, and sides. Or try high-protein, earthy dried peas in split pea soup and Indian dal, a spicy legume stew with endless variations.

KEGEL EXERCISES

Delivery requires more than nutrition alone. You can also help strengthen your abdominal muscles during your pregnancy with Kegel exercises. Kegel exercises strengthen the pelvic floor muscles, which support the uterus, bladder, and bowel. Not sure whether you're contracting your pelvic muscles or your abdominals? Try to stop the flow of urine while you're going to the bathroom. If you succeed, you've got the basic move. Three times a day, try to contract those muscles for periods of 3 seconds flexed, 3 seconds relaxed. Move up to 10 seconds as you get stronger. As your muscles become stronger—and you become more experienced with the exercises—this movement will be more pronounced. And it will pay off when you're bearing down during delivery.

gain during pregnancy, but it can also help control how big your baby grows before birth. And that's great news, because the idea of having to give birth vaginally to a baby larger than eight pounds is frightening. So avoid sugary foods: They offer you little nutritional value and encourage outsize babies. Another trick is to eat foods that are a good source of fiber, like peas, since they can help stabilize your blood sugar levels.

We can thank research on people with diabetes for knowing that peas, grains, and other high-fiber foods are good for us. A study from University of Gottinger in Germany asked people with type 2 diabetes to consume either a low-glycemic index (GI) meal of legumes or a high-glycemic meal of potatoes. Eating the legume meal resulted in delayed increases in the diabetics' blood sugar and insulin levels. Researchers concluded that people with type 2 diabetes *may* not need to count the carbohydrates in dried peas, the type of legume used in this study, because the carbohydrates in legumes appear to be released slowly into the bloodstream. This is amazing, since 70 percent of the calories in beans are from the carbohydrates!

Worried about the sugar content of peas and other vegetables? Don't be! The sugars we're talking about here are the bad sugars known as refined sugars that you find in soda pop, packaged foods, candy, and baked goods. It's also the white sugar you may be spooning into your cups of coffee and tea. Avoiding white (bad) sugar is a healthy way to eat every day during pregnancy and after.

Herring

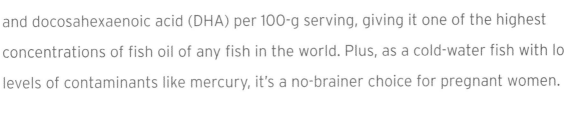

BY NOW, YOU'VE PROBABLY GOTTEN THE IDEA that we think fish is essential to a healthy pregnancy diet. Herring isn't the most commonly consumed fish we recommend, but it should be. Herring contains 2 g of eicosapentaenoic acid (EPA) and docosahexaenoic acid (DHA) per 100-g serving, giving it one of the highest concentrations of fish oil of any fish in the world. Plus, as a cold-water fish with low levels of contaminants like mercury, it's a no-brainer choice for pregnant women.

HERRING AT A GLANCE

Serving Size: 1 fillet (143 g)	Calcium: 10%
Calories: 290	Vitamin A: 3%
Saturated Fat: 4 g	Vitamin C: 2%
Protein: 33 g	Iron: 9%
Fiber: 0 g	

Avoiding Preterm Labor

There are so many reasons to include fish in your diet. Early in your third trimester, you may be concerned with giving birth too early. Luckily, modern medicine can do great things to help your baby survive if he or she happens to deliver earlier than may have been ideal. Plus, a healthy diet can help. Eating healthy foods can help you stay strong and will give your baby the best start at life, no matter how early that may come. Certain foods like fish are thought to be particularly helpful in improving gestation.

A healthy diet that includes fish may also be a great way to ward off early labor. Researchers from Denmark set out to investigate these issues in a study of 8,729 women whose seafood intake in early pregnancy was assessed by a questionnaire. They tested whether a low intake of seafood in early pregnancy was a risk factor for preterm delivery and low birth weight and whether it was associated with lower fetal growth. The group found that 1.9 percent of women who ate fish at least once a week had a premature birth, but this increased to 7.1 percent among women who never ate fish. The researchers concluded that low consumption of fish was a strong risk factor for preterm delivery and low birth weight. Eating fish like herring and salmon may be an easy way to reduce your risk of giving birth too early.

Jonny's Tasty Tips

If you've ever tasted herring, it's probably been pickled in sandwiches, the most popular way to eat it (especially in Britain). And creamed herring was a staple at my Jewish grandmother's table and is still popular at delis everywhere! But you can also find *fresh* herring at your local fish store. The bones are soft and easy to remove. Fresh herring is great grilled or baked with acidic flavors like white wine and lemon. (Remember, the wine's alcohol content burns off during cooking so it's perfectly safe.)

TO EAT, OR NOT TO EAT?

There is a lot of conflicting information out there about the safety of consuming fish during pregnancy. For example, the Food and Drug Administration and the Environmental Protection Agency in the United States recommend that pregnant and nursing women consume only five ounces of fresh fish a week. This can make it difficult to get sufficient DHA into your bloodstream. Fish oil supplements are tested for heavy metals such as mercury and PCBs, therefore offering you another option to help you get higher levels of DHA into your bloodstream without worrying about toxins. It is important to note that experts in the field suggest that the benefits of fish consumption far outweigh the risks.

When More Is Better

Even more fish in your diet is considered very healthy. Higher dietary intakes (more than 2 g a day) of DHA during pregnancy has been found by scientists to support your baby's brain development in the womb. Plus, eating more foods that contain DHA means more DHA is available to you, the mother, which reduces your risk of postpartum depression.

Baby Brain Food

Your baby's brain will appreciate the fish oil in herring, too. A study published in the *American Journal of Clinical Nutrition* found that pregnant women who ate more fish gave their babies a better chance at brain development. The researchers found that women with higher blood levels of fish oil had babies with better sleep patterns in the first 48 hours following delivery compared to women with lower blood levels of fish oil. Experts have hypothesized that an infant's sleep patterns are thought to reflect to the maturity of a child's nervous system, so adding fish into your diet can help your baby's brain mature and help you get some much-needed sleep after labor.

Eat Fish, Stay Happy

During pregnancy and lactation, a woman's level of DHA is low because her body is giving the nutrients to her baby. So after giving birth, a woman is often left depleted of omega-3 fatty acids. Ongoing research has found that women with low levels of DHA may be at an increased risk of developing the condition known as "baby blues" or postpartum depression. Approximately 15 to 20 percent of women who give birth in the United States develop postpartum depression, according to the Mother and Child Foundation. Help ensure that you're not one of them by eating plenty of DHA-rich fish like herring.

Molasses

MOLASSES IS AN INGREDIENT THAT USUALLY SITS at the back of your pantry until the holidays, when it gets pulled out to make Grandma's famous gingerbread cookies. But in a few short weeks, Grandma's going to get another type of holiday treat: a new grandbaby. Celebrate the latest addition to your family with some of those delicious cookies, because molasses is not just all sugar. It has nutrients, too. Lots of them!

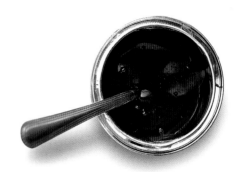

MOLASSES AT A GLANCE

Serving Size: 1 Tbsp (20 g)	Calcium: 4%
Calories: 58	Vitamin A: 0%
Saturated Fat: 0 g	Vitamin C: 0%
Protein: 0 g	Iron: 4%
Fiber: 0 g	

FAST FACT

Constipation is a common problem for pregnant women. One of your grandmother's solutions for constipation was to dissolve two tablespoons of unsulphured blackstrap molasses in a glass of warm water and drink it down. Try this natural home remedy if you need some help.

Sticky Sweet Nutrition

Sweet, sticky, and packed with sugar, molasses is not the type of food you want to start spooning onto every dish. But molasses has a few hidden nutritional gems that are helpful during your third trimester, like magnesium and manganese. Magnesium is an essential nutrient that can help you feel more energized. It will help you get through those seemingly simple yet totally exhausting events in your day, like trying to roll that big belly of yours out of bed. It can be quite the feat to negotiate that much of a front load from a lying to a standing position. Magnesium is a catalyst for your metabolism of energy sources; in other words, it helps you get energy out of food faster. You'll find 48 mg of magnesium in just 1 tablespoon of molasses.

Manganese is an essential mineral that plays a role in normal bone development, and that's important for your growing baby. There is 0.3 mg of manganese in 1 tablespoon of molasses, which is 15 percent of your daily needs. And for pregnant women, manganese helps maintain sex-hormone production, the same hormones that are magically keeping all of the physical changes in your pregnancy going perfectly on schedule.

Jonny's Tasty Tips

Blackstrap molasses is very dark and has a robust, somewhat bitter-tart flavor. I think it's delicious! I use it in recipes that range from baked beans to soy-based sauces. If you like barbecue, it makes a yummy barbecue sauce for pork or chicken. And yes, it's great with ginger, even if you'd rather try it in a curry or Chinese seasoning sauce rather than in the famous gingersnap cookies. Check it out as a sweetener in ginger tea, too!

Shoe Solution

Molasses is a great source of a few nutrients that may be the solution your swollen ankles are looking for. Vitamin B6 (pyridoxine) is one of those nutrients you just can't live without. It plays a key role in your body's ability to get energy out of fats, proteins, and carbohydrates, helping you get more steps into your day. Plus, it helps keep your levels of homocysteine—a fat that is linked to arteriosclerosis—low.

But the real bonus to including foods like molasses in your diet in the third trimester of pregnancy is that it just may help shrink those swollen feet and ankles of yours. Vitamin B6 plays a role in your sodium/phosphorus balance (i.e., your electrolytes) and they play a big role in how much water you have in your body. Potassium is another mineral involved in water retention, and there is some potassium in molasses to help your body try to get the balance back, allowing you to fit into those cute shoes again. Molasses has about 290 mg (8 percent of your daily needs) of potassium and 0.1 mg (7 percent of your daily needs) of vitamin B6 per tablespoon.

Choose Blackstrap Molasses

Blackstrap molasses is the healthiest choice. It is rich in many nutrients, including calcium and iron, two nutrients you're still in great need of during your third trimester. If possible, look for organic, unsulphured blackstrap molasses, which will contain fewer unwanted contaminants. And for ways to include molasses in your diet beyond gingerbread, gingersnaps, and snickerdoodles, try it as a sweetener for your oatmeal, in smoothies or yogurt, and in breads and other baked goods.

Nuts

MANY SIZES, SHAPES, COLORS, AND FLAVORS OF nuts are available at your local market. And each one is packed with healthy nutrients like minerals, protein, fiber, good fats, and vitamins. From trail mix to a handful of sliced almonds on your salad, there are so many ways to add nuts to your meals, and they're a healthy addition to your diet during your third trimester.

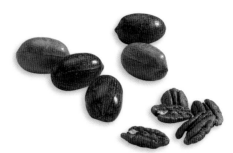

NUTS AT A GLANCE - Almonds/Pecans/Peanuts

Serving Size: 1 oz (28 g)

Calories: 170/200/165

Saturated Fat: 1g/2g/2g

Protein: 6g/3g/7g

Fiber: 3g/3g/2.5g

Calcium: 7%/2%/2%

Vitamin A: 0%/1%/0%

Vitamin C: 0%

Iron: 6%/3%/3%

Who's the Nuttiest?

Believe it or not, all nuts have about the same number of calories (about 150 calories per ounce). On the higher end, at about 200 calories per ounce, are macadamia nuts, pecans, and Brazil nuts, which are all higher in fat. But a lot of the fat in nuts is considered good fat, or monounsaturated fat. As for fiber, pine nuts, almonds, and pecans top the list with about 3 g per ounce. All types of nuts are a great source of protein and contain many vitamins and minerals that are healthy for you and your baby.

PASS ON THE PEANUTS?

We know you've heard of people with peanut allergies. And some experts believe that avoiding known allergens, such as peanuts, during pregnancy can reduce the risk of allergic reactions developing in your child. However, there is a lack of evidence that this approach actually works, and until further research is carried out, there are no guidelines about peanut consumption during pregnancy.

Jonny's Tasty Tips

Are you nuts for nuts? I know I am! You don't need to eat a lot of them to get their health benefits, either: One 1-ounce serving a day or 5 ounces a week from a variety of nuts gives you all of nuts' goodness without a calorie overload. Here are some of my favorite ways to enjoy them, many courtesy of Melissa Stevens, the nutrition program coordinator for preventive cardiology and rehabilitative services at the Cleveland Clinic:

- Add cashews or peanuts to a stir-fry (when cooking with nuts, add them at the end of cooking so they'll keep their crunch).

- Toss roasted pine nuts into marinara sauce.

- Add slivered almonds to yogurt.

- Toss walnuts, pecans, or slivered almonds into a spinach, strawberry, and red onion salad.

- Create your own trail mix. (I love nuts, dates, raisins, and oats.)

- Put pine nuts, basil, olive oil, and Parmesan in a food processor and make your own pesto.

And, of course, there's the snack that I've been recommending for years: natural peanut or almond butter smeared on an apple or a few sticks of celery.

FAST FACT

Peanuts are the most popular nut. But they're not really nuts at all. Instead, peanuts are legumes, relatives of peas and beans. Nut or not, peanuts have about 165 calories per ounce and 2.5 g of fiber, making them a good nutritional choice.

Handful of Health

Nuts are a source of the important trace mineral selenium. Grabbing a handful of nuts as a snack during your pregnancy may be a good way to help reduce your risk of preeclampsia. Research suggests that having low levels of selenium in your diet during pregnancy may be associated with pregnancy complications, including preeclampsia. In fact, research from the United Kingdom in 2004 found that women with low levels of selenium raised their risk of developing preeclampsia as much as four times over women with normal selenium levels. Brazil nuts are the best source of selenium of all foods, with 544 mcg an ounce (6 to 8 nuts).

Papaya

A WELL-RIPENED PAPAYA IS RICH IN VITAMINS
and nutrients, and we recommend it for pregnant
women in moderate amounts. A ripe papaya is
rich in vitamin C, and it's effective in preventing
and controlling constipation and heartburn. Just
one cup of papaya contains more than your daily
needs of vitamin C (about 85 mg).

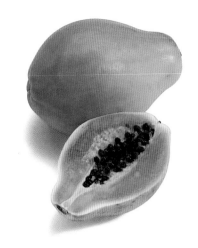

PAPAYA AT A GLANCE

Serving Size: 1 cup (140 g)	Calcium: 3%
Calories: 55	Vitamin A: 25%
Saturated Fat: 0 g	Vitamin C: 130%
Protein: 0 g	Iron: 1%
Fiber: 3 g	

Papaya also contains lots of fiber, potassium, vitamin
A, and folate. Fiber is helpful for your digestive tract,
potassium can help fight swollen ankles, vitamin A is
needed for the growth of your baby's eyes, and folate
is needed for the last-minute cell growth your growing
baby is experiencing now. So slice up some fresh, ripe
papaya as a tropical snack or try blending it with
some milk and honey for a delicious smoothie.

Happy Digestion

Papayas contain an enzyme called papain. This enzyme
can help you digest foods, a process that can become
daunting as your uterus continues to grow and your
intestines are squeezed into the remaining space in
your belly. According to experts at the Hospital for
Sick Children and founders of the Motherisk Program,
papain is effective for indigestion and heartburn, both
of which can be a problem during pregnancy. Enjoying
some ripe papaya is a tasty way to get some papain
into your diet. Papain is also available in supplement
form. But be sure to talk to your obstetrician or midwife before taking papain supplements.

FOOD SAFETY

Papaya is yet another food that some people will argue you shouldn't eat while you're pregnant. But if we were to put down all the foods that the Internet says you shouldn't eat during pregnancy, you'd find it hard to eat at all! There would hardly be anything left. In fact, while writing this book, we would type each food into an Internet search engine to see what popped up in relation to pregnancy. And without a doubt, most times there was some chat room where people were discussing why that food might pose a risk to women during pregnancy.

But ladies, let's think this through. What is the real risk of eating a food? It *is* a food, after all, and is probably eaten traditionally somewhere in the world. We need to assess the true risk of these food rumors. Plus, most of these questionable foods would be difficult to eat in large enough amounts to cause the effects people are worried about. It is very unlikely that you'll have a miscarriage or cause your baby serious distress from eating a certain food.

For example, the concern with papaya is that an unripe or even a semiripe papaya is rich in concentrated latex, which may cause uterine contractions. The latex affects oxytocin and prostaglandin levels, which can cause your uterus to contract. But you would have to eat a *lot* of unripe papaya to get these types of results. Plus, green papaya salad is a common dish in Thailand, and it's made with unripe papaya. To be safe, we recommend sticking with ripe papaya and eating it in moderation, so you can enjoy its health benefits without worrying about risk.

Jonny's Tasty Tips

When I was growing up in New York, I remember going into the hot dog and papaya stands known as Orange Julius and discovering the taste of this exotic fruit, which the guys behind the counter would actually throw fresh into blenders that were churning 24/7. I didn't know anyone who didn't like the taste of it then, and I still don't. It wasn't for nothing that Christopher Columbus called papaya "the fruit of the angels."

Papayas with reddish flesh have a different taste than the orange-fleshed types, which are sweeter. For eating raw, choose fruit that's free of black spots and skin damage. The spreading yellow color on the peel indicates that the fruit is softening and shows how far along it is in ripening. By the way, the black seeds inside are edible—they have a slightly bitter peppery taste. Slice a papaya into your next fruit salad, make your own smoothie, or just sit back, close your eyes, and enjoy a ripe piece or two. Angelic!

Parsley

LISTING THE NUTRIENTS FOUND IN THIS common garnish is like writing out the label of your prenatal vitamin: It's got almost everything! Don't pass up this green super-power on your plate just because it was put there as a decoration. Parsley is packed with a wide variety of vitamins and minerals that are great for you and your baby.

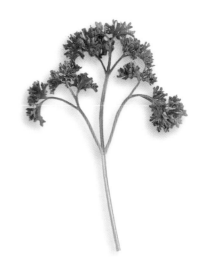

PARSLEY AT A GLANCE

Serving Size: 2 Tbsp (10 g)

Calories: 4

Saturated Fat: 0 g

Protein: 0 g

Fiber: 0 g

Calcium: 1%

Vitamin A: 25%

Vitamin C: 18%

Iron: 2%

FAST FACT

Not all parsley is the curly kind that usually ends up as a garnish on your plate. Flat-leaved or Italian parsley is considered even higher in nutrients than the curly-leaved kind. But curly or flat, you can't go wrong eating parsley!

Your Green Multi

Parsley contains a wide variety of important nutrients, making it one of the healthiest foods to eat during your pregnancy. Parsley is a source of vitamin E, vitamin A, vitamin C, and vitamin K (200 percent of your daily needs) and contains a small amount of the B vitamins thiamin, folate, riboflavin, niacin, pantothenic acid, and vitamin B6. This herb also contains some minerals including phosphorus, zinc, calcium, iron, magnesium, potassium, copper, and manganese. Phew—that's a lot of nutrients! Each of these plays a role in your health during your third trimester.

Help During Labor

Perhaps the most important nutrient in parsley is calcium: You need one calcium molecule for every muscle contraction you make. Imagine how much calcium you'll need to get enough muscle contractions to deliver your baby! Choosing to chomp on that parsley instead of tossing it aside sure is starting to sound like a good idea. You'll find 14 mg of calcium in 2 tablespoons of parsley—that's not bad for a little mouthful of green garnish!

Jonny's Tasty Tips

Parsley's not just another pretty face on your plate. Up your intake of this delicious herb by thinking of it not as a garnish but as a staple like basil or cilantro: Add it to green salads; mix it liberally into egg, chicken, and tuna salad; use it to replace some or all of the basil in pesto; or make a beautiful salad of sliced tomatoes, parsley, and cottage cheese. Add parsley to hummus and refried beans. Don't be afraid to add a whole half-cup of minced fresh parsley on cooked carrots or new potatoes. You'll find that it adds a great flavor punch!

More Than Vitamins

This green, leafy herb contains some lesser-known nutrients too. Parsley contains the flavonoid luteolin. Luteolin has been shown to function as antioxidant. It combines with highly reactive oxygen-containing molecules (called free radicals) and helps prevent damage to cells. In addition, scientists have found that parsley is an effective way to increase your blood levels of antioxidants, your best way to defend against aging and disease. During your third trimester though, your interest in antioxidants may center on their ability to free up your body's energy and attention from repairing damage caused by free radicals so it can focus on your impending labor.

SAY NO TO PARSLEY OIL

The green, fresh stems and leaves of parsley have all the health benefits we've discussed here. But oil made from parsley does not have the same benefits. Parsley oil is sometimes sold as a supplement. It is not a healthy option for pregnant women. When consumed in large amounts, parsley oil can stimulate contractions of the uterine muscles and possibly result in preterm labor. Skip the oil and stick with the fresh herb.

Peppermint

NOTHING BEATS THE REFRESHING SMELL OF A peppermint leaf. A perfect finishing touch to a meal, a peppermint is a common end-of-dinner treat not just because it freshens your breath but because it is known to soothe the digestive system. But rather than sticking your hand in the candy jar, try chewing a fresh peppermint sprig or brewing a cup of peppermint tea. In fact, you may want to reach for a sprig of peppermint more often once you realize that it's packed with nutrients.

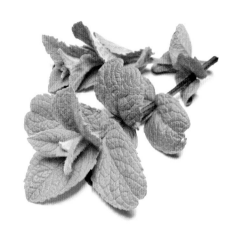

PEPPERMINT AT A GLANCE

Serving Size: 2 Tbsp (3 g)	**Calcium:** 1%
Calories: 2	**Vitamin A:** 3%
Saturated Fat: 0 g	**Vitamin C:** 2%
Protein: 0 g	**Iron:** 1%
Fiber: 0 g	

Healthy Teeth and Skin

Peppermint is a good source of niacin, phosphorus, and zinc. Niacin is a B vitamin that helps your skin stay young. Niacin helps the skin repair DNA that can be damaged by sunlight. Niacin also helps your skin look more youthful and healthy by encouraging skin cell turnover (newer skin cells are more beautiful than old, dry, dying cells). With all of the stretching it's experiencing in these last few months of pregnancy, your skin will appreciate the help. There is about 0.1 mg of niacin in 2 tablespoons of peppermint. Phosphorus works with calcium to build your baby's teeth and bones. And zinc plays a role in your immune cell activity.

A Spoonful of Health

You will also find fiber, vitamin A, vitamin C, calcium, iron, magnesium, potassium, copper, manganese, riboflavin, and folate in mint. But these nutrients aren't present in values that are anything to gawk at (only about 1 to 2 percent of the recommended daily amount for pregnant women in 2 tablespoons of peppermint). But peppermint is still considered a very nutrient-dense food: After all, 2 tablespoons is not a lot of food.

Jonny's Tasty Tips

Mint's not just for drinking or decorating lemon tarts. I love to add peppermint sprigs into an herb-rich green salad to give it a little bite, and of course it's a natural in fruit salads. You can add peppermint sprigs as a garnish in iced tea or lemonade (be sure to eat that sprig when you've finished your tea). And mint plays a major role in Middle Eastern and Mediterranean dishes like couscous and tabbouleh salads. Mint jelly is a natural with lamb and mutton—try fresh mint sprigs instead and enjoy the flavor without the sugar. Add peppermint sprigs to a dish of fresh raspberries or strawberries for a refreshing dessert. And don't forget to chew a mint sprig or two after supper. It not only aids digestion, it will work wonders on that after-dinner breath!

Your Cup of Tea

A soothing cup of peppermint tea is so cozy and warming on a cold day. And a glass of iced peppermint tea is amazingly refreshing when it's hot. Peppermint tea is touted for its ability to soothe the digestive tract, an effect that you may be craving if your uterus is putting extra stress on your digestive tract's ability to work. It's important to mention that, unlike ginger tea, which is well documented for its ability to safely alleviate digestive complaints during pregnancy, there are no studies on the safety of spearmint or peppermint tea in pregnancy. In the United States, peppermint as an herb has "generally recognized as safe" (GRAS) status. Health Canada advises that pregnant women use peppermint in moderation, which means about 1 or 2 cups per day.

Peppermint Oil

Research studies have found that peppermint oil may be helpful for irritable bowel syndrome (IBS) due to its antispasmodic effects. It seems to reduce slow-wave frequency in the small intestine, which slows peristaltic movement. If you have IBS, talk to your obstetrician about the safety of taking peppermint oil during pregnancy.

Red Raspberry Leaf Tea

RED RASPBERRY LEAF CONTAINS MANY
compounds well known to offer your body
antioxidant protection, including beta-
carotene (vitamin A), vitamin E, glutathione,
chlorogenic acid, anthocyanidins, ellagitannins,
and flavonols (quercetin, kaempferol, catechins, and phenolic acids). As you can imagine,
red raspberry leaf tea is considered a great source of antioxidants.

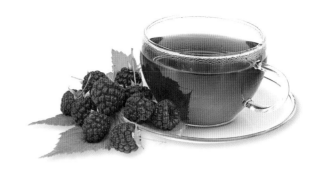

RED RASPBERRY LEAF TEA AT A GLANCE

Serving Size: 5 fl oz	Calcium: 0%
Calories: 1	Vitamin A: 0%
Saturated Fat: 0 g	Vitamin C: 0%
Protein: 0 g	Iron: 0%
Fiber: 0 g	

Antioxidants help keep your body free from damage caused by free radicals, so it stays healthier and spends more time feeling great and less energy repairing cell damage. Red raspberry leaf tea is also thought to support healthy blood vessel dilation (vasodilation) and may help promote uterine contractions, helping to promote a healthy labor and the general health of the uterus.

Easy Labor

A national survey of 500 members of the American College of Nurse-Midwives found that of midwives who use herbal preparations to stimulate labor, 63 percent used red raspberry leaf. That's a great reason to consider serving up a cup of this tea during your third trimester, but it's also a caffeine-free, nutrient-rich drink to help keep you hydrated. Never fear—you won't go into labor from a cup of this tea! It can safely be consumed during pregnancy. In fact, my pregnant girlfriends and I use it as our tea of choice for our afternoon tea visits.

Many women drink raspberry leaf tea during their pregnancies in the belief that it shortens labor and makes labor "easier." Drinking the tea is perfectly safe and will not cause labor to start. But used in a supplement form, red raspberry leaf may be very helpful during labor! A group of Australian researchers decided to look a little further into the effects of red raspberry leaf on pregnancy in a double-blind, randomized, placebo-controlled trial that involved 192 women with low-risk pregnancies. The women consumed red raspberry leaf in a tablet form from week 32 of their pregnancy.

There were no adverse effects, but it did not shorten the first stage of labor. Yet it did shorten the second stage of labor by about 10 minutes and resulted in a lower rate of forceps deliveries. Unfortunately though, the results were not significant enough, and the researchers concluded that red raspberry leaf needs more investigation (particularly regarding the ideal dosage).

In 2001, the journal *Midwifery and Women's Health* reported that taking red raspberry leaf orally does not seem to reduce the length of labor or decrease the need for analgesics in the perinatal time period. More research in the future will help us determine how effective red raspberry leaf tea is in helping with labor and pregnancy.

Is It Safe?

Red raspberry leaf tea is considered safe for use by pregnant women when used orally in amounts commonly found in foods, such as a few cups of tea a day. According to the Natural Medicines Comprehensive Database, red raspberry leaf is considered safe when used orally and appropriately in medicinal amounts during late pregnancy and under the supervision of a health-care provider. Red raspberry leaf is commonly used in higher dosages by midwives to facilitate delivery. Talk to your obstetrician or midwife about red raspberry leaf tea before using it.

STAGES OF LABOR

We've been discussing the effects of red raspberry leaf tea in shortening the second stage of labor. But how can you tell when you've entered the second stage? Here's how labor breaks down.

Stage one of labor is when the cervix dilates and thins to allow the baby to move into the birth canal. This is the longest stage of labor and is divided into three subphases: early labor, active labor, and transition. Early labor involves mild to moderately strong contractions, and your cervix will dilate to 3 centimeters. This stage can last for a few hours or days. In active labor the cervix dilates to 7 centimeters and the contractions become longer and stronger. This stage of labor usually lasts between 3 and 8 hours. The last subphase is transition, when your cervix dilates to 10 centimeters. This is often the shortest (15 minutes to a few hours) but most difficult stage of labor.

The second stage of labor is the actual delivery of the baby. It can take a few minutes to a few hours and requires pushing with each contraction. There's a final stage of labor as well. The last stage of labor is the delivery of the placenta.

Rhubarb

DURING YOUR THIRD TRIMESTER, RHUBARB IS
one of the healthiest foods you can eat. Rhubarb
is a good source of magnesium, calcium, potassium,
manganese, vitamin C, vitamin K, silica, and fiber.
While rhubarb's leaves are toxic, its stalks are enjoyed
for their great taste and beautifying benefits. That's right—
rhubarb is great for your skin. And with each additional week into your
pregnancy, your skin is being asked to stretch even farther. Keep your skin looking
its best with the help of rhubarb.

RHUBARB AT A GLANCE

Serving Size: 1 cup (122 g)	Calcium: 10%
Calories: 26	Vitamin A: 2%
Saturated Fat: 0 g	Vitamin C: 14%
Protein: 1 g	Iron: 1%
Fiber: 2 g	

FAST FACT

Fruit or vegetable? Confusing as it is, some
of our favorite vegetables, like peppers and
tomatoes, are technically fruits, while rhubarb,
which we enjoy as a dessert, is actually a
vegetable.

Scaffolding Support

In this delicious vegetable, you'll find vitamin C (about
10 mg in a cup), an important antioxidant. Vitamin C
protects all of the areas in your body that are primarily water (it's a water-soluble antioxidant), helping
you prevent damage from free radicals. Having more
antioxidants in your body will free up time and energy
from damage repair so your body can focus on baby
growth and delivery. Plus, vitamin C is a necessary
component of healthy skin. The scaffolding of your
skin is collagen, which can't be made without vitamin
C. Keep your skin strong and resilient with the help of
vitamin C-rich foods like rhubarb.

Jonny's Tasty Tips

Rhubarb is a treat I eagerly anticipate each spring. Sweet and sour at the same time, rhubarb is a perfect addition to Grandma's famous apple crisp or strawberry pie. But I'd rather eat my rhubarb with yogurt or applesauce. Stew it first with a little honey and then stir it in. It will turn your applesauce a beautiful pink!

Silica for Skin, Hair, and Bones

Silicon (silica) may be the second most abundant mineral on earth, but it is probably not a nutrient you've thought about before reading this book. You can find silica in stringy vegetables like asparagus, celery, and rhubarb. Silica binds 300 times its own weight in water. So it helps your skin retain water, helping it stay hydrated and healthy while it stretches over your growing uterus. Your bones, teeth, and hair (and your baby's too) use silica to stay strong, healthy, and hydrated. Unfortunately, silica is very difficult for your body to absorb, and you excrete between 10 and 40 mg of it every day. Rhubarb can help you and your baby get enough of this mineral to enjoy beautiful skin and hair and healthy teeth and bones.

Sesame Seeds

WHEN YOU'RE THINKING OF HEALTHY FOODS
for your third-trimester diet, seeds probably
don't spring to mind. But they're very nutritious,
offering you many of the nutrients you so
desperately need during your pregnancy, such as
calcium, iron, and fiber. Sesame seeds have a delicious,
nutty flavor. And they're so convenient: It's easy to sprinkle them on salads and
stir-fries, or just enjoy them as you munch on your favorite breakfast or snack bar.

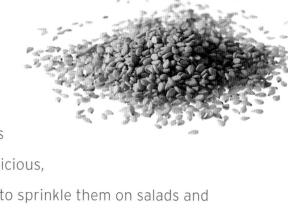

SESAME SEEDS AT A GLANCE

Serving Size: 1 ounce (28 g)	**Calcium:** 25%
Calories: 160	**Vitamin A:** 0%
Saturated Fat: 2 g	**Vitamin C:** 0%
Protein: 5 g	**Iron:** 20%
Fiber: 3 g	

FAST FACT

Milk can interfere with iron absorption. Drink
water rather than milk with your meal when
you're eating iron-rich foods like meat, green
leafy vegetables, and sesame seeds.

Minerals and More

Sesame seeds are a very good source of copper and
manganese, and they're also a good source of magnesium and phosphorus. And a 1-ounce serving (about
28 g) contains about 10 percent of your daily needs of
three B vitamins: thiamin, vitamin B6, and folate. All
three Bs are helpful both for your baby's development
and for keeping your energy levels up. Sesame seeds
are also packed with protein—they contain more protein than any other nut or seed. Those 5 g of protein in
your serving of sesame seeds will help keep you fueled.

Calcium for Baby's Nerves

During the last trimester of pregnancy, your baby's
body is fine-tuning his or her nervous system, and
his or her brain is creating important pathways that
will eventually help him or her laugh, walk, and read.
Nerves send messages from your brain to all of the
parts of your body, and every message requires calcium. You already know that calcium is important for
your baby's teeth and bones, but it is also needed for
nerve transmission and muscle contractions. Luckily,

Jonny's Tasty Tips

I like to bring out the nutty flavor of sesame seeds by toasting them in a dry skillet over medium heat until they're golden brown. But eating the whole seeds is just one way to enjoy them. Sesame butter is a great alternative to peanut butter and is usually made of whole roasted sesame seeds. Tahini is made from hulled sesame seeds and is therefore a more refined, less fiber-rich product, though it's still delicious. Two of my favorite Middle Eastern appetizers are both sesame based: hummus, which is made from ground chickpeas, garlic, and tahini, and baba ghanouj, which has a base of roasted eggplant seasoned with tahini, lemon juice, garlic, and salt. Enjoy them with whole-wheat pita or use them as dips for celery and carrot sticks.

RICH IN GOOD FATS

Concerned about the fat in sesame seeds? Sure, sesame seeds are considered a fatty food, but they are a source of good fat, making them an excellent choice for your pregnancy diet. The fats in sesame seeds are mostly monounsaturated and polyunsaturated fats. Of the 13 g of fat found in a 1-ounce serving of sesame seeds, 11 are these good fats.

a healthy diet can help provide you with the extra calcium you need during your third trimester. Sesame seeds are a calcium-rich choice: one serving (1 ounce) provides about 25 percent of your daily needs of calcium. This is an impressive amount of calcium, when you consider that a cup of milk contains about 30 percent of the daily recommended value.

Iron for Mom

Women in general tend to be iron deficient, and during your pregnancy, your body has had even greater iron needs. Not only are you producing more blood but your baby's own bloodstream is also growing and developing. And blood cells can't develop without iron. If you don't get enough iron, you can develop anemia (a condition involving a deficiency of iron in the blood) during pregnancy. Sesame seeds are an excellent dietary source of iron. One ounce of sesame seeds provides your body with close to 20 percent of your daily recommended amount.

Fiber for Digestion

You never imagined you'd get this big. Everyone told you it would happen, but you never really thought you wouldn't be able to see your own feet. Packed in that growing belly of yours is a uterus that now resembles a small watermelon. In the meantime, your intestines have had to move over and try to function despite the diminishing space. As a result, you may be having some trouble with your bowel movements. Eating fiber is a healthy way to help keep your intestines moving during your pregnancy. Sesame seeds are a good source of fiber: just 1 ounce provides 3 g of fiber. You can also try adding flaxseeds (ground flaxseeds or flaxmeal) to your salads and smoothies for a nutty taste, extra fiber, and some healthy omegas to boot.

Swiss Cheese

SWISS CHEESE IS NOT ONLY A DELICIOUS
food to include in your third trimester of
pregnancy; it also has lots of healthy benefits
for you and your baby. Like all cheeses, Swiss
cheese is a great source of calcium, a very important
you'll be needing a lot of over the next few months.

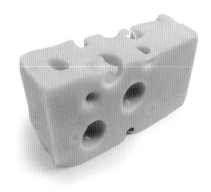

SWISS CHEESE AT A GLANCE

Serving Size: 100 g	Calcium: 75%
Calories: 380	Vitamin A: 15%
Saturated Fat: 18 g	Vitamin C: 0%
Protein: 27 g	Iron: 1%
Fiber: 0 g	

Why You Need Calcium

As we've said often in this book, calcium is a very
important nutrient for pregnant women. It is needed
for the development of your baby's bones (all 300 of
them) and to keep your own bones healthy and strong.
Teeth need calcium to grow and stay strong. Every
muscle contraction requires calcium; every little kick or
wave your baby gives you from inside your belly uses
calcium. And in order for your body to deliver that
baby, your uterus will make some amazing contractions, each of which will require lots of calcium.

Still not convinced? Then consider this: If you don't
provide your body with enough calcium in your diet,
it will pull calcium from your bones. If you do this too
often, your bones become weak. Be nice to your bones—
treat them to calcium-rich foods like Swiss cheese.

Calcium versus Preeclampsia

The calcium in your piece of Swiss cheese may also
be good for your blood pressure, and it may help
you reduce your risk of developing preeclampsia.
Preeclampsia is an extremely dangerous condition that
can occur in pregnancy and can cause illness or death
in the mother and/or baby. It is rare (5 to 8 percent of
pregnancies) and is characterized by high blood pressure and protein in the urine. When a group of British
researchers reviewed twelve studies in the Cochrane
Database, they found an association between calcium
and preeclampsia.

The researchers found that calcium supplementation appears to cut the risk of preeclampsia in pregnant women almost in half. It may also help to prevent
preterm labor. Most prenatal vitamins include calcium,

Jonny's Tasty Tips

I don't really have to tell you how to enjoy Swiss cheese, do I? My favorite way to eat it is also the simplest: a wedge of Swiss cheese, a handful of almonds or hazelnuts, and an apple, pear, or bunch of grapes. Or go fancy by melting it and dipping vegetables in it for a yummy, healthy fondue. And by the way—Swiss cheese is an even better source of calcium than milk!

and many of the healthiest foods for pregnancy in this book are chosen because of their high calcium content.

You really need plenty of calcium from the moment you become pregnant—or even before—through delivery and breast-feeding. The researchers recommended that pregnant women should try to get adequate dietary calcium before they become pregnant and in early pregnancy, since it may be needed to prevent the underlying cause of preeclampsia.

WHAT MAKES THOSE HOLES?

Ever wonder what gives Swiss cheese its holes? *Propionibacteria freudenreichii* is used in Swiss-cheese manufacturing to produce its flavor and characteristic holes. *Propionibacteria* is a type of probiotic (microbes that offer you healthy benefits). In a clinical trial, *P. freudenreichii* was able to decrease symptoms of constipation in a group of elderly people—good news for your squashed intestines!

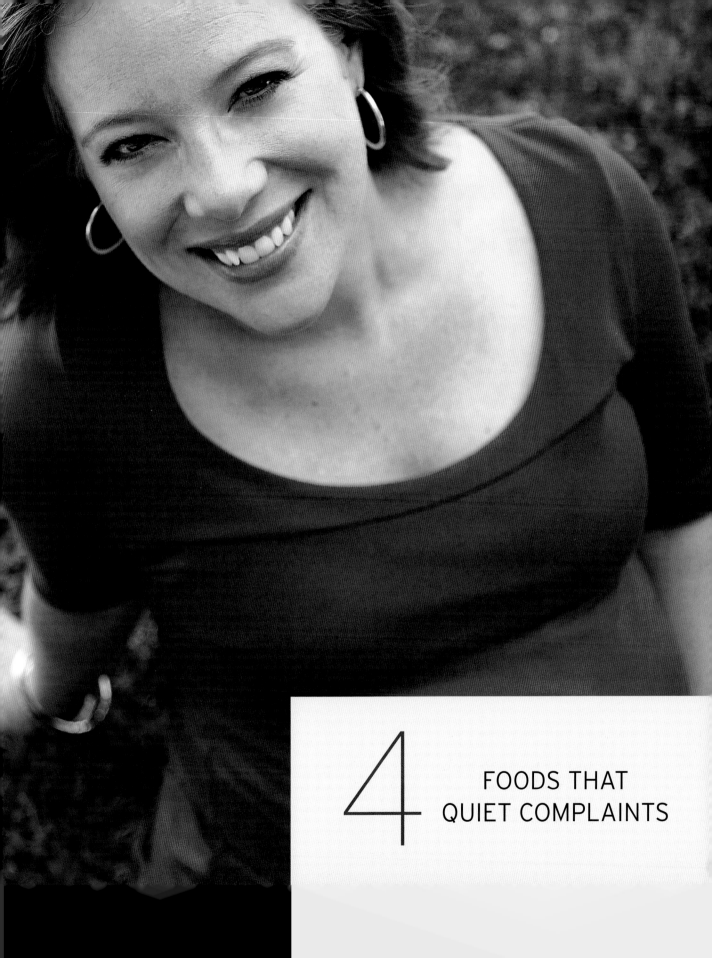

4

FOODS THAT
QUIET COMPLAINTS

CONVINCED THAT YOU'RE DESTINED TO SPEND the rest of your days coping with insomnia, back pain, and all the other pregnancy aches and pains? Luckily, we all know that pregnancy is just a 40-week event, so you certainly won't be suffering forever. But that knowledge may not be enough to get you through. Here's the good news: You can eat your way through most of your complaints. Believe it or not, you've got an arsenal of foods that you can use to help relieve some of these symptoms.

Food affects your mood, and it can affect the symptoms of pregnancy too. Whether it's constipation, acne, gas, leg cramps, backaches, breast tenderness, or that nagging lack of energy, there are foods that may help ease your misery. Let's talk about some of the most common complaints during pregnancy and the foods you can eat to help quiet them. Then we'll focus on the top foods for pregnancy complaints.

ACNE

You may start to feel like you're back in high school when you look at your reflection in the mirror each morning. Red bumps keep popping up overnight. Despite all of your attempts to cleanse, tone, and moisturize appropriately, your skin is still breaking out in pimples. For the same reason you had acne during puberty, you're having acne during pregnancy: hormones. Luckily, this round of acne will not last as long as your previous encounter! Most women find that their acne disappears shortly after delivery. Eating foods that help prevent inflammation like fish and fermented foods like yogurt and kefir can help reduce the redness of your acne.

BREAST TENDERNESS AND STRETCH MARKS

It is absolutely amazing how much your breasts grow during pregnancy. If you have ever complained that you have a flat chest, then never fear; your new bosom is here. By the end of the first trimester, your breasts will have increased about one cup size, and by the end of your third trimester, they'll have grown another size. For some women, it's like getting a sneak peak at what you might look like with implants. But feeling like Pamela Lee Anderson comes with a price: tender breasts.

Soon after your pregnancy test comes back positive, your breasts start to become more sensitive, to the point that even taking a shower can be painful. The increase in blood flow to your breasts can cause them to swell, become sensitive, and even cause the area around your nipples to become darker in color. Some women's breasts are so tender that the idea of lying on their stomachs is ludicrous.

Sadly, there is no perfect food for alleviating the breast tenderness associated with pregnancy. Your best move is to support your breasts with a good-quality bra to help reduce pain.

A good bra can help reduce stretch marks, too, but this time, you can do more: There are foods that can help you keep your breasts beautiful by preventing stretch marks. As your breasts grow, your skin is stretched. To help prevent stretch marks on your breasts, be sure to include healthy sources of good fats in your diet like fish and flax seeds and foods like asparagus, rhubarb, and kiwis, which contain special nutrients that support skin health. It's also important to drink plenty of fluids to support your growing breasts and stretching skin.

CONSTIPATION

There are many reasons why a pregnant woman may suffer from constipation, but the two most obvious culprits are surging hormone levels and the ever-decreasing space available in your gut for your intestines to function in. High levels of the hormone progesterone cause the muscles of the intestine to function far less efficiently than normal, resulting in dry, hard stools and infrequent bowel movements.

Drinking plenty of water is one of the easiest ways to quiet this pregnancy complaint. Regular exercise and visits to the bathroom whenever the urge arises are two great lifestyle strategies to quiet constipation.

You can even eat your way through this complaint. Foods that are high in fiber can help soften stool and keep your bowels moving. There are two types of fiber: insoluble and soluble. Soluble fiber forms a gel-like substance in your gut that softens your stool. Insoluble fiber can't be digested by your body, so it helps push everything through your intestines and out the other end. You will need both types of fiber to get your colon moving. Luckily, most of the healthy foods in this book (including nuts, vegetables, whole grains, and fruits like prunes) contain a mixture of both fibers, giving your colon the attention it needs.

HOME REMEDY

According to Grandma, blackstrap molasses is known to help alleviate constipation. Just dissolve 2 tablespoons in a glass of warm water and you're good to, uh, go.

FAST FACT

Iron supplements commonly cause constipation. You may find them less of a problem if you take them on a full stomach and drink plenty of fluids.

LOW ENERGY

Some women are surprised and demoralized when they feel an ongoing lack of energy during pregnancy. It shouldn't come as a surprise: Your body's making a baby, after all, and that's its energy priority right now. But it can still be daunting, especially if you're used to high energy levels.

The good news is that, while fatigue is a major problem during the first trimester, you'll usually feel more energetic during the second and third trimesters. But don't be surprised if carrying around that close-to-full-term baby in your third trimester doesn't leave you winded and in need of a pregnancy catnap. Not only is your body using a vast amount of energy to make a baby—it's actually sedating you. You read that right: Your body is producing a lot more progesterone, which is a natural sedative. It's Mother Nature's way of saying "Slow down!"

But slowing down and dragging are two different things. Eating healthy foods is a great way to help boost your energy levels. Complex carbohydrates (we prefer the more modern term *low-glycemic carbs*) are great providers of energy, as they offer you a slow supply of fuel to keep you going throughout your day. You'll find low-glycemic carbohydrates in most of your healthy foods like nuts, seeds, high-fiber whole grains, vegetables, and fruits. Protein is another great energy provider. Enjoy eating your way through this pregnancy complaint.

Various minerals and vitamins are involved in the metabolism of energy, helping you convert the energy in the food you've eaten into fuel you can use. Nutrients like the B vitamins, magnesium, antioxidants, iron, and amino acids can help you get your oomph back. Let's take a closer look at these natural energizers.

B-lieve in Bs for Energy

B vitamins are one of your best friends when it comes to making energy. But the names of B vitamins can be confusing, since some go by simple numbers (like B12) while others go by names that aren't B-related (like folate). To make sure you're getting all your Bs, here are their names and numbers: thiamine (vitamin B1), riboflavin (vitamin B2), niacin (vitamin B3), pyridoxine (vitamin B6), biotin (vitamin B7), folate (vitamin B9), and cyanocobalamin (vitamin B12).

B vitamins support energy metabolism. They play a role in the metabolism of fats, carbohydrates, and proteins into energy. The most important of the B vitamins for extra energy is vitamin B12. Most of these energizing B vitamins are found in grains, mushrooms, and some vegetables, but vitamin B12 is only found in good quantities in meat, dairy products, and eggs (that's why vegetarians are notoriously deficient in B12). Luckily, some of the foods discussed in Chapters 1, 2, and 3 are packed with B vitamins, like eggs, chickpeas, and multigrain cereal.

Mineral Mobilizers

Iron is not directly energizing, but it helps the true driver of energy: oxygen. Oxygen is carried in the blood from your lungs to the rest of your body. Red blood cells contain hemoglobin, and hemoglobin contains iron. Without iron, your body couldn't carry oxygen to your cells, which need it to make energy. Pregnant women commonly have low iron levels. To help enhance your body's ability to take up iron, be sure your multivitamin also includes vitamin C and bioflavonoids, since both these nutrients will improve iron absorption. And eat your way to higher iron levels with iron-rich foods like spinach.

If you are short on magnesium, your body will have an increased need for oxygen. That means you'll have to expend more energy to get the laundry done, make dinner, or even climb the stairs. Low levels of magnesium in your diet can cause you to tire easily. There are lots of great food sources of magnesium in our list of the 100 healthiest foods for pregnancy, including halibut, soybeans, almonds, spinach and oatmeal. Time to add some magnesium into your diet and enjoy more energy!

Antioxidants and Amino Acids

Antioxidants protect your internal batteries so they can keep recharging and producing energy. How? Antioxidants like lutein, selenium, and bioflavonoids neutralize free radicals. Free radicals are damaging compounds that form in your body as a byproduct of your daily activities. Free radicals cause damage to healthy cells by stealing electrons from parts of the cell. The ribosome is the part of your cell that makes energy like an internal battery. The ribosome relies on its structure to be able to make energy. If free radicals damage the structure of a ribosome, it can't make energy. Antioxidants can protect your cells and ribosomes from free radicals. Make sure your diet includes plenty of antioxidant-rich fruits and vegetables like acerola cherries and kiwi.

Amino acids are the building blocks your body needs to make proteins. Most of us think of amino acids as a requirement for body builders and athletes. However, did you know that enzymes and hormones are also proteins? Yes, you need amino acids to make the enzymes that drive your metabolism. Hormones that make you feel happy and energetic are also made from amino acids. Thus, to keep your energy levels high, be sure to look for foods that contain amino acids, like aged Cheddar cheese, trout, and yogurt.

GAS

Those increased progesterone levels cause havoc to your body, including increasing gas and bloating in some women. Progesterone slows down your digestive tract, which means your food sits around in your intestines a little longer. This can be a benefit, since it allows your food more time to be absorbed, but it also means the microbes in your gut have more time to ferment food, causing higher levels of gas than you are probably used too.

Luckily, you can use a few tricks while eating that will help. First, try not to swallow a lot of air. (Gulping air is a successful strategy some women use to control the nausea that comes with morning sickness, so weigh the benefits and drawbacks of this technique.) If you typically drink soda, iced tea, and other beverages through a straw, skip the straw during pregnancy—you're taking in a lot of extra air with every sip, and that can lead to gas. Try not to sip hot beverages or soup, which can also cause you to swallow a lot of air. Instead, drink your liquids from the lip of the cup or even drink your soup from the bowl's edge (or drink your soup from a cup instead of a bowl if it makes you too self-conscious).

Here are more ways to get gas under control: Try to drink plenty of water, since this will help ensure that things keep moving in your intestines. And reach for lots of high-fiber foods, because they'll help push and

GET UP AND GO

Lacking a little oomph in your day? Pregnancy is a major life change, and to make that baby requires a lot of energy, which may have you feeling sluggish. Remember that exercise is always a great way to help you feel more energized. But take it easy and listen to your body while exercising. Pregnancy is not the time to start training for a marathon, but it's also not the time to stop exercising all together. Regular exercise is part of a healthy pregnancy.

propel your food through your 20-plus feet of increasingly cramped intestines. Nuts, seeds, vegetables, fruits, and grains are all great ways to add fiber to your diet, and they contain lots of other healthy nutrients for you and your baby. You can also try to avoid gas-producing foods like cabbage, high-fat foods, and carbonated beverages. A healthy digestive system is host to a high number of probiotics (good microbes that live in your digestive tract). You can eat your way through constipation, gas, and bloating with the help of fermented foods like kefir and yogurt that contain probiotics.

LEG CRAMPS AND BACKACHES

During pregnancy, some women will suffer from cramps in their legs, most often in their calves and usually in the middle of the night. This cramping can be incredibly painful. Many experts believe that calcium is related to muscle cramps. Including cheese, yogurt, milk, grains, nuts, and dark leafy greens in your diet are great ways to help make sure your muscles have enough calcium to keep them relaxed.

During your last trimester, it is common to suffer from back pain. This is caused by the increased weight in your belly pulling on your back muscles, changes in your posture, relaxation of the ligaments in your back, and overstretching of your abdominal muscles.

Some tricks can help you protect your back: Avoid picking up heavy objects, and if you have to lift something, be sure to lift with your legs and not with your back. Support your back with pillows while you sleep and try not to sit or stand in one position for too long during the day.

Ensuring that your diet has enough protein can help your abdominal and back muscles stay as strong as possible. Minerals such as magnesium and sodium found in vegetables and grains can help your muscles have the tools they need to work optimally and can help keep your muscles hydrated.

MORNING SICKNESS

The stomach-churning, hung-over sensation of morning sickness is one that most women experience early in their pregnancies. Caused by the increase in hormones that occurs during the early stages of pregnancy, morning sickness can really wreck your day. Many foods can help you quiet this pregnancy complaint, including oatmeal, ice chips, and ginger. (See chapter 1 for details on these helpful first-trimester foods.) Plus, eating in general can help fend off morning sickness. Take a read through chapter 1 if you find that you're fighting the urge to hug the toilet every morning. We've given you lots of tips for fighting this miserable side effect.

WEIGHT GAIN

It's all part of pregnancy, that ever-climbing number on the scale. But many of us have struggled for decades to maintain a perfect weight, a toned body, and a healthy body image. Unfortunately, all of those goals need to go out the door for the next year. Pregnancy is a full-body experience, and no matter what, you *will* gain weight. It's simply part of the process.

The best thing you can do is stay active and eat well. If the foods you are eating are healthy, full of nutrients, and satisfying, then you'll only gain the weight your body needs to have a healthy pregnancy. (Desserts, fat-filled treats, and buttery baked goods don't count as healthy foods, in case you're wondering.)

Go ahead, ladies, eat! Eat and enjoy it. You can't drink, you probably can't skydive, and heck, you can't even take cold medicines. So you might as well eat, as long as you eat smart. And that's where this book comes in.

Top Foods for Pregnancy Complaints

Bleeding gums, carpel tunnel, itching, hemorrhoids, headaches, and many other complaints are all part of the marvel of pregnancy. Luckily, many of the most common complaints can be quieted with the help of a healthy diet, exercise, and some simple lifestyle tricks. You really *can* eat your way through pregnancy complaints. Let's take a closer look at the healthiest foods you can eat during your pregnancy that may help you quiet some of those complaints.

HERE ARE THE 15 HEALTHIEST FOODS TO QUIET THE COMPLAINTS OF PREGNANCY:

- ACEROLA CHERRIES
- AGED CHEDDAR CHEESE
- ARTICHOKES
- CAROB
- FLAXSEED

- KEFIR
- KIWI
- PRUNE JUICE
- PUMPKIN SEEDS
- RAINBOW TROUT

- SPINACH
- SUNDRIED TOMATOES
- WHEAT GERM
- WHOLE-GRAIN PASTA
- YOGURT

Let's look at each of these healthy foods and see why they're so great when those aggravating pregnancy complaints are wearing you down. And once again, Jonny's ready to come to the rescue with great ways to use less-familiar foods like acerola cherries, kefir, and flaxseed in "Jonny's Tasty Tips."

Acerola Cherries

YOU MAY NOT FIND ACEROLA CHERRIES IN the local market, but they're worth combing the health food stores for. These cherrylike fruits are the richest known natural source of vitamin C on earth. As a result, they have become popular in North America and Europe as a natural source of vitamin C in supplements. Offering a wide variety of minerals and antioxidant, acerola cherries are one of the healthiest foods for pregnancy.

ACEROLA CHERRIES AT A GLANCE

Serving Size: 1 cup (98 g)	Calcium: 1%
Calories: 31	Vitamin A: 12%
Saturated Fat: 0 g	Vitamin C: 2500%
Protein: 0 g	Iron: 1%
Fiber: 1 g	

* The nutritional facts data provided in this book are approximations based on the food's nutrient value and a pregnant woman's RDA.

Quieting Acne

Your skin may be affected by acne thanks to your higher hormone levels during pregnancy. What causes acne, anyway? When dirt, oil or bacteria clogs a pore in your skin, your body responds with an inflammatory reaction to try to clear the area of the infection. Inflammation in your skin is what causes the red, puffy appearance of pimples. Here's where vitamin C comes in. Vitamin C is an antioxidant that protects your skin from damage from free radicals. Free radicals form in your skin when it is exposed to sunlight, chemicals in cosmetics, and inflammation. Eating foods that contain vitamin C, like acerola cherries, may help protect your skin from free radical damage caused by acne inflammation.

In fact, vitamin C is your skin's best friend. When sailors traveled from Europe to the New World in the 18th century, they realized the importance of vitamin C in their diet. Without vitamin C from fresh fruits on these long trips, some sailors' skin would start to deteriorate, a condition called scurvy. Your skin needs vitamin C to make collagen, one of the two main structural compounds that make it strong and elastic.

Better Than Oranges

Acerola cherries typically contain about 1,500 mg of vitamin C per gram, and they can contain much more, up to 4,000 mg. By comparison, a navel orange contains just 60 mg of vitamin C per 100 g, making acerola cherries the king of vitamin C-containing fruits. And there's more to acerola than vitamin C. Acerola cherries are an excellent source of other powerful antioxidants such as anthocyanins, carotenoids, selenium, zinc, and proanthocyanidins. All of these nutrients can support healthy skin, a healthy body, and a healthy pregnancy. Plus, they are a source of iron and calcium, two nutrients your body has greater needs for during pregnancy.

Hold Off on the Supplements

In Barbados, the West Indies, and South America, cherrylike, sweet-sour acerola fruit are commonly eaten fresh or made into jams or jellies. In North America and Europe, acerola cherries are harder to find fresh but can be found in dried or powdered form at health food stores and are also used in juices. But since taking acerola cherry supplements (such as powdered acerola) during pregnancy has not yet been proven safe, you should consult your obstetrician or midwife before taking it (or any item) in supplement form. We suggest sticking with the dried fruit, fruit juice, or—if you're lucky enough to find them—fresh fruit.

Jonny's Tasty Tips

In Southern California, bushy acerola cherry trees produce multiple crops from March through December, so I can enjoy the bright red, cherry-shaped fruits fresh almost year-round. (They're also grown in South Texas and other hot-climate areas, as well as in Mexico and Puerto Rico.) My favorite variety, Manoa Sweet, produces big, 1-inch bright red "cherries." I love the sweet-tart flavor of the fresh fruit. If you're lucky enough to find fresh acerola cherries, just remember that they may look like cherries, but they have their own texture and flavor (not to mention three hard, dark seeds). So enjoy them for what they are, not what they're named for!

FAST FACT

The best food sources of vitamin C are acerola cherries, bell peppers, broccoli, kiwi, gogi berries, oranges, and strawberries.

Aged Cheddar Cheese

CHEDDAR CHEESE—MMMM: A TASTY HUNK
of cheese is one of the best snacks in the
world. Plus, you can eat it knowing that
it's a healthy choice for your baby. Cheese
contains some of a pregnant woman's most-
needed nutrients: calcium and protein. Choosing
aged Cheddar ups its flavor and safety.

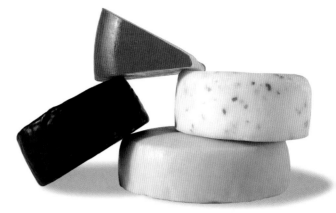

AGED CHEDDAR CHEESE AT A GLANCE

Serving Size: 100 g (about ¾ cup)	Calcium: 70%
Calories: 400	Vitamin A: 18%
Saturated Fat: 20 g	Vitamin C: 0%
Protein: 25 g	Iron: 3%
Fiber: 0 g	

Looking for aged Cheddar will help you stay away from
the processed cheeses that are lower in nutrients.
Plus, if you reach for aged cheese, you'll find you eat
less: Its potent buttery flavor can help satisfy your
cravings before you eat more calories than you need.
Add some Cheddar cheese to your diet and eat your
way through leg cramps, backaches, and digestive
complaints.

Building Blocks

Cheese may not spring to mind as a good source of
protein, but it is: One cup of Cheddar cheese (an easy
amount to eat on a plate of nachos) contains 33 g of
protein. That's a lot of protein. And, as we've told you

WHICH CHEESES ARE SAFE?

When you're pregnant, it can be hard to keep
the safe foods straight from the not-so-safe
foods. But hard cheeses like Cheddar are generally safe. Stay away from moldy cheeses like
blue cheese and be wary of soft cheeses like
Brie and Camembert, since some are on the
"no" list. See chapter 5, beginning on page
210, for a complete list of foods to avoid
during pregnancy.

many times, protein is an essential part of a pregnant
woman's diet. Most women don't eat enough protein
even when they're not pregnant. It's especially important to eat plenty now.

Here's why: Your body breaks down protein into
its building blocks, the amino acids. Then it can use
these amino acids to build enzymes, hormones, and
muscles as needed. Right now, your body is producing

a lot of hormones, and you're also building a baby, so you need more protein. Plus, as your pregnancy progresses and your weight increases, there will be more stress on your muscles. Strained muscles require more protein to repair and rebuild. Backaches and other muscle aches can be relieved with a healthy diet that contains good sources of protein like aged Cheddar cheese.

Calcium for Muscle Cramps

Cheese is a great-tasting source of calcium. Aged Cheddar cheese is packed with calcium—one cup contains all the calcium an adult needs in a day. But as a pregnant woman, your calcium needs are higher, which is why most prenatal supplements contain calcium to augment the calcium you're getting from a healthy diet. We all know that calcium is needed for healthy bones and teeth. But did you know that calcium plays a role in preventing muscle cramps? Eating foods that are rich in calcium, like Cheddar cheese, may help prevent leg cramps, a common pregnancy complaint.

Digestive Health

Cheddar cheese is a source of the good bacteria called *probiotics*. Probiotics may be one of the most important foods for your body. The work done by probiotics in your digestive tract in a day is equivalent to the work done by your liver. It's amazing! Probiotics help you digest and absorb food, they make vitamins, they prevent infections like diarrhea, they boost your immune system, and they can fight those plagues of pregnant women—constipation, gas, and bloating. Keeping your digestive system healthy during pregnancy will keep you feeling great. Grab some cheese and eat your way through your digestive pregnancy complaints.

Jonny's Tasty Tips

There are thousands of ways to include cheese in your diet, but some are healthier than others. One of my favorites is snacking on an apple with a few slices of Cheddar cheese. Or try adding a few slices to your next whole-grain sandwich. (Make sure you top that Cheddar with tomatoes and plenty of dark greens like romaine lettuce, arugula, and/or spinach to make a good sandwich great.)

Try shredding some Cheddar cheese on your broccoli or Brussels sprouts to boost your daily calcium intake. Shredded Cheddar can make almost any dish more nutritious, from baked potatoes to apple pie, but I especially enjoy it on bean dishes, soups, and salads. And you can make a super dip from plain yogurt mixed with shredded Cheddar and dried or fresh herbs like oregano, basil, chives, or cilantro. Try it with veggies like celery and carrot sticks, cherry tomatoes, radish slices, and bell pepper strips.

One last thing: Never, ever think that "processed cheese food" is the same as real cheese. Processed cheese food bears the same relationship to *real* cheese as a Twinkie does to real food. If you see "cheese food" on the label, for goodness' sake, put the package down and step away from the counter!

Artichokes

RICH, BUTTERY ARTICHOKES TASTE SO DELICIOUS they seem like a decadent treat. But these big buds (they're actually the immature stage of a giant thistle-like flower) are not only easy to prepare, they're packed with nutrients that may help quiet some of your pregnancy complaints. And their guilt-free fatty texture is hard to beat.

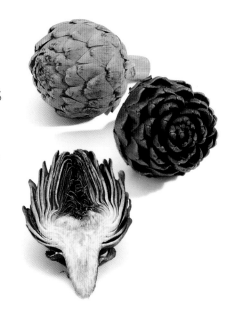

ARTICHOKES AT A GLANCE

Serving Size: 1 medium artichoke (120 g)	Calcium: 3%
Calories: 64	Vitamin A: 0%
Saturated Fat: 0 g	Vitamin C: 13%
Protein: 3 g	Iron: 12%
Fiber: 10 g	

Energizer

Are you feeling sluggish? Reach for an artichoke. Artichokes are a great nonmeat source of iron, which is an energizing nutrient. Iron is used to make hemoglobin in your red blood cells. Hemoglobin is what carries oxygen from your lungs to your baby and your muscles. And oxygen is the ultimate energizer. Breathe deeply often and you'll notice a difference. Your baby will appreciate it, and you'll start to feel refocused and vitalized. A medium boiled artichoke has about 1 mg of iron (about 12 percent of your recommended daily intake).

There's another energizing nutrient in artichokes: folate. In fact, there's a whopping 100 mcg of folate in a medium-size artichoke. That's about an eighth of your daily folate needs. Folate helps your body metabolize proteins, which are the building blocks for the hormones and enzymes that help your body keep going and feeling energized.

Get Unstuck

Eating artichokes has another benefit as far as pregnancy problems are concerned. During your pregnancy, you may suffer from constipation, which can be alleviated with some extra fiber in your diet. Artichokes are wonderful sources of fiber, with 10 grams of fiber per artichoke (pregnant women need about 28 grams a day). Biting into an artichoke is a fiber-packed way to eat your way through constipation. And they're often recommended to soothe indigestion, another common pregnancy complaint.

There's More

Artichokes are one of the healthiest foods for you to eat during pregnancy because they're packed with nutrients you really need during pregnancy like iron, folate, and fiber. But they also contain niacin, magnesium, phosphorus, potassium, copper, vitamin C, vitamin K, and manganese.

FAST FACT

Artichokes may taste rich and buttery, but they're actually fat-free, with only 64 calories for a medium artichoke.

Jonny's Tasty Tips

I think of artichokes as the lobsters of the vegetable community—you have to really work to get at the good parts. The part that contains the meat is called the "heart," even though it's located at the bottom of the bud. And it takes some digging to get there. Is it worth it? Definitely!

So how do you cook this vegetable lobster? Simply trim the tops and stems and steam them for about half an hour. When they're tender, work your way to the heart by pulling off the outer leaves, which often have a bit of rich, fatty flesh at the very base. Stick the base in your mouth and scrape off the flesh with your teeth, tossing the rest of the tough, fibrous leaf on a saucer (you really need one for all the extra pieces), and then go on to the next leaf. Eventually, you'll work your way to the center of the artichoke, which is where the "choke" part comes in. Above the tender, delicious artichoke heart is a bunch of soft but prickly fluffy-looking stuff called the choke. It may look soft, but don't eat it! Scoop it off with a spoon and add it to that growing pile in your saucer, until you reach the flat part underneath. Now you've struck gold—the rich, creamy heart of the artichoke. Use your spoon to scoop it out and enjoy, tossing the very bottom of the bud on that overloaded saucer. Like eating lobster, eating an artichoke is not a dainty, polite process. But it's fun to get primal sometimes!

Want to up the flavor ante even more? Again, as with lobster, lemon juice brings out artichokes' rich, buttery flavor. So, for that matter, does butter. For a truly decadent delight, melt a little organic butter while your artichoke is steaming, stir in some freshly squeezed lemon juice, and dip each leaf base into the melted butter before putting it in your mouth. But remember how naturally rich artichokes taste and don't overdo it: Go heavy on the lemon juice and light on the butter or you'll lose those stomach-soothing benefits.

What about jarred and canned artichoke hearts and bases? They are no fuss, no muss, right? Right. But sometimes it seems there's a cloud to every silver lining, and this is no exception: Jarred artichokes usually come in oil—so much for their naturally low calorie count!—and while canned artichokes are almost always canned in water, they have a lot of added sodium. And too much sodium can lead to fluid retention (as in swollen ankles), another pregnancy complaint. Of course, you can always rinse those canned artichoke hearts before you eat them. And here's a little trick: If you use the oil-based jarred artichokes, enjoy them in a salad and use the oil as the salad dressing.

Carob

GOT PREGNANCY-INDUCED ACNE? GET carob. If you enjoy baking, then you probably already know about carob. Naturally sweet and made from the dried pods of the carob tree, it can be used instead of cocoa or sugar as a healthier alternative in many recipes.

Carob (also known as locust bean gum) is a great ingredient, rich in copper, riboflavin, calcium, potassium, and manganese. And it offers you a unique way to quiet your acne while satisfying your sweet tooth.

CAROB AT A GLANCE

Serving Size: 1 oz (28 g)	Calcium: 8%
Calories: 150	Vitamin A: 0%
Saturated Fat: 8 g	Vitamin C: 0%
Protein: 2 g	Iron: 2%
Fiber: 1 g	

Skip the Sugar

Acne can be aggravated by sugar. You may remember being told as a teenager that if you wanted clear skin, stop eating those chocolate bars. But it's not the chocolate in the bars that's the problem—it's the sugar. Eating sugar causes an inflammatory reaction in your body, and acne is inflammation based. By reducing the amount of white sugar in your diet, you can help reduce the severity of your pregnancy acne. Carob is a low-sugar alternative to chocolate. And you can feel good about eating it, because carob is a very healthy food. Ounce for ounce, it has more fiber and calcium than cocoa and fewer calories too.

Copper Fights Acne, Too

Carob is also offers your skin a good source of copper. Copper is a great addition to your acne-fighting diet, since it acts as an antioxidant in your skin, protecting it from damage and reducing the severity of acne's redness and puffiness. Copper also works like a natural UV protectant, preventing sunlight from causing damage that may further irritate your skin.

Cramping Your Style

Carob also contains indigestible fibers, which are extremely helpful to your intestines during pregnancy. High levels of progesterone produced during pregnancy cause your intestines to relax and slow, which can lead to constipation. Eating carob and other foods high in indigestible fibers is a great way to help your intestines keep moving and keep your colon from putting a cramp in your style.

Jonny's Tasty Tips

Carob looks chocolaty, and it has a rich, milk chocolate feel in your mouth. But don't expect it to taste like chocolate! If you were ever given a "chocolate" bar or cookie made from carob and were expecting that chocolate taste, you probably were disappointed. This time, think of it as a whole new flavoring—it actually tastes more like honey—and enjoy it for its own sake. Try it (again)—you'll like it!

You can enjoy carob in chip or powder form. If your recipe calls for chocolate or cocoa, you can replace it with the same amount of carob. You can also use carob chips instead of chocolate chips or just snack on them when your sweet tooth starts begging. You can even use carob as a sugar replacement. Carob powder is almost 50 percent natural sugar and can be used instead of sugar in virtually all bread and pastry products.

Flaxseed

FLAXSEEDS ARE ONE OF TODAY'S
most popular health foods because of their
unique nutritional content. Known for their
ability to reduce hot flashes during menopause,
flaxseeds are also packed with healthy compounds
that can help quiet pregnancy complaints.

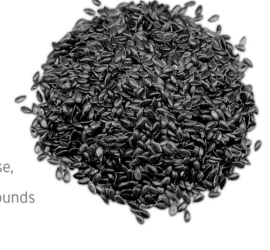

FLAXSEED AT A GLANCE

Serving Size: 1 tbsp (1 g)	Calcium: 0%
Calories: 37	Vitamin A: 2%
Saturated Fat: 0 g	Vitamin C: 0%
Protein: 1 g	Iron: 2%
Fiber: 2 g	

FAST FACT
Flaxseeds are also known to help alleviate
symptoms of PMS, making them a healthy
addition to your post-pregnancy diet too.

Fatty Seeds

Flaxseeds are best known for their healthy fat content.
Flaxseeds are a good source of the omega-3 fatty acid
alpha linoleic acid (ALA): There are over 3 grams of
omega-3 fatty acids in two tablespoons. This fatty acid
can be converted in your body into the essential fats
docosahexaenoic acid (DHA) and eicosapentaenoic
acid (EPA). These two essential fats are vital to your
baby's brain and eyes. The bad news is that the conversion of alpha-linolenic acid (ALA) to DHA and EPA
is very inefficient (some estimates say it's as low as
10%). The good news is that ALA is great for clear
skin. And flaxseeds are easy to find in any health
food store.

Clear Skin Solution

Quiet that acne with the help of omega-3 fats in flaxseed. According to Dr. Alan Logan, author of *The Clear
Skin Diet*, eating sufficient omega-3 fatty acids can
help fight acne. That's because omega-3 fats acts as
an antioxidant in the skin. Your pimples are red and
puffy, a sign of inflammation. Inflammation is a process that involves your white blood cells, which unfortunately produce free radicals that damage your skin.
ALA can reduce inflammation, inhibiting the production of free radicals by white blood cells and helping
your skin recover from acne faster. That's great news!
No one likes a pimple that sticks around longer than
it has to.

Pregnancy acne is caused by hormones that cause your skin to produce more oil; the oil clogs your pores, which forms pimples. So you can't "cure" pregnancy acne, since you need those hormones to stay pregnant. The best you can do is keep your skin clean and feed it with nutrients that will help it heal as fast as possible. Add flax to your diet and enjoy clearer skin sooner.

Flax for Fiber

Flaxseeds are a great source of fiber. There are 4 grams of fiber in just two tablespoons of milled flaxseed. That's an easy amount to add to your cereal or yogurt every morning! As you know, constipation is a common pregnancy complication. Eating foods like flaxseed that are a good source of fiber can help quiet this complaint.

More Energy, Stronger Muscles

All seeds, including flaxseeds, are great low-fat, vegetarian sources of protein. You'll find 1 gram of protein in each tablespoon of flaxseed you add to your diet. Protein is a great source of energy, which may help you feel less fatigued. Plus, protein is good for your muscles. Your back muscles are having the workout of a lifetime. Including protein in your diet will offer your muscles the amino acids they need to rebuild and repair, helping keep them strong.

Jonny's Tasty Tips

Wondering how to eat those little seeds? The best way is to grind them in a food processor or blender into flaxseed meal because most of the complaint-fighting nutrients are found inside the seed. (You can also buy pre-ground flaxseed meal at your health food store; look for it in the refrigerated section.) For added texture and crunch, I like to sprinkle organic flaxseed meal on cereal, veggies, or salads or stir it into yogurt, oatmeal, and smoothies. Just remember to keep flaxseeds and flaxseed meal in the fridge to prevent their healthy oils from going rancid.

FAST FACT

You may have pregnancy-induced acne and think that everybody's staring at that pimple. But adult acne is not just a pregnancy thing. According to a 2002 study in the *Archives of Dermatology,* in western populations of men and women older than 25, 40 percent to 54 percent have some degree of facial acne, and clinical facial acne persists into middle age in 12 percent of women and 3 percent of men. So there's no reason to feel self-conscious about your pimples: At least they'll soon be gone!

Kefir

SOMETIMES CALLED "DRINKABLE YOGURT,"
kefir is a traditionally fermented milk drink that has
similar benefits to yogurt. (See page 208 for more
on yogurt.) Kefir "grains" (the starter) are mixed with
milk, and healthy microbes grow, creating an enzyme-
and probiotic-rich drink. Kefir is a great food for your
digestive system and may help quiet your pregnancy-
related complaints like bloating, gas, and constipation.

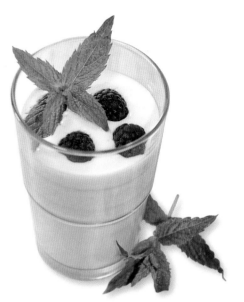

KEFIR AT A GLANCE

Serving Size: 100 g	Calcium: 0%
Calories: 48	Vitamin A: 0%
Saturated Fat: 0 g	Vitamin C: 0%
Protein: 6 g	Iron: 0%
Fiber: 1 g	

FAST FACT

Traditionally, kefir was made in skin bags that
were hung near a doorway. Anyone passing
through would knock the bag to keep the milk
and kefir grains well mixed. Today, there are
easier ways to make kefir at home, or you can
buy it ready to eat from the store.

Probiotics for Pregnancy

Your intestinal tract is host to trillions of microbes:
some good, some bad. The helpful ones are called
probiotics. Two main families of probiotics live in
your small and large intestine: *Lactobacilli* and
Bifidobacteria. Probiotics, especially *Bifidobacteria*,
can help with digestive problems like constipation,
a frequent complaint during pregnancy.

Scientists have found that as infants we have a
lot of *Bifidobacteria* in our colons, but as we age, their
numbers decrease. The result is an increasing problem of constipation in adults. A study in the *Journal
of Health, Nutrition and Aging* released in 2007 found
that in a study involving more than 200 elderly people,
eating food containing *Bifidobacteria*, like kefir, was
effective at normalizing bowel movements. Since you
may be suffering from constipation right now, put this
research to work for you.

As a pregnant woman, you also have high progesterone levels, which slow your digestive tract. In
addition, your growing uterus is telling your colon to

move over and make room for baby. Eating foods that contain probiotics can support a healthy digestive tract and may help keep you regular. Kefir also contains *Lactobacilli*, probiotics that are known to help reduce gas and bloating in your digestive tract, other common pregnancy complaints.

"B" Vitalized

Kefir contains valuable B vitamins. When you eat food, the carbohydrates, fats, and proteins need to be broken down so your body can use them to create energy. In order to break down your food and metabolize energy, you'll need B vitamins. Having lots of B vitamins in your body will ensure that you can make energy whenever you need it. But B vitamins are water soluble, so you can't store them in your body. That means you need to consume foods like kefir that contain B vitamins throughout your day to help keep your energy metabolism going.

Beat Lactose Problems

The beneficial yeast and bacteria in kefir actually consume most of the lactose (or milk sugar) in the milk used to produce it. So if you're lactose intolerant (a condition caused by insufficient amounts of the enzyme lactase in the body), you'll find kefir easy to digest. Plus, many probiotics can produce lactase in your digestive system, helping you break down any lactose in the foods you eat.

Jonny's Tasty Tips

Even if you've never tasted kefir, you may have enjoyed a mango lassi at an Indian restaurant. Lassis are delicious yogurt-based drinks that can be sweet or salty (with cumin and chile peppers instead of the fruit). If you've had one, you know how filling and refreshing they are. Kefir is too. Culturing kefir at home may be more than you want to take on right now, but if you buy your kefir at the grocery or health food store, follow my rule for all yogurt-like products: Get kefir with the fewest possible ingredients (plain is best—you can always add fruit at home) and make sure the label says that it contains live cultures.

FAST FACT

Probiotics only live in the body for a handful of days, which is why you need to eat them regularly to get their health benefits.

Kiwi

THOSE PRETTY GREEN SLICES ON THE FRUIT

plate look innocuous, but kiwis are actually
one of the healthiest foods on earth and one
of the tastiest foods to help you quiet your
pregnancy complaints. Did you know that kiwis
are an excellent source of vitamin C? In fact,
kiwis have more vitamin C in them than oranges.
One cup of tasty kiwi offers you about 275 percent
of your recommended daily needs of vitamin C (an orange has 200 percent).

KIWI AT A GLANCE

Serving Size: 1 medium fruit without skin (76 g)	Calcium: 3%
Calories: 46	Vitamin A: 1%
Saturated Fat: 0 g	Vitamin C: 110%
Protein: 1 g	Iron: 1%
Fiber: 2 g	

Skin Savvy

The vitamin C in kiwis can support your skin, offering it the building blocks it needs to build collagen, the molecule in your skin that allows it to stay strong and stretch into your new shape. Researchers have found that kiwi fruit can double collagen production in the skin. To a lesser degree, it can also stimulate fibroblast growth (fibroblasts are cells in the skin that produce collagen and elastin), all of which translates into stronger, more beautiful skin.

Here's another benefit: The healthier your skin is, the less it will itch. Itchy skin is a common complaint for pregnant women. It's caused by the stretching that happens when your skin has to stretch around your newly enlarged breasts and growing belly. Support your skin by eating foods that are skin-healthy, like kiwis, and you'll find you can quiet this itchy complaint.

Kiwis offer your skin yet another level of support. Polysaccharides in kiwi fruits have been found to stimulate skin cell growth by up to 30 percent. That means your skin can grow, repair, and stretch faster. So grab a kiwi and help your skin rejuvenate and stay beautiful.

Complaint Department Manager

Packed in these little green fruits are lots of nutrients to support your pregnancy. Kiwis are a good source of dietary fiber (3 grams per kiwi), vitamin E (1.3 mg per kiwi), and potassium (284 mg per kiwi). Eating lots of dietary fiber can help alleviate gas, bloating, and constipation, which are all common complaints during pregnancy. Vitamin E is a fat-soluble antioxidant which can help your body stay strong and energized. Potassium is helpful in regulating your water levels, helping to reduce your risk of accumulating too much fluid and causing your ankles to swell.

Jonny's Tasty Tips

Sliced kiwi is a refreshing, delicious, low-calorie snack. Add kiwi to your fruit salad, include it in a spinach salad, or eat it as a low-calorie dessert. For the best fruit, select kiwi fruit that are firm with no signs of decay. Here's the easiest way to eat a kiwi: Instead of peeling and slicing it, just cut it in half and spoon out the green flesh. (The little black seeds are completely edible, by the way.) I love to toss a kiwi, fuzzy skin and all, into my juicer with other fruits and veggies. The skin adds healthy enzymes (but not fuzziness) to the fresh juice. Yummy!

FAST FACT

Vitamin C is water-soluble, so your body can only store so much before it passes through your system. It's important to include foods like kiwis that are rich in vitamin C in your diet throughout the day.

Prune Juice

WHEN YOU THINK ABOUT PRUNE JUICE, YOU probably think of constipation. And that's why we've included this food as one of the healthiest choices to help quiet your pregnancy complaints. Constipation is a problem that many pregnant women suffer. Serve up a glass of prune juice and quiet this complaint.

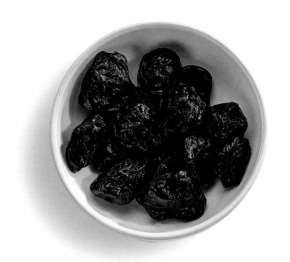

PRUNE JUICE AT A GLANCE

Serving Size: 1 cup (256 g)	Calcium: 3%
Calories: 182	Vitamin A: 0%
Saturated Fat: 0 g	Vitamin C: 15%
Protein: 2 g	Iron: 14%
Fiber: 3 g	

FAST FACT

What *are* prunes, anyway? They are nothing more than dried plums. Some plums dry better than others, and those are called prune plums. But if you see "dried plums" making their way onto your supermarket shelves, they're just a face-lift for that old standby, prunes. Buy them and their juice and enjoy!

Internal Plumber

Prunes are well known for their ability to clean out your internal pipes. Fiber is very helpful to your digestive tract, providing bulk and softening the stool to help keep it all moving. A glass of prune juice contains about 3 grams of fiber. During pregnancy, the high hormone levels that give you that tranquil feeling also affect your digestive tract. The food you eat will travel through your digestive tract a little more slowly during pregnancy, making fiber an even more important aspect of your diet.

Be sure to include lots of sources of fiber in your diet to help ensure that your digestive tract stays on track. A poorly moving digestive tract is prone to constipation, hemorrhoids, gas, and bloating. Plus, the longer food sits in your colon, the longer bad bacteria have a chance to flourish. Bad bacteria produce toxins that can be absorbed by your colon into your bloodstream. Get some fiber into your diet and keep things moving for a healthy gut and a healthy you.

Beware of Sugar

The downside: Prune juice also contains a startling amount of sugar. One glass of prune juice can contain up to 42 grams of sugar. Good as prune juice is for your digestion, you should limit consumption of simple sugars like this. If you eat foods that are high in simple sugars throughout the day, you'll cause your blood sugar levels to spike, which is hard on your body and may be linked to overweight babies at birth. So, if you find that prune juice is a helpful way to get some extra fiber into your diet, just be sure to drink it in moderation, like a cup a day, as opposed to switching it for your daily glasses of water!

Iron Mom

There's more to that glass of prune juice than fiber. In fact, prune juice is a great source of iron. As you drink down that glass of prune juice, you're offering your body 3 mg of much-needed iron. Many women suffer from anemia during pregnancy. Anemia is a condition in which the body doesn't have enough iron, causing the blood to have problems carrying oxygen efficiently. The result is fatigue. If you're suffering from a lack of energy, try increasing your iron intake by including foods like prune juice in your diet and eat your way through this pregnancy complaint.

So pour yourself a glass of prune juice and enjoy the fiber and iron it contains. Prune juice is also a source of vitamin B6, magnesium, and potassium. It's a healthy way to bypass fatigue, constipation, and other pregnancy-related digestive complaints.

Jonny's Tasty Tips

What's the first thing you think of when I say "prunes"? Half the people I know think of shuffleboard courts, retirement colonies, and their great-aunts sipping prune juice for "regularity." But these dried plums (an attempt to spin prunes to something more acceptable by changing their name) are a great pregnancy food. They're delicious, and they're one of the best and easiest ways to get more soluble fiber into your diet. Yes, you can drink a glass of prune juice every morning. But I also love the flavor of whole dried prunes and really enjoy snacking on them with almonds when I need a pick-me-up. If you've avoided prunes because of their "old folks" reputation, try some "dried plums" today. You and your body will love 'em!

Pumpkin seeds

MOST WESTERNIZED COUNTRIES DON'T have diets that are rich in seeds. Despite our need for quick, on-the-go foods, unless we're in the habit of snacking on sunflower seeds, this portable and delicious food doesn't make it onto our grocery list. But it should! Seeds are packed with vitamins, minerals, fiber, and protein. One of the best is pumpkin seeds.

PUMPKIN SEEDS AT A GLANCE

Serving Size: 1 oz (about ½ cup)	Calcium: 2%
Calories: 125	Vitamin A: 0%
Saturated Fat: 1 g	Vitamin C: 0%
Protein: 5 g	Iron: 4%
Fiber: 2 g	

North Americans may only roast and enjoy pumpkin seeds once a year, when we're carving a pumpkin for Halloween. But in the Southwest and South of the Border, roasted pumpkin seeds, aka pepitas, are a treasured treat. You'll want to start a pumpkin seed-eating tradition of your own once you discover that eating these delicious, nutritious seeds can help quiet some common pregnancy complaints.

Fuel-Efficient

Pumpkin seeds are a good source of magnesium: a half-cup contains more than 25 percent of your recommended daily intake. Magnesium helps speed up your ability to use carbohydrates, fats, and proteins as sources of energy. Food is your fuel, and magnesium helps you turn this food into energy your body's cells can use. So if you're feeling a little fatigued during your pregnancy, reach for a handful of magnesium-rich pumpkin seeds. Plus, pumpkin seeds are a great vegetarian source of iron, with about 2 mg of iron per cup of seeds. Dietary iron is also a great energy booster. You can definitely eat your way through the fatigue that's a frequent pregnancy complaint.

Repair Shop

It may seem strange to speak of healing in a book about pregnancy, but with all of the pulling, stretching, and other changes happening to your body, there is always a need for small repairs. One of the most important minerals involved in healing is zinc. Pumpkin seeds are an amazing source of zinc. In just 1 cup of pumpkin seeds, you'll find close to half your daily zinc needs.

Seeds for Muscle Strength

Part of the healing that occurs on a regular basis in your body during pregnancy is the repair of muscles. As your uterus grows, your back, abdominal, and hip muscles are required to carry an extra load and to stretch in new ways. Luckily, these muscles are very quick to adapt. With the help of protein in your diet, these muscles will be better armed to keep up with their new tasks. Protein is an important part of a pregnancy diet, but it needs to come from the right sources. High-fat sources of protein like hamburgers and fried chicken are not the best choices. Seeds, nuts, and beans are great sources of protein: They're low in bad fat and much higher in other nutrients like vitamins and minerals. Include foods like pumpkin seeds in your diet to help boost your intake of protein—there are 5 g of protein per half-cup of pumpkin seeds.

These tasty seeds also contain sodium, potassium, phosphorus, calcium, and many other minerals that are involved in muscle health and hydration. Buy a bag of roasted pepitas and enjoy eating your way out of pregnancy complaints.

Jonny's Tasty Tips

Usually, I'm all for eating foods in as close to their natural state as possible. But in the case of pumpkin seeds, research has shown that roasted seeds have far more protein, minerals, and fiber than raw seeds. They can also have lots more calories and salt. I'd suggest a happy medium: Buy pumpkin seeds raw and roast them at home. It's easy: Melt some organic butter or heat macadamia nut oil or olive oil and toss the pumpkin seeds in to coat. Spread the pumpkin seeds in a single layer on a baking sheet and season them with turmeric, garlic, or cayenne pepper, and then bake them till they're crisp. You can snack on these nutritious seeds as is or add them to trail mix, sautéed veggies, or salads, not to mention my favorite—oatmeal.

FAST FACT

During pregnancy, zinc deficiency has been linked to impaired cognitive function and motor activity in the infant.

Rainbow Trout

FISH IS ONE OF THE HEALTHIEST FOODS ON EARTH,
and it's definitely a great choice for pregnant women,
particularly if you'd like to quiet some of those pregnancy
complaints. Rainbow trout and other fish contain a type of
fat called omega-3 fatty acids.

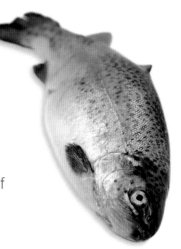

RAINBOW TROUT AT A GLANCE

Serving Size: 1 fillet (71 g)	Calcium: 6%
Calories: 120	Vitamin A: 4%
Saturated Fat: 1 g	Vitamin C: 4%
Protein: 17 g	Iron: 1%
Fiber: 0 g	

Omega-3 fats are associated with lower cancer risk
rates and improved heart and brain health, good reasons for all of us to eat them. Plus, omega-3s are great
for your skin and mood—two things that may be suffering during your pregnancy. In a fillet of rainbow trout,
there are about 900 mg of omega-3 fatty acids, of
which 300 mg is eicosapentaenoic acid (EPA) and
600 mg is docosahexaenoic acid (DHA).

Cleaning Up

Eating fish like rainbow trout may help you reduce the
acne you've been sporting during pregnancy. Omega-3
fatty acids are involved in your skin's health on several
levels. Eating good fats helps control the moisture
level in your skin: Too much moisture can lead to acne;
and aggravating as it is, too little moisture can lead to
irritation and acne. So a perfect moisture balance is
key to clear skin. Secondly, omega-3 fats are immunomodulatory, which means that they help regulate (or
even "boost") the immune system. Pimples start with
a reaction by your immune system to dirt, bacteria,
or oil that has become trapped in a skin pore. Then
inflammation enters the pore, forming that typical red
bump we call a pimple. The inflammation will clean
out the pore eventually, but the process can damage
the skin. Omega-3 fats can reduce the severity of the
inflammation, keeping your pimples to a minimum and
reducing the damage your skin has to endure.

Brain Food

In high school, tuna was touted as a brain food, causing many of us to grab a tuna fish sandwich in the hope that it might get us through the trigonometry final. The reason, it turns out, is that your brain fat is made up of mostly omega-3 fatty acids, the kind found in fish like tuna and rainbow trout. Research has shown that having higher levels of omega-3s in your diet has been linked to better cognitive function. These fats are "essential," which means that your body can't make them and you have to get them from food or supplements. If you don't eat fish, you probably aren't getting enough of them.

Mood Food

If pregnancy is causing mood swings, blame it on your hormones. During pregnancy, some women feel like they've gone crazy. Your feelings and mood can be uncontrollable at times, thanks to your raging hormone levels. And there are a lot of emotional changes going on: After all, you're about to be a mom! Thank goodness, omega-3 fatty acids are well known for their ability to improve your mood. So add some fish like rainbow trout to your diet during pregnancy and eat your way through mood-related pregnancy complaints.

Jonny's Tasty Tips

Grilled, baked, or poached—rainbow trout is one delicious fish. But you may be worrying about the safety of eating fish like trout because you've heard about the possibility of contaminants. It's true that fresh fish caught in contaminated rivers and lakes close to cities can have high levels of mercury, PCBs, and other contaminants that if eaten in huge amounts could be harmful to your baby's health. But here's the good news: The rainbow trout at your local market is required to meet government safety standard levels. Estimates show that you would need to eat more rainbow trout than any one person could ever eat in a week to get high enough levels of these contaminants in your blood. So relax and enjoy the delicious flavor and health benefits of trout without worrying about contaminants.

FAST FACT

Women with higher blood levels of omega-3 fats have a lower risk of developing postpartum depression.

★ Spinach

SPINACH IS THE STAR SALAD GREEN IN ANY BOWL.
Romaine and iceberg lettuce are no competition
for this nutritional heavyweight. Spinach has four
times more potassium, 18 times more vitamin A, and
20 times more vitamin K than iceberg lettuce. Adding
spinach to your diet will not only make you feel good
about the valuable nutrition you're offering your baby, it
can also help quiet some of your pregnancy complaints.

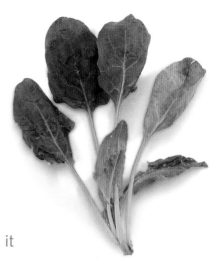

SPINACH AT A GLANCE

Serving Size: 1 cup (30 g) raw	Calcium: 3%
Calories: 7	Vitamin A: 50%
Saturated Fat: 0 g	Vitamin C: 12%
Protein: 1 g	Iron: 4%
Fiber: 1 g	

LOWERING BLOOD PRESSURE

Spinach contains a lot of vitamins and minerals
that support cardiovascular health. In a study
published in the *Journal of Agriculture and Food
Chemistry*, researchers found that four peptides
(protein components) in spinach inhibit angiotensin I-converting enzyme. This is the same
enzyme blocked by ACE inhibitor drugs, which
are used to lower blood pressure. High blood
pressure during pregnancy can lead to complications like preeclampsia, so eating heart-
healthy foods like spinach now is a smart idea
for your health and your baby's.

Popeye Was Right

Spinach contains 1 mg of iron per cup and about
60 mcg of folate, which is close to seven times more
than you'll find in iceberg lettuce. Iron and folate are
both key nutrients for helping you fight that fatigue
you've been complaining about. Iron will help you
carry more oxygen from your lungs to the cells in your
body that need it to make energy. And folate is needed
to help you get energy from the foods you're eating.
Switch to spinach and eat your way through fatigue.

A Better View

Hopefully, we've already convinced you that spinach can knock the socks off iceberg lettuce nutritionally, but here's even more evidence: It contains 44 times more lutein and zeaxanthin, These two antioxidants are vital to eye health and color perception, and your growing baby needs plenty of them right now as his eyes develop. Your baby may not have a lot to look at in your uterus, but healthy eating during pregnancy can help him one day enjoy the dark greens of ferns in the forest, the dark red of fresh tomatoes on the vine, and the clear blue of the ocean.

Jonny's Tasty Tips

To get the most from spinach, you need to eat it with fat. Yes, you read that right. The lutein that promotes good vision can't be absorbed unless fat is also present. I suggest that you enjoy your spinach steamed, sautéed, or fresh in spinach salad with a little olive oil and a topping of chopped hard-boiled eggs (another great source of lutein). One of my all-time favorite ways to eat spinach is to stir-fry it in some coconut oil. Even if you think you hate spinach, you'll find that it's absolutely delicious when cooked that way. And spinach is one of the lowest-calorie foods on the planet. You'd have to eat barrels of the stuff to equal the calories in even one small serving of french fries.

Whether you like your spinach by the barrel or the bowl, I recommend that you buy organic spinach. The Environmental Working Group put spinach on its 2003 list of twelve foods most contaminated by pesticides. Better safe than sorry!

FAST FACT

It's time to skip the iceberg lettuce and reach for more nutritious greens like spinach. Not only is spinach nutrient-dense, but some of those nutrients can help relieve your pregnancy complaints. Kale, collards, Swiss chard, and arugula are other healthy greens to add to your pregnancy diet.

Sun-Dried Tomatoes

THIS GOURMET FOOD SHOULD BE ONE OF your pregnancy pantry staples. Chopped up and added to a salad dressing, tossed into pasta, or in a starring role on a whole-wheat pizza, sun-dried tomatoes are a great addition to your diet. Beyond their delicious flavor, they contain many nutrients than may help relieve your pregnancy complaints.

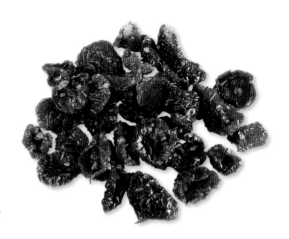

SUN-DRIED TOMATOES AT A GLANCE

Serving Size: 1 oz (28 g), about ½ cup	Calcium: 3%
Calories: 72	Vitamin A: 4%
Saturated Fat: 0 g	Vitamin C: 15%
Protein: 4 g	Iron: 12%
Fiber: 3 g	

Digestive Disturbance

Need a little push? Constipation coupled with a slow-moving digestive tract can be a problem during pregnancy. Luckily, the answer to this complaint is easy: Eat more fiber. Sun-dried tomatoes are a gourmet way to increase your fiber intake. A half-cup of sun-dried tomatoes contain about 3 g of fiber.

A Salty Solution

A half-cup of sun-dried tomatoes contains over 500 mg of sodium and 900 mg of potassium, two minerals that help your body maintain its fluid balance. When your body's fluids are properly balanced, your kidneys have an easier job and your bladder may find the demands on it are more manageable despite its pregnancy-cramped location. Plus, a proper fluid balance can help reduce swelling in your feet and ankles, a common pregnancy complaint. Craving something salty? You may just need more sodium, and in that case sun-dried tomatoes are a nutrient-packed way to get some extra sodium into your diet much better than that traditional salty snack, bag of potato chips. But whether you're eating chips or sun-dried tomatoes, you don't want to overdo it. Too much sodium can cause your body's fluid balance to falter. Half a cup of sun-dried tomatoes per serving is plenty.

Muscle Support

It may be hard to believe, but there is protein in sun-dried tomatoes. In fact, there are 4 g of protein in just a half-cup of these salty, delicious dried treats. Protein supports your muscles, which is especially important during pregnancy. Considering that your muscles are being asked to stretch and carry around an extra 25 to 40 pounds of weight, you may find that your muscles ache. Eat your way through this pregnancy complaint with the help of protein in healthy foods like sun-dried tomatoes.

"B" More Energetic

Is fatigue dragging you down? Eat your way to energy with the help of the iron and energizing B vitamins—thiamin, riboflavin, and niacin—found in every bite of sun-dried tomatoes. And there's more to this wrinkly food: Sun-dried tomatoes are a good source of magnesium, phosphorus, vitamin C, vitamin K, copper, and manganese.

Jonny's Tasty Tips

Sun-dried tomatoes are usually preserved in olive oil. That's really good news because oil promotes maximum absorption of the powerful carotenoid lycopene, and tomatoes are a super-rich source of this protective phytochemical. So enjoy your sun-dried tomatoes *and* their olive oil in your next salad, sauté, or sandwich.

Wheat Germ

EVER WONDER HOW THEY TURN THE GOLDEN brown wheat in the fields into that fluffy white bread we love to slather with jam, butter, or cheese? When wheat is processed, the bran and germ are removed, and what's left is used to make white flour and bread. But the germ is where you'll find the highest concentration of nutrients. Luckily, the nutritious part is packaged up and sold as those jars of wheat germ you see in the cereal aisle at the store.

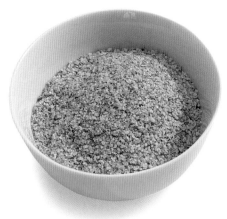

WHEAT GERM AT A GLANCE

Serving Size: 1 oz (about ¼ cup	Calcium: 1%
Calories: 100	Vitamin A: 0%
Saturated Fat: 0 g	Vitamin C: 0%
Protein: 6 g	Iron: 8%
Fiber: 4 g	

With just a little sprinkle, you can add some nourishment back into your diet. Not only is wheat germ a good source of fiber, it's a great source of B vitamins, iron, and other nutrients to support a healthy, complaint-free pregnancy. It may even help you eat your way out of that pregnancy fatigue.

Fighting Fatigue

There are fantastic amounts of iron in wheat germ (about 8 percent of your recommended daily intake in a quarter-cup). Iron is considered an energizing nutrient. It does not energize your body directly the way B vitamins work to help metabolize energy itself (worth noting that a quarter-cup of wheat germ contains over 20 percent of your daily needs of thiamin, vitamin B6, and folate, and about 10 percent of your riboflavin and niacin needs). Iron is needed to make hemoglobin, the compound in your red blood cells that carries oxygen from your lungs to the rest of your body. Oxygen is the ultimate energizer, and eating foods that contain iron can help you fight fatigue. Low levels of iron in your diet can lead to a type of anemia, a condition in which you feel fatigued because your red blood cell count is low. Grab some wheat germ and eat your way out of pregnancy fatigue.

Skin Stretching

When your skin's asked to stretch to accommodate your new shape, it needs some extra nutritional support. Wheat germ contains some great nutrients for your skin: vitamin E and protein. Vitamin E is an important antioxidant in the fatty part of your skin that can help keep the skin hydrated and free of irritation, like the itching pregnant women often experience as their skin stretches. A half-cup of wheat germ contains about half of your daily needs of vitamin E. With close to 6 g of protein in a quarter-cup of wheat germ, it's a great way to offer your skin some extra protein. Protein is needed to support the production of enzymes that help your skin grow and repair. Eat your way to healthier and happier skin with the help of wheat germ.

Jonny's Tasty Tips

I'll tell you right now, I'm not a huge fan of wheat. But I am a big fan of wheat germ. Wheat germ has a nice nutty flavor and a crunchy texture and is great in shakes or sprinkled on all kinds of things, from cereal and yogurt to veggies and salads. If you use flour in recipes, consider replacing ½ to a whole cup of it with wheat germ to increase both fiber and nutrients.

Wheat germ is a nutritional powerhouse, but because it's high in oil (good oil, but still oil), it can easily go rancid if it's not stored properly. A jar of vacuum-packed wheat germ is fine for up to a year, unopened, but opened jars should be refrigerated and used within a few months.

FAST FACT

Wheat germ is a great source of folic acid (folate), which is needed for your baby's healthy development and to prevent spina bifida.

Whole-Grain Pasta

IT'S TIME TO DITCH THE WHITE PASTA AND choose from the wide variety of whole-wheat and whole-grain pastas now available in markets around the world. Like white bread, white pasta has had the nutritious parts of the wheat grain stripped away, so it's a nutritional wimp! Pick up some whole-wheat pasta and eat your way through your pregnancy complaints like constipation, bloating, and gas.

WHOLE-GRAIN PASTA AT A GLANCE

Serving Size: 1 cup (140 g)	Calcium: 2%
Calories: 174	Vitamin A: 0%
Saturated Fat: 0 g	Vitamin C: 0%
Protein: 7 g	Iron: 7%
Fiber: 6 g	

Double Action

Whole-grain pasta is definitely richer in fiber than your traditional white pasta. Plus, it contains both soluble and insoluble fiber, and you need both to keep your digestive tract healthy. Soluble fiber forms a nice soft stool that is sponge-like. It can trap extra cholesterol and sugar to help keep your blood as healthy as possible. Plus, it keeps your visits to the bathroom running smoothly. This is also where insoluble fiber comes in. Insoluble fiber is not broken down by the digestive tract, so it helps push your food through the system, preventing backlogs. Working together, insoluble and soluble fiber can help you reduce the gas and bloating that are common complaints during pregnancy. And with enough fiber in your diet from sources like whole-grain pasta, you'll also find you can eat your way through any constipation problems.

Probiotic Boost

The fiber in whole-grain and whole-wheat pastas isn't just helpful in keeping your digestive system going—it can also help support your probiotic population, which keeps your digestive system running smoothly. Probiotics are the healthy microbes that live in your digestive tract. They live on certain fibers that your body can't use, called oligosaccharides. Feeding your good microbes will help you digest your food, can alleviate constipation, and will reduce the production of gas, which causes bloatingKeep your probiotics happy and ditch those digestive pregnancy complaints.

SKIPPING CARBS IS BAD FOR YOUR BABY

Low-carb diets are popular and one of us—Jonny—has written extensively about the many benefits to be had by lowering your intake of carbs (see "Living Low Carb"). But a very strict low-carb diet is not the way to go while you're pregnant. While we still feel strongly that sugar does you little or no good (during pregnancy or any time!), don't cut out valuable carbs like vegetables, beans, fruits, and moderate amounts of whole grains. A little pasta isn't going to kill you, especially if it makes you feel good and even more especially if you surround it with vegetables (pasta primavera), smother it in tomato sauce, and lose the Italian bread as an accompaniment. If a stricter low-carb diet works for you, there's no reason not to go back to it later on. But the Atkins Induction Phase isn't the way to go—at least not while you're pregnant or nursing!

Jonny's Tasty Tips

You've finally made the switch to pasta that's good for you, as opposed to white pasta that's full of soft, squishy empty calories. Now don't ruin it by pouring on gobs of gooey sauce! Enjoy your pasta with a spicy marinara sauce full of the good lycopenes in tomatoes and all the benefits of onions, garlic, and herbs. Or sauté some veggies in organic extra-virgin olive oil and use them to top your pasta, with a sprinkling of shredded Parmesan or Asiago if you like.

Another great way to go is to stir some pesto into the hot pasta just before serving. Or cook veggies like snow or snap peas, snap beans, or asparagus and toss lightly with organic butter, and then fold them into your pasta. How does a "sauce" of artichoke hearts, kalamata olives, and sun-dried tomatoes sound? Don't be afraid to experiment—anything goes, as long as it's good for you. And don't forget that big, veggie-rich salad on the side!

Feeling Full

Whole-wheat and whole-grain pastas are also filling. They help you feel full sooner, preventing the overeating that you may be prone to during your pregnancy. Plus, whole-grain pastas contain higher amounts of B vitamins, iron, and protein—other nutrients known to help quiet pregnancy complaints.

★ Yogurt

YOGURT IS BACK IN FASHION AND FOR good reason. Research suggests that it can help your body build healthy bones, muscles, and teeth, keep your skin beautiful, and improve your digestive-tract health. With acne, skin itchiness, leg cramps, constipation, gas, and bloating as common complaints during pregnancy, yogurt may be the ultimate pregnancy food, since it helps relieve all these complaints.

YOGURT AT A GLANCE

Serving Size: 1 cup (140 g)	Calcium: 42%
Calories: 174	Vitamin A: 0%
Saturated Fat: 0 g	Vitamin C: 0%
Protein: 7 g	Iron: 7%
Fiber: 6 g	

Bones, Muscles, and Teeth

You are in serious need of calcium these days. That baby is pulling calcium out of your bloodstream like crazy, leaving your muscles, teeth, and bones in short supply. So be sure to seek out lots of foods that contain calcium during your pregnancy. Yogurt is a great source of calcium, with close to 500 mg (about half your daily needs) in just 1 cup.

Cramped

The calcium in yogurt can help out with another pregnancy problem, too: muscle cramps. Experts think that a lack of calcium in your diet can lead to muscle cramps. Those tight, pulling sensations you get in your calves in the middle of the night are leg cramps. You may be able to prevent them by adding more calcium to your diet. Grab a cup of yogurt and dig in!

A Happy Digestive Tract

Being a fermented food, yogurt is a great source of probiotics, those healthy microbes that live in your digestive tract. A healthy digestive tract is host to trillions of probiotics that keep it moving, digesting, and free of gas and bloating. Ditch those digestive pregnancy complaints of gas, bloating, and constipation with the help of the probiotics in yogurt.

Beautiful Skin

Researchers believe that probiotics may improve overall health by helping to keep inflammation in check, thereby preventing inflammatory disorders from intensifying. While there is no proof that eating yogurt can reduce inflammation in the skin, probiotics are known to reduce inflammation in other parts of the body, including the intestinal tract and lungs. Since both acne and itching are problems in your skin that are related to inflammation, yogurt is a healthy food choice if you're fighting these pregnancy complaints.

Energized and Calm

Yogurt is a good source of riboflavin, with 1 cup providing you with 30 percent of your recommended daily value. This B vitamin helps protect cells from oxygen damage and supports cellular energy production. When you are deficient in riboflavin, inflammation can occur, causing irritation, itchiness, and damage. Eating yogurt may help prevent these pregnancy complaints.

BE A SMART YOGURT SHOPPER

To get the benefits of yogurt's probiotics, the yogurt you eat must contain live cultures. To determine whether the yogurt you buy contains living bacteria, check the labels for "active yogurt cultures," "living yogurt cultures," or "contains active cultures." Look for the LAC (Live and Active Cultures) seal in the United States. Don't be fooled by the words "made with active cultures." All yogurts are made with active cultures, but no live cultures survive heat treatments. Try to stick with yogurts that don't contain added sugar or artificial sweeteners since these additives can have toxic effects to your body. Better yet, go organic! Some new yogurts have added probiotics that may offer you even more relief from pregnancy discomforts.

Jonny's Tasty Tips

Not all yogurts are created equal. The best nutritional deal is plain yogurt, which has only two ingredients: live cultures and milk. The longer the ingredient list, the more calories you get and the less yogurt nutrition. In some highly sweetened containers of yogurt, you're getting more calories in the sweetener than you are in the yogurt. Be sure to read the protein and sugar values on the nutrition panel. The higher the protein and the lower the sugar content, the more actual yogurt you're getting in the container. Buying plain yogurt gives you the options of adding your own fruit, blending it into smoothies, making dips for veggies, or using it as a savory side dish like a raita (the most popular version of this Indian dish combines chopped cucumber, cumin seeds, and plain yogurt) to accompany spicy food.

One more thing: I'm not a fan of no-fat foods, including nonfat yogurt. Many vitamins and minerals—including calcium—are better absorbed with some fat. Yogurt with some fat in it fills you up and is much more satisfying than the no-fat kind and generally contains a lot less sugar to boot.

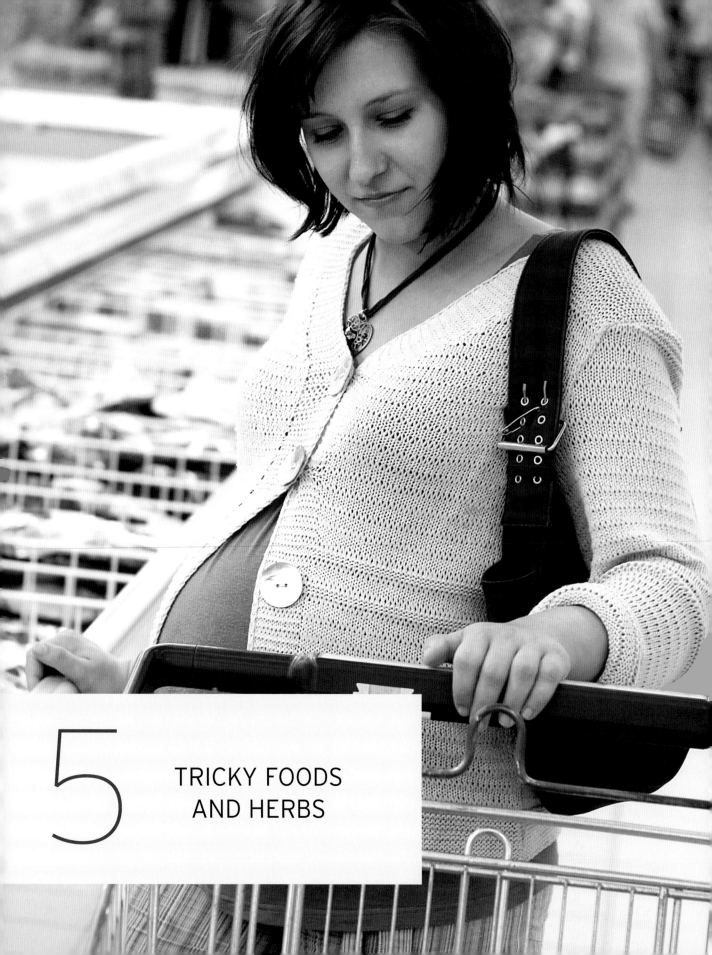

5

TRICKY FOODS
AND HERBS

WARNING: PREGNANT AND LACTATING
women should not eat this, drink that, or do anything. These days, everywhere you turn there are warnings for pregnant women. When you're pregnant, it can start to feel like you should live in a bubble, and even then, you can't eat or drink *anything*. It seems every food supposedly poses a risk to you and your baby's health. And then there are the warnings about drinks you should avoid, supplements you should fear, and pharmaceuticals that might harm you.

Is it all true? What are the real risks of eating and drinking during pregnancy? Let's help relieve the anxiety associated with choosing your next meal with some careful investigation of the facts behind some foods your might find tricky during pregnancy.

THE EARLY SCARES

One of the scariest things about pregnancy is that most women don't even know that they're pregnant until they're about four or five weeks in. In the first few weeks, your baby has already started to form some of his most important structures, like the spinal cord. In those few first weeks, you may have exposed yourself to any number of questionable foods, beverages, pills, and the like. That's why eating a healthy diet and taking folic acid supplements *before* conception is so important.

But this is no time to panic about the half-bottle of wine you and your girlfriend drank the other night when she came over to announce her engagement or the medicine you've been taking daily at your doctor's recommendation. Remind yourself that many generations of perfectly healthy babies made it into the world while their mothers were eating, drinking, and even smoking with abandon, as they didn't know any better.

Of course you want to give your baby the best possible care even before he or she is born! But instead of blaming yourself, arm yourself with informa-

tion: Look up the food, drink, etc., that's worrying you on a reliable health database, such as your local government's websites, the U.S. Department of Health and Human Services, or the Centers for Disease Control; or try some Canadian sites like Motherisk or Health Canada, or BabyCentre out of the United Kingdom, and talk with your obstetrician or midwife about any risks you and your baby may have been exposed to during those "I didn't know I was pregnant" weeks. Together you can monitor any potential problems as your baby develops.

Worries for That Baby Bump

Once you've reached your thirteenth week of pregnancy, your baby is officially into his second trimester and no longer in the embryonic stage. Now officially called a fetus, your baby is working hard to grow and perfect many of the systems he or she laid down in the first trimester (including his brain, heart, digestive system, etc.). During this period of pregnancy, your baby is at slightly less risk from contaminants. Plus, by this stage, you not only know you're pregnant, you're aware of the risks of exposure to nicotine, alcohol, and potentially harmful chemicals.

THE TRUTH ABOUT TERATOGENS

The bad news is that exposure to certain substances can cause problems in your baby's development. Such substances are called teratogenic. Teratogenic substances can disturb the growth and development of an embryo or fetus. Here's a list of some possible teratogens. Bear in mind that not all of these are proven teratogens, nor is this list complete, but it's a useful starting point.

Some Common Teratogenic Drugs, Substances, and Diseases

- Acetaldehyde
- ACE inhibitors
- Aflatoxin
- Aluminum chloride
- Alcohol
- Anticonvulsants
- Chlamydia
- Cigarette smoke
- Cocaine

- HIV
- Lithium
- Methadone
- PCBs
- Penicillin
- Pesticides
- Radioactivity
- Retinol
- Rubella

- Syphilis
- Tetracycline
- Thalidomide
- *Toxoplasma gondii* (causes toxoplasmosis)
- Tricyclic antidepressants
- Valium
- Warfarin
- X-rays

Now, wait: Before you close this book, completely terrified that anything you touch may cause harm to your baby, a few facts about teratogens will help put your potential exposure in perspective:

- A teratogen can cause an effect only after a certain level of exposure is reached.
- The effect of teratogens depends upon the timing of exposure.
- Although teratogens may increase the risk for birth defects, they do not necessarily cause problems in all cases.

So, yes, if you think you've been exposed to a teratogen while you were pregnant, by all means discuss it with your obstetrician or midwife. If you're a smoker, heavy drinker, recreational drug user, or live or work in an environment that's known for heavy metals or other toxic contaminants, it's especially important to inform yourself of the risks.

Now that we know more about health, it's important to do the best you can to give your baby a healthy start through sound lifestyle choices. So drop those bad habits the minute you realize you're pregnant and make an effort to give your baby (and yourself) a healthy nine months!

In the second trimester, you can relax and enjoy focusing on foods that will help fuel your pregnancy, promote your baby's healthy development, and pose the least risk to your baby's health. As your belly grows in your second trimester and you start to feel the baby moving, you'll probably react like most women and start to find your fears of contaminant exposure fading away as your desire to eat well takes center stage.

THE WARNING LIST

Focusing on foods may seem like an easy task, but unfortunately there are a lot of tricky foods during pregnancy. According to the American Pregnancy Association, pregnant women should avoid eating all of the following foods: raw meat, deli meat, fish with mercury, smoked seafood, raw shellfish, soft cheeses, unpasteurized milk, caffeine, alcohol, and unwashed vegetables. Most of the concerns about these foods are based on the potential for harmful bacteria in high quantities in these foods or their potential to contain contaminants like heavy metals, pesticides, and other harmful chemicals.

It's a pain to have to remember this list all day, every day. And the tricky part is that some of these foods aren't easy to identify—maybe you're not sure which cheeses are considered soft, and how can you tell which fish have mercury contamination?—while others are large groups of foods, some of which are actually good-for-you foods like fish and vegetables. It can be hard to keep it all straight.

There are many foods that we classify as tricky during pregnancy. Some of these foods are well-known no-nos for pregnant women, while others are surrounded by confusion. Let's dig a little deeper into some of the most tricky foods and beverages you'll encounter during your pregnancy and find the facts about which ones to avoid, why they might pose a risk, if it's safe to consume even a small amount of some of them, and if so, how much. Then we'll tackle the whole issue of herbal supplements, beginning on page 235.

Top Tricky Foods for Pregnancy

As you look at the list of risky foods for pregnancy, you'll see why they can be so confusing. We've already suggested that you eat fish, eggs, and cheese and that you drink herb teas in moderation and make sure you get plenty of water. Yet it looks like all these foods are on the no-no list too!

The keys are what kinds of food or drink you're having and when and how much. Eggs are fine. Raw eggs are not. Cheese is fine. Soft cheese is not. Peppermint tea is fine in moderation; nettle tea is not. Trout, salmon, tuna, herring, anchovies are fine in moderate portions. Mussels and scallops will have to wait till after delivery.

HERE ARE THE TOP 11 TRICKY FOODS DURING PREGNANCY:

- ALCOHOL
- ARTIFICIAL SWEETENERS
- CAFFEINE
- DELI MEATS
- HERB TEAS
- HOT DOGS
- RAW EGGS
- SEAFOOD
- SOFT CHEESES
- TRANS FATS
- WATER

Let's take a closer look at these foods and separate the good, the bad, and the ugly. (And if you just *have* to skip ahead to water on page 233 and see what could possibly be wrong with it, we don't blame you!)

ALCOHOL

People have been drinking alcohol since the dawn of civilization. (In fact, a popular current theory is that cities came about so people could cultivate grain to make beer rather than bread, as had been previously thought.) The damaging effects of alcohol on the unborn baby may have been known almost as long.

In Ancient Rome, couples were forbidden to drink alcoholic beverages on their wedding night to prevent conceiving a child with birth defects. And in 1736, the College of Physicians in London reported that drinking during pregnancy was "a cause of weak, feeble and distempered children."

But it wasn't until 1968 that a French physician reported distinct birth defects in a group of children born to alcoholic mothers. A few years later, an American physician, Dr. K. Jones, described a similar pattern of characteristics, which he named fetal alcohol syndrome (FAS). Today, FAS is still a leading known cause of significant cognitive deficits in children. Worldwide, it is estimated that one in every 1,000 babies is born with FAS. No wonder alcohol is not recommended for pregnant women!

Risk of Fetal Alcohol Syndrome

Fetal alcohol syndrome (FAS) occurs in babies born to women of every age and ethnicity. The risk of FAS and the severity of damage caused by it are related to how much alcohol is consumed during pregnancy and the stage of pregnancy in which the alcohol is consumed. Any beverage containing alcohol (beer, wine, or spirits) can put the baby at risk. When a mother drinks alcohol, it is absorbed into her bloodstream and then it crosses the placenta, easily entering the baby's blood. The alcohol then reaches vital organs such as the brain and heart. It is then eliminated, sent out of the baby and into the amniotic fluid, creating an alcoholic bath for the baby.

CHARACTERISTICS OF FETAL ALCOHOL SYNDROME

If you drink too much during pregnancy, here are some of the potential symptoms and complications your child may have to endure:

Brain Damage

- Small head size due to poor brain growth
- Behavioral problems
- Hyperactivity, learning disabilities
- Cognitive deficits

Poor Growth

- Decreased weight and length at birth
- Poor growth throughout life
- Possible heart defects

Abnormal Facial Features

- Narrow eye slits
- Short nose, turned upward
- Smooth, thin upper lip
- Small chin
- Cleft lip and/or cleft palate are possible

The concern for the baby's health goes beyond the effect alcohol can have on organ development—we're talking about the overall survival of the baby. A 2002 study at the University of Pittsburgh found that children of mothers who drank at least one drink a day during their first trimester weighed, on average, sixteen pounds less at the age of fourteen than those with no exposure to alcohol in the womb. Birth weight has been shown to be lower in babies born to women who have fifteen drinks or more each week during their pregnancy, according to the Royal College of Obstetricians and Gynecologists. A healthy birth weight is associated with better survival and overall health of a baby, making these effects of alcohol very scary.

Keep the Bar Closed

The damaging effects of alcohol are not limited to the crucial first three months of pregnancy when the baby's organs are being formed. Maternal alcohol consumption during the second and third trimesters can cause even more brain damage and behavioral problems. Children who were exposed to alcohol while in the womb are also known to be less effective at suckling and more likely to show disturbed sleep patterns.

There are worries that even fairly modest regular drinking can have effects on the baby that may not become apparent for several years after birth. One study in the United States found that children exposed to alcohol in the womb were more likely to display behavioral and conduct (reaction and response) disorders at the age of six than children from non-drinking mothers. Heavier drinking (consuming more than twenty drinks each week) has been associated with intellectual impairment, according to the Royal College of Obstetricians and Gynecologists. Childhood behavior could be influenced by any level of alcohol exposure, but the larger the "dose," the greater the risk becomes.

There is no safe amount or safe time to consume alcohol during pregnancy. The risks are simply not worth it. Switch your favorite alcoholic beverage for a healthy nonalcoholic option. If you love beer, caffeine-free ginger ale is available in glass bottles that are just like beer bottles. Alcohol-free sparkling grape and apple juice can be a fun substitute for wine. Or try a "mocktail," where you can enjoy the cranberry juice and orange juice combination used to make your favorite cocktail but skip the booze.

So why not just switch to nonalcoholic beer or wine instead? The best food and drink choices for you to make during pregnancy are ones that offer your baby nutritional benefits, and let's face it, nonalcoholic beer and wine are definitely *not* nutritional superstars. You'd be better off drinking milk, juice, or water. For something bubbly, try sparkling mineral water with a splash of juice in it. You can even top it with a slice of orange or an umbrella if you'd like a special treat.

Artificial Sweeteners

The name *artificial sweetener* already suggests that you'd be best off steering clear of this food. Artificial never means healthy. But skipping the artificial sweetener pack at the coffee shop is not enough to keep this bad food out of your diet. Artificial sweeteners are used in many everyday food products, including soft drinks, yogurt, desserts, fruit spreads, chewing gum, salad dressings, and candy. You'll need to start reading your food labels carefully to find if any of these are hiding in your favorite munchies.

There are many artificial sweeteners, including aspartame, cyclamates, sucralose, and saccharin. Some are considered safe for consumption during pregnancy, while others are not. The government considers the artificial sweetener aspartame safe for pregnant women but recommends that saccharin and cyclamates be avoided. Sucralose, a relatively new artificial sweetener on the market, does not currently carry a precautionary claim for pregnant women.

Now, here's the thing: The government says a lot of things are "safe," but many of us are not nearly as sanguine. The alternative and integrative medicine journals are filled with stories about "aspartame responders" who have very bad reactions to aspartame (Equal/NutraSweet), and neurologist Russell Blaylock, M.D., has gone so far as to call aspartame an *excitotoxin*, meaning it has the potential to harm brain cells. So our feeling is that the more you can avoid artificial chemical sweeteners—even the ones the government has declared "safe"—the better off you are. There are plenty of good sweeteners like xylitol (a sugar alcohol), erythritol (also a sugar alcohol), and stevia that have absolutely no health concerns.

All in all, we recommend that you skip the artificial sweeteners and foods that contain them. Instead, find more natural alternatives like sugar, turbinado sugar, maple syrup, cold-pressed organic honey, stevia, or the sugar alcohols (xylitol and erythritol). Now let's take a closer look at the most common types of artificial sweeteners.

ASPARTAME

Aspartame, sold in the United States as Equal and NutraSweet, is a chemical made in a laboratory. It isn't natural. In fact, it was accidentally discovered by a chemist doing lab work on an anti-ulcer drug. Two amino acids, phenylalanine and aspartic acid, are put together to make aspartame. It tastes sweet and therefore is used as an artificial sweetener in foods around the world. The acceptable daily intake (that is, the amount experts in North America feel is safe to consume each day) is 40 mg per kilogram of body weight per day (that's about 0.1 ounce per 100 pounds of body weight). For an average woman (weighing 60 kilograms, or just over 132 pounds) to consume that much aspartame, she would have to consume sixteen cans of a diet soft drink.

HOW SWEET IT IS

When compared to sucrose, found in everyday white sugar, some of these artificial sweeteners pack a serious punch. Cyclamates are 30 times sweeter than sucrose (sugar). Aspartame is 200 times sweeter, saccharin is 300 times sweeter, and sucralose is 600 times sweeter than sugar. But the real winner is neotame, an aspartame derivative that is 8,000 to 13,000 times sweeter than sugar!

Evidence *may* show that aspartame is safe for pregnant women, but that's only true if it's consumed in moderation. And aspartame is one of the most popular artificial sweeteners used in food products, making your daily consumption higher than you may think. It's a good idea for all people but particularly for pregnant women to avoid excessive consumption of food products that contain aspartame—and not just because of the artificial sweetener: After all, these foods are probably replacing nutrient-dense, energy-yielding foods.

Saccharin and Cyclamates

Many countries won't allow the artificial sweeteners saccharin and cyclamates to be added to foods. They are, however, commonly available in these countries in sugar-like packets as table-top sweeteners. (Cyclamates have been banned entirely in the United States since 1970, though this is currently under review; saccharin is still marketed as Sweet'N Low.)

Like aspartame, saccharin was inadvertently discovered by a chemist who was working on coal tar derivatives. Yum!

There are careful regulations about the labeling of these sweeteners. It is a good idea to carefully read any precautionary statements on all foods you consume, particularly since these sweeteners are not recommended for pregnant women.

Sucralose

Sucralose, marketed in the United States as Splenda, probably tastes more like sugar than the other available artificial sweeteners. It's even stable when heated, unlike the others, so you can bake with it and buy it bagged in bulk as a white or brown sugar substitute. Baked goods with no sugar calories? What's not to love?

Plenty—usually, all it takes is an explanation of what is in sucralose to turn someone off of it. Sucralose is made by combining a sugar and chlorine molecules. It tastes sweet and cannot be absorbed by the body, meaning it's calorie free. But you're still putting the same chemical you put in your swimming pool into your mouth! As with all artificial sweeteners, there is some debate as to whether or not sucralose can cause cancer; however, to date the science is not conclusive, and sucralose is considered safe by most governments for use in food products.

The Last Word

The bottom line: Just say no to artificial sweeteners. They don't offer you or your baby any nutritional benefit and are often in junk foods; so if you're eating them, you're cheating your body and baby of more nutritious foods. Plus, there is some debate as to the effect of these sweeteners on your appetite. Since they don't act like sugar in your body, your brain may not properly register that you've eaten, so you still feel hungry and may overeat. In other words, you may end up consuming more calories than you truly need and gaining weight. Recent research correlating diet soda consumption and weight gain showed that consuming artificially sweetened products was counterproductive. After all, we choose the artificially sweetened products because they're labeled "diet" or "calorie-free," and we assume they would promote weight loss, not weight gain.

As for the debate about the safety of artificial sweeteners, perhaps it's easiest if we take a step back and look at the bigger picture. A few decades ago, smoking was considered to pose little risk to health. Today we know how wrong we were, to the point that in some countries smoking in a car if children are present is illegal. We learn new things each day, and one day we may discover that artificial sweeteners are dangerous. In the end, the safest choice for all pregnant women to make about what they consume is to always reach for natural foods, the foods we've eaten for centuries.

Sweetening Agents

Many sweetening agents are also commonly found in products: isomalt, lactitol, maltitol, mannitol, sorbitol, thaumatin, and xylitol. These sweeteners (also called sugar alcohols) are naturally found in fruits and vegetables in small amounts. They cause a low glycemic response in the body, which means that they are slower to enter the bloodstream than sugar. This means that although they're not calorie free, they are slightly easier for your blood-sugar control system to deal with, and that's a healthy effect.

Sugar alcohols are definitely less sweet than white sugar (sucrose), which makes them a little less palatable and not likely to be found in a sugar-like packet at the local coffee shop. A true benefit of sugar alcohols is that they can't be broken down by bacteria in your mouth, making them a great choice for chewing gums, since they may prevent tooth decay. On the other hand, eating too much of these sweeteners can cause abdominal cramps and diarrhea. Sugar alcohols are thought to pose little risk to pregnant women, but often products that contain these ingredients are unhealthy food choices (aka junk foods that contain other "added" things like bad fat and preservatives).

High-Fructose Corn Syrup

While we're on the topic of sweeteners, it's impossible not to include the biggest offender of all: high-fructose corn syrup. Have you ever taken a moment to realize how many foods you eat that contain this troublesome additive? Most noticeably, you can find high-fructose corn syrup in many everyday foods like soda, candy, cookies, some crackers, cereals, and condiments.

High-fructose corn syrup has been the cornerstone of the food and beverage industry in North America since its large-scale production began in the late 1970s. High-fructose corn syrup is made from corn. After it's milled, the resulting starch is processed into a syrup. Added enzymes convert the syrup into fructose. Glucose syrup is then added to the mix to make high-fructose corn syrup. The most common form of the syrup contains 45 percent glucose and 55 percent fructose.

FAST FACT

Those pink, blue, and yellow "sugar" packets at the local coffee shop are packed with different artificial sweeteners. Cyclamate is what you'll find in SugarTwin. Saccharin is in Sweet'N Low. Aspartame is the ingredient in Equal and NutraSweet. And Splenda is made from sucralose.

What's the big deal? Well, research is suggesting that consuming high-fructose corn syrup may be linked to diseases like obesity and diabetes. In August 2007, at the American Chemical Society conference, U.S. researchers suggested that soft drinks containing high-fructose corn syrup may be linked to the development of diabetes, especially in children. Their study found that drinks sweetened with high-fructose corn syrup contained "astonishingly high" levels of reactive carbonyls (highly reactive compounds believed to cause tissue damage). People with diabetes tend to have elevated levels of reactive carbonyls in their blood. These harmful reactive carbonyls are not present in table sugar.

Your appetite may also be affected by this sugar alternative. Usually after eating, your appetite decreases, but according to some studies, appetite does not decrease as much after drinking fructose-sweetened beverages. There is also concern that drinking beverages containing high-fructose corn syrup may cause increased triglyceride levels in the blood, an indicator of risk for cardiovascular disease. Once again, it pays to read food and drink labels and skip the products that contain this questionable sweetener.

CAFFEINE

It's time to ditch that cup of joe. Concerns about the risks of caffeine consumption during pregnancy are growing, with new research showing that it may have negative effects on the pregnancy. The trickiest part about caffeine is that like artificial sweeteners it may be hiding in many food sources that you do not realize, including brownies, chocolate chips, chocolate pudding, coffee, espresso, hot chocolate, lattes, ice cream containing chocolate, soda, tea, and yerba mate. The amount of caffeine in food products will vary based on the serving size, product type, and preparation method. The chart on page 219 offers some insight into how much caffeine is in commonly consumed products.

Place Your Order

How much caffeine should you have in a day? On average, an adult in the United States consumes about 120 mg of caffeine a day, which is 3 cans of caffeinated soda or about 1.5 cups of coffee (and yes, many of your friends probably consume way more than this). Currently, government and health organizations suggest that pregnant and lactating women should restrict their daily caffeine intake to 300 mg, the equivalent of three coffee cups (not mugs) of coffee a day. But new research is suggesting that as little as 200 mg of caffeine—about two coffee cups or one mug of coffee—may be a better daily maximum for pregnant women.

Since caffeine is not an essential nutrient for your health and it commonly comes in foods that are not very healthy, it may be best to minimize or even eliminate caffeine from your diet during pregnancy. Plus, removing caffeine from your diet can help improve your sleeping patterns.

A Scientific Brawl

You'd think there would be one, single, clear-cut answer about caffeine intake during pregnancy. But there's not. The problem is that studies on caffeine and pregnancy are not producing consistent results. Some studies are suggesting that caffeine has no significant effect on miscarriage risk, while other studies have reported alarming results.

A study done in the United Kingdom first advised women to avoid caffeine during pregnancy. The study involved 474 pregnant women, who were questioned about their coffee, tea, and cola consumption before and during pregnancy. Women who consumed more than 300 mg of caffeine per day (about three cups of coffee) during pregnancy had double the risk of miscarriage compared to women who consumed less than 150 mg of caffeine per day.

Less Is Best

A more recent study suggests that 300 mg of caffeine per day is too much. In the January 2008 issue of the *American Journal of Obstetrics and Gynecology*, caffeine is shown to be a problem even at low levels. The study looked at 1,063 pregnant women in San Francisco from October 1996 through October 1998 who did not change their pattern of caffeine consumption during their pregnancy. They then looked to see how the women fared for the first twenty weeks of their pregnancies.

The researchers found that women who consumed 200 mg or more of caffeine per day had a miscarriage rate double that of women who consumed no caffeine. To put this into perspective, 200 mg of caffeine is about 1.5 cups of coffee or five cans of caffeinated cola. The most alarming conclusion of this study was that even low levels of caffeine may increase miscarriage risk in pregnant women. It's time to skip the caffeine.

It's the Caffeine, Not the Coffee

Let's be clear: We're not just talking about coffee here. In the *American Journal of Obstetrics and Gynecology* study, researchers found that it didn't matter what caffeinated beverage was consumed by the pregnant women. Once a woman consumed 200 mg of caffeine, the miscarriage rate increased. This helps confirm that it's caffeine that's the culprit, not a chemical in coffee.

CAFFEINE AMOUNTS IN COMMONLY CONSUMED FOODS

PRODUCT	Serving Size (oz)	(ml) (unless otherwise stated)	Milligrams of Caffeine (ml) (approximate value)
COFFEE			
Brewed	8	237 (1 cup)	135
Roasted and ground, percolated	8	237	118
Roasted and ground, filter drip	8	237	179
Roasted and ground, decaffeinated	8	237	3
Instant	8	237	76-106
Instant decaffeinated	8	237	5
TEA			
Average blend	8	237	43
Green	8	237	30
Instant	8	237	15
Leaf or bag	8	237	50
Decaffeinated tea	8	237	0
COLA BEVERAGES			
Cola beverage, regular	12	355 (1 can)	36-46
Cola beverage, diet	12	355	39-50
COCOA PRODUCTS			
Chocolate milk	8	237	8
1 envelope hot-cocoa mix	8	237	5
Candy, milk chocolate	1	28 g	7
Candy, sweet chocolate	1	28 g	19
Baking chocolate, unsweetened	1	28 g	25-58
Chocolate cake	2.8	80 g	6
Chocolate brownies	1.5	42 g	10
Chocolate mousse	3.2	90 g	15
Chocolate pudding	5.1	145 g	9

Values in table referenced from the following sources: Harland, B.F., 2000. "Caffeine and nutrition." *Nutrition* 16(7-8):522–526. Shils, et al., 1999. *Modern nutrition in health and disease*. 9th edition. Williams and Wilkins. Waverly Company, Baltimore.

DOES COFFEE STUNT GROWTH?

There's a fear that caffeine consumption has the potential to impair fetal growth (low birth weight and short gestation length). However, some studies have failed to find a clear-cut connection between the two. But enough studies have indicated a connection for you to be extremely cautious about caffeine intake during pregnancy. Just say no to that cuppa joe!

Decaffeinated Coffee, Tea, and Cola

Reaching for a product labeled "decaffeinated" may seem like a healthy alternative, but it's not. First, decaffeinated does not mean caffeine free. There is still caffeine in these products that when added to that chocolate bar or glass of chocolate milk can move your daily caffeine consumption into the high range without your noticing.

Second, the process of decaffeinating tea, coffee, and soda is questionable from a health perspective. The chemicals used may still be present in the drink and may pose some health risks. At a meeting of the American Heart Association in late 2007, a study was reported in which drinking decaffeinated coffee increased the levels of cholesterol and apoprotein B, both risk factors for heart disease, in the blood. In the study, three groups were compared: one group drank three to six cups of regular caffeinated coffee, a second consumed three to six cups of decaffeinated coffee, and the third drank no coffee.

Bottom Line

The evidence suggests that caffeine is one of those tricky foods that you should avoid during your pregnancy. Keep in mind that caffeine is found in all products made from coffee beans and cocoa (yes, this means chocolate), as well as tea and colas. So keep an eye out for "hidden" sources of caffeine in your diet, like that candy bar or chocolate chip cookie that's calling your name.

DELI MEATS

You may have to give up ordering your favorite Cold Cut Trio at the local sandwich shop during your pregnancy. Many health and government agencies are warning women about the dangers of eating deli meats. Deli meats are not the healthiest foods on earth anyway, since they contain sulfates and added fat. But it's not these ingredients that are an issue for pregnant women; it's the potential for something to be *on* that meat. And it's something you can't see: bacteria. Pregnant women, the elderly, and people with compromised health are all advised to avoid deli meats, because they may contain harmful bacteria that can cause serious illness like listeriosis and toxoplasmosis.

Little Buggers

No matter how sanitary your local sandwich shop or kitchen counter is, improper food handling or cross-contamination of food can occur at any stage of its processing. Strict regulations in most countries control the growth of bacteria in deli meat, but no system is perfect. In 2008, a major outbreak of listeriosis occurred in Canada when a major manufacturer of deli meats and other processed meats realized the bacteria was on some of its packaging equipment at higher levels than are considered safe. Many people became sick, some even dying.

Listeriosis is caused by the bacterium *Listeria monocytogenes*. Listeriosis is generally considered a rare disease, but it's obviously not that rare. And it's a very serious disease. Symptoms of listeriosis (nausea, vomiting, stomach cramps, diarrhea, fever) may be mistaken for stomach flu. Pregnant women and their unborn children are at particular risk. During the first three months of pregnancy, listeriosis may cause miscarriage, and later in pregnancy, it may cause acute illness or stillbirth. Early diagnosis and effective treatment are crucial to the survival of the infected fetus.

Heat Helps

Keeping your deli meat cold is not enough when it comes to listeriosis. Unlike other bacteria, *Listeria monocytogenes* can survive cold temperatures and sometimes grows on foods stored in the refrigerator. The best way to prevent exposure to this little bugger is either to avoid susceptible foods like deli meats or heat your deli meat if you can't bear to give it up.

Parasite Problems

Toxoplasmosis is caused by the parasite *Toxoplasma gondii*. Pregnant women can contract this disease by eating contaminated raw meat or handling used cat litter. Toxoplasmosis can cause few or mild symptoms in you, but can have severe results in a fetus. Usually, infection during the first two trimesters is less common, but if it happens, it can lead to severe effects, such as eye or brain damage. Most exposed infants are born without symptoms, yet are at risk of developing blindness or mental disability later in life. Infection in the third trimester is less of a concern, since most of the fetus's development has already occurred.

FAST FACT

The bad bacterium *Listeria monocytogenes* can be found in a variety of dairy products, leafy vegetables, fish, and meat products. Making sure your meat is properly cooked, choosing pasteurized dairy products, and carefully washing produce can help reduce contamination risk.

Early diagnosis and treatment of toxoplasmosis during pregnancy can reduce the severity of fetal infection. Your doctor can do a simple blood test to tell you if you have been infected. Symptoms could include mild flu-like symptoms (tender lymph nodes, muscle aches, etc.).

Since toxoplasmosis can harm your child, it's best to change your lifestyle habits so you don't come into contact with this parasite. Do not change your cat's litter (get your spouse or partner to do it or if that's not possible, wear disposable gloves and wash your hands afterward), cook your meat thoroughly, and wash your fruits and vegetables to remove any potentially contaminated soil. As for sushi, if you can't kick the craving, instead of eating the raw fish and putting yourself at risk of getting infected, choose vegetarian sushi.

Food Poisoning

The three bacteria commonly associated with food poisoning in the general population are *Salmonella*, *Campylobacter*, and *Escherichia coli* (E. coli). Luckily, the presence of these bacteria, as well as *Listeria* and the parasite *Toxoplasma gondii*, can be minimized with proper food handling techniques and safe food handling at home. Heating meats and other foods that might possibly be contaminated can also help reduce the risk of exposure. But during pregnancy, you should resist the temptation to eat deli meats and other prepared meats to reduce the risk of exposure to these nasty little buggers.

HERB TEAS (AND REAL TEA)

Perhaps one of the most confusing food-related concerns during pregnancy is tea. Herb teas are considered the safest of the teas since they usually don't contain caffeine, but even that is not a steadfast rule. Some so-called herb teas contain caffeine. It can be tricky to know which herb teas are safe and which aren't.

Next time you're standing in line at the local coffee shop, remind yourself that it's okay to ask what's in the tea you're thinking about ordering: They won't look at you like you've lost your marbles. You may be surprised what's in your tea bag. Some teas that sound herbal are really made with green or black tea, both of which contain caffeine. Others will contain some herbs you had no idea were in there, and those herbs may not be safe for pregnant women. It's a good practice to always read the ingredients of your herb tea, particularly if it's a combination of various plants.

The Safe List

It was a real challenge to come up with a "safe list" of herb teas. That's because every resource seems to contradict the others. Even teas that are renowned for helping pregnant women combat the side effects of pregnancy, like chamomile and red raspberry leaf, can end up on some people's unsafe lists. That's because some lists don't take into account the difference between drinking a cup or two of herb tea and gulping down capsules of concentrated, medicinal-level herbs. In moderation (2 or 3 cups a day), most herb teas are thought to be safe. These herb tea ingredients are most often found on the safe list: citrus peel, ginger, peppermint, lemon balm, orange peel, and rose hips. Red raspberry leaf, chamomile, and peppermint teas were discussed in our list of healthiest foods in chapters 1, 2, and 3. Let's look more closely at a few popular herb teas.

Red Raspberry Leaf Tea

Nicknamed the pregnancy tea, red raspberry leaf is a tea that's often recommended to pregnant women. It is rich in iron, a nutrient you and your baby desperately need during your pregnancy. Red raspberry leaf tea is also thought to help tone the uterus, increase milk production, decrease nausea, and ease labor pains. But some controversy exists as to whether red raspberry tea should be used throughout pregnancy or just in the second and third trimester due to its uterine effects. Today many health-care professionals suggest avoiding this tea in the first trimester until more information is gathered on its safety. For more on the benefits of red raspberry leaf tea, see page 165.

Peppermint Tea

Peppermint is well known to ease the stomach, and peppermint tea may help alleviate nausea in the first trimester. (Ginger is another tea that is wonderful for easing nausea.) Peppermint is also thought to help relieve flatulence, a problem common in pregnant women as their elevated levels of progesterone can slow digestive movement, allowing more gas to form. Peppermint tea is almost always caffeine-free, making it an excellent choice when you're at a restaurant and need an after-dinner alternative to coffee. Some mint teas are a combination of various mints, such as peppermint and spearmint, and these combo teas are also generally considered safe. For more on the benefits of peppermint tea, see page 164; for more on ginger tea, see page 49.

Chamomile Tea

Chamomile is a popular caffeine-free, relaxation tea. It is high in calcium and magnesium and can even help promote a feeling of sleepiness, which is great when you're tossing and turning with pregnancy-induced insomnia. Just drink it in moderation. One cup a day is considered safe, but we're still waiting on research studies to confirm there is no risk if you drink multiple cups a day.

"Maybe" Teas

A number of herb teas have less clear-cut data for safe use during pregnancy. Dandelion tea is rich in vitamin A, calcium, and iron, and it's nourishing to the liver. But the safety information available on drinking dandelion tea during pregnancy is considered insufficient, so dandelion tea is on the maybe list.

Rose hips are also on the maybe list. They are a common ingredient in many combination herb teas. They're a very good source of vitamin C. But while some resources say rose hips are okay, others recommend avoiding them during pregnancy. If you enjoy rose hip tea or jam, discuss their safety with your obstetrician or midwife before drinking another cup or spreading that jam on your biscuit or English muffin. If they give you the go-ahead, we say go ahead!

Different sources place these teas on either side of the safe and not-safe line. It's smart to speak with your obstetrician or midwife about any herb tea you'd like to drink during pregnancy. And if you have favorites that you drink already, again, please check the labels! Some blends contain as many as a dozen herbs. Better safe than sorry.

The No List

We hope we don't have to tell you not to drink any "diet" teas or detox teas while you're pregnant. Not only do these teas cause diarrhea and other dehydrating effects, pregnancy is *not* the time to focus on dieting or detoxing! But some herb teas seem harmless or are even recommended for pregnancy, and yet we've put them here as nos. Nettle, alfalfa, and yellow dock are three herb teas you will find on most no lists. These teas have raised some concerns, because there's no proof of their safety for consumption by pregnant women.

Nettle is used in many pregnancy teas, as it is thought to be a good all-around pregnancy tonic. It is even recommended by many midwives and herbalists. The concern is about which part of the nettle plant is used, the root or the leaves, and how much is used. If you want to try nettle leaf tea, be sure to talk to your obstetrician or midwife before buying or drinking it to ensure that the product you are using is safe for you.

Alfalfa tea may be good later in pregnancy and is thought to help prevent postpartum hemorrhage. But alfalfa is also commonly placed on no lists because of concerns about its safety when used in high dosages.

As for yellow dock tea, it is thought to help treat anemia in pregnant women due to its high levels of iron but is also considered a laxative. Therefore, it's also placed on many no lists for pregnant women.

Black, White, and Green

What about "real" tea made from leaves of the tea plant *Camellia sinensis*? Most of the world's tea is black, white, or green tea, all made from the leaves (and sometimes buds) of this small shrub. (The difference is how the leaves and/or buds are treated before drying; for example, black tea leaves are fermented, but green tea leaves aren't.) All of these teas contain caffeine, a compound that we know is best avoided during pregnancy. So before you reach for a cup, be sure you know if you're drinking caffeine-free herb tea or caffeinated black, white, or green tea. And remember that just because a tea is labeled decaffeinated does not mean it's caffeine free.

Safety First!

All in all, women are advised by most health and government agencies to use herb teas cautiously and to critically examine any information about their proposed benefits. Discuss them with your obstetrician or midwife for some additional direction. And remember: If you're still not sure about which tea is safe, you can always order hot water with lemon, or many coffee shops will gladly steam you up some frothy milk, which tastes great with a touch of honey or a sprinkle of cinnamon.

HOT DOGS

Processed meats like hot dogs are a tricky food during pregnancy. For many women, processed meats are an easy way to get protein into their diet while on the run during the day. However, processed meats can contain bacteria, like the ones that cause listeriosis, and parasites that can harm your baby, as we saw in the section on deli meats beginning on page 222. Food-borne illnesses like listeriosis can lead to miscarriage, premature delivery, fetal infection, and even fetal death. Properly heating hot dogs (to 160 °F, 60 °C) can help reduce the risk of contamination. But there are also other reasons to ditch that 'dog.

Ballpark Frank

Hot dogs are almost as American as apple pie. According to the National Hot Dog and Sausage Council, U.S. consumers buy about 1.5 million pounds of hot dogs per year. They note that during "hot dog season," Memorial Day to Labor Day, Americans typically consume 7 *billion* hot dogs. But hot dogs are definitely not healthy food. They are very high in saturated fat and sodium. Up to 80 percent of some hot dogs' calories come from fat, which is well over what is considered a healthy amount. Your diet should never exceed intakes of saturated fat greater than

10 percent. Salt and fat are linked to an increased risk of heart disease. Plus, hot dogs contain nitrates (a preservative) and color enhancers, both of which are unhealthy for you or your baby. In fact, nitrate-related substances have been reported to cause cancer in animals.

What's in There?

Despite common hype, hot dogs typically contain muscle meat trimmings from pork or beef. They typically do *not* contain animal eyeballs, hooves, or genitals, according to the National Hot Dog and Sausage Council. But it's worth noting that the U.S. government does allow them to contain pig snouts and stomachs, cow lips and livers, goat gullets, and lamb spleens. If a hot dog contains these by-products, the manufacturer is supposed to list them on their label.

RAW EGGS

You're probably thinking, who would eat raw eggs? Well, raw eggs themselves may not be a main dish in your repertoire of dinner meals, but you may be eating them and not realizing it. Do you eat soft-boiled eggs or Caesar salad? How about mayonnaise or eggnog? Raw eggs are sometimes hiding in foods, making them a tricky food during pregnancy.

To be safe, avoid soft-boiled eggs and foods that may contain raw eggs, including mayonnaise, homemade ice cream or custard, Hollandaise sauce, eggnog, mousses, and Caesar dressings. By avoiding these foods, you can help reduce your exposure to salmonella—and if you've ever had salmonella poisoning, you'll agree that it's worth every effort to avoid it.

LISTERIOSIS: THE REAL RISK

According to the Centers for Disease Control and Prevention (CDC), an estimated 2,500 persons become seriously ill each year in the United States with listeriosis. Pregnant women account for 27 percent of these cases. The CDC claims that pregnant women are 20 times more likely to become infected than healthy, nonpregnant adults. The risk may be small, but you owe it to your baby to try to eliminate any foods from your diet that might result in his death. Surely you can bring yourself to give up hot dogs, deli meats, and raw meat for nine months!

THE LONG-TERM RISK

Eating hot dogs and deli meats could potentially have a long-term impact on your health as well. In November 2007, the World Cancer Research Fund reported the results of a five-year project that looked at more than 7,000 clinical studies on diet and cancer. They concluded that eating processed meats (like deli meats and hot dogs) on a regular basis can significantly increase the risk of colon cancer. Eating 50 g (one hot dog, or about the amount of cold cuts on half a sub) a day of processed meats for several years increases colorectal cancer risk by 21 percent. The results were part of the 2007 *Food, Nutrition, Physical Activity and the Prevention of Cancer: a Global Perspective*.

Salmonella is a bacterium that lives on food. Eating food contaminated with salmonella can cause you to feel flu-like symptoms: stomach cramps, nausea, vomiting, diarrhea, and fever. Symptoms usually appear about 12 to 72 hours after exposure and can last up to 7 days. Those groups at a higher risk, such as pregnant women, the elderly, and immunosuppressed people (such as people with HIV or AIDS), can have more severe complications.

Fighting Back

The best defense is to avoid foods with a high risk of salmonella contamination. Next, make sure the food you're eating has been properly cooked. Like many other harmful bacteria that can be found on food, salmonella can be destroyed when the food is cooked to a safe internal temperature. Use a meat thermometer to make sure meat gets hot enough in the center to kill salmonella: that's 140 °F (60 °C) for beef and fish, 165 °F (74 °C) for chicken, and 160 °F (71 °C) for pork. Obviously, you're not going to use a thermometer to measure the temperature of your breakfast eggs. But while you're pregnant, make sure your hard-boiled eggs are cooked completely through, your scrambled eggs are set (not runny), and your fried eggs are "fried hard," not sunny side up.

SEAFOOD

Seafood can be a great source of protein and iron, and the omega-3 fatty acids in many fish can help promote your baby's brain development. In fact, a British study suggests that skimping on seafood during pregnancy may contribute to poor verbal skills, behavioral problems, and other developmental issues during childhood. However, some fish and shellfish contain mercury, PCBs, and other contaminants, which is why seafood is on our list of tricky foods during pregnancy. Do the risks outweigh the benefits? Let's find out.

Mercury

Many women are worried about eating fish because it may contain mercury. Too much mercury may damage your baby's developing nervous system. But here's the good news: It's almost impossible for you to eat too much mercury if you're eating a healthy, balanced diet. Even the Food and Drug Administration (FDA) of the United States says that pregnant women can safely eat two meals of canned tuna a week (and tuna is rumored to be mercury-containing fish). Plus, the benefits of the good fats, called omega-3 fatty acids, in fish far outweigh the risks of including this food in your diet.

If you're still worried, here are a few ways to reduce your concerns about your mercury intake. First, avoid bigger and older fish, since they tend to have more mercury in them. Swordfish, shark, king mackerel, and tilefish are big fish that have longer life spans, so avoid them during pregnancy. Instead, choose salmon, canned tuna, pollock, shrimp, and catfish, which are all on the FDA list of acceptable fish for pregnant women to eat. But of this list, only the salmon and tuna are good sources of the important omega-3 fats your baby needs for proper brain and eye development. (Both salmon and tuna have made our list of 100 healthiest foods for pregnancy; read more about them on pages 135 and 118.)

Sushi

Sushi is a great way to get fish into your diet, but not when you're pregnant. Raw fish can contain harmful bacteria, parasites, and/or viruses. Pregnant women are advised to avoid eating sushi and any other raw fish. Refrigerated smoked seafood is also off-limits, unless it has been heated (for example, if it's cooked in a casserole or other dish). Canned or shelf-stable smoked seafood is thought to be a lower-risk smoked-fish food, if you're really craving it. And if you can't shake that craving for sushi, try ordering vegetarian sushi, which will calm your craving without putting you at risk of infection.

Raw Shellfish

As with most animal products, eating raw shellfish is not a good idea during pregnancy, because it may be contaminated with bacteria that can make you and your baby sick. The majority of seafood-borne illness is caused by undercooked shellfish (oysters, clams, and mussels). Cooking shellfish is a great way to prevent infection. But cooking won't prevent algae-related infections that are associated with red tides.

Purchase your seafood from a reputable vendor. Ask about red tides if you are buying shellfish and never eat them if they don't open during cooking. Most important, if your seafood smells really fishy, that probably means it isn't fresh. Err on the side of safety and throw it out!

The Best Fish

The best way to eat fish is fresh. When you're buying fresh fish, look for fish that are free of brown spots and don't have a shiny film. Fish should be cooked to an internal temperature of 140 °F (60 °C). When the fish separates into flakes, it's done. If you're cooking salmon, watch for drops of white fat to start gathering on the top to let you know it's done. Salmon is one

HIDDEN TROUBLE

Raw eggs aren't the only foods that may be contaminated with salmonella. Salmonella is usually found on foods that have not been handled properly during preparation. Here is list of foods that have been blamed for salmonella poisoning:

- Raw and undercooked meat, especially poultry
- Sprouts and cantaloupes
- Raw or undercooked eggs
- Unpasteurized dairy products, like raw milk and raw milk cheeses, cream-filled desserts, and creamy toppings
- Pet treats (we know you wouldn't eat these, but you might handle them)
- Fish and shrimp
- Sauces and salad dressings

FAST FACT

Cheese really is one of the trickiest foods for pregnancy. Remember that dairy products such as milk, mozzarella cheese, and cottage cheese can be a healthy part of your pregnancy diet. But it's best to avoid any cheese that could be contaminated with harmful bacteria or milk that is unpasteurized.

of the healthiest fish for you, since it contains high amounts of the omega-3 fatty acids required by your body and your baby. Tuna, mackerel, sardines, and anchovies are also great sources of these fats, and some of these are small fish, which means they will have lower levels of mercury. (For more on sardines and anchovies, which are also on our list of 100 healthiest foods, see pages 281 and 33.)

SOFT CHEESES

Cheese is one of the healthiest foods for your pregnancy. So why are some cheeses on the tricky list? Because some cheeses can host harmful bacteria, including listeria, that can make you and your baby sick. Listeria, as we've seen, can lead to miscarriage, premature delivery, fetal infection, and even fetal death. That's not something you want to mess around with!

Avoid Cheeses Made with Unpasteurized Milk

According to the Mayo Clinic, any food containing unpasteurized milk is a big no-no during pregnancy. So read your cheese label carefully and make sure the label indicates that it was made with pasteurized milk to reduce your risk of exposure to food-borne illnesses like listeriosis. Cheeses to watch for include Brie, Camembert, blue cheese, and Mexican-style cheeses like queso blanco, queso fresco, queso de hoja, queso de crema, and queso asadero.

Skip the Mold

It is recommended that pregnant women also avoid cheeses that are soft-mold-ripened (including Brie, chèvre, and Camembert) or blue-veined (such as Danish blue, gorgonzola, and Stilton). These cheeses are more moist and less acidic than other cheeses, which creates a perfect environment for bacteria to grow. But again, thorough cooking should kill any listeria or other bacteria that may be living in the cheese.

Safe Cheeses

For cheese lovers who are starting to worry they'll be spending nine months deprived of their favorite food, let's take a moment to point out some cheeses that you *should* indulge in. Cheese is actually a very healthy pregnancy food—you just need to make sure you're eating the right ones. Hard cheeses like Babybel, Cheddar, Austrian smoked, Double Gloucester, Emmental, feta, Gouda, Havarti, Orkney, Parmesan, Swiss, and provolone are safe and delicious, so dig in!

There are even some soft cheeses that are safe to eat during pregnancy, including cottage cheese, cream cheese, boursin, mascarpone, mozzarella, and ricotta. Several of these have made the list of the 100 healthiest foods. Read more about Cheddar on page 182, Swiss on page 171, and cream cheese on page 46.

TRANS FATS

Trans fats are the big, bad, and ugly of bad fats. Over the last few years the health impacts of these fats have hit home, and people of all ages and health conditions are being advised to steer clear of trans fats. So of course trans fats made our list of tricky foods for pregnancy. Even though you know they're not healthy, you may still be eating them. That's because they are hiding in all sorts of foods—more than you may have imagined.

Where They Came From

When saturated fat was labeled as a cause of heart disease a few decades ago, food manufacturers worked to find another solution to improve the shelf life of their products. By hydrogenating plant oils, a process in which the oil is made more stable and less likely to go rancid, they were able to increase the shelf life of the products. This is why those crackers last a few months on your shelf. Plus, the process made liquid oils into a semisolid state, offering manufacturers new opportunities to improve packaged food texture. Puddings and margarines are great examples of the semisolid state that hydrogenating fats can help create.

However, the process of hydrogenation has its downside. First, it reduces the amount of good fat in the product (monounsaturated and polyunsaturated fat). But worse, hydrogenating fats can cause trans fats to form. Trans fats also exist naturally in small amounts in some foods. These bad fats can sit around in your blood vessels and organs (liver, heart, and kidneys) and promote problems, including heart disease.

The Problem with Trans Fats

In their efforts to improve the fat content of our foods without affecting shelf life, food manufacturers created a new problem. Consuming too much trans fat raises the level of bad cholesterol in the blood, a risk factor for heart disease. In the Harvard Nurses' Health Study,

involving over 80,000 women, those women who consumed the most trans fats were 50 percent more likely to develop heart disease and were almost 40 percent more likely to develop type 2 diabetes.

Way Too Much

We all eat too much trans fat. Statistics from Canada show that the consumption of trans fats has increased 40 percent over the past decade. Meanwhile, the World Health Organization recommends that a person's daily intake of trans fats should not exceed 1 percent of their total daily energy (caloric) intake, and that's being conservative. In July 2002, the National Academy of Sciences released a report concluding that the only safe intake of trans fat from the diet is zero.

Part of the problem is that trans fats are hiding in all sorts of foods. Any food product that is deep-fried will contain trans fats, including doughnuts, fries, potato chips, corn chips, and chicken fingers. But they also lurk in foods you may not have thought of, like margarine, hot chocolate mix, microwave popcorn, infant foods, instant cake mixes, crackers, and cookies. Yikes!

Luckily, many countries around the world have required trans fats to be listed on the Nutrition Facts panel of foods. Plus, many fast food outlets and food manufacturers have taken steps to lower their use of hydrogenated fats and replace them with nonhydrogenated fats. In the meantime, fresh and natural is always best when making a food choice. Fresh foods are less likely to have trans fats, while almost all processed foods do.

Get the Good Fats

Thank goodness, not all fats are bad, since we all need to eat fat to survive. Fat in your diet allows the body to absorb fat-soluble vitamins such as vitamins A, D, and E. Good fats, like the monounsaturated fats that you'll find in olive oil and foods like avocados, nuts, and seeds, promote your health and your baby's. Another group of healthy fats, called polyunsaturated fats, are essential for healthy skin and hair and promote proper brain and eye development. Polyunsaturated fats are found in good quantities in flax, hemp, and fish, and in smaller amounts in most oily plants. As for saturated fats, don't exclude them from your good fat list—remember there are good saturated fats in lots of foods, including coconut oil and nuts.

Feeling Fat?

If you're worried about the amount of fat accumulating on your body during pregnancy, it's time to trust your body. Your body has taken stock of your fat stores and already made a decision if you are fat enough. If you're putting on some extra fat around your midsection, than your body decided you don't have enough fat to carry this baby to term and to breast-feed.

HIDE AND SEEK

How much trans fat are you eating? Check your food labels carefully to see if you're eating trans fats. But even if the label says there's no trans fat, it may not be telling the whole story. Many countries have regulations that allow a Nutrition Facts panel to say zero trans fats, even if there are some in there—it's a rounding rule that makes this one tricky food.

How do you know how to avoid trans fats? Simple. Read the ingredients. If the ingredients contain "partially hydrogenated" or "hydrogenated" oil of any kind, put the product down and step away from the grocery shelf! And unfortunately, you can't always trust the "no trans fats" sticker—government regulations contain a loophole that allows manufacturers to say "no trans fats" if there is less than a half-gram of trans fats per serving. By making the "serving size" unrealistically small, some manufacturers are able to get away with the "no trans fats" sticker. But eat a realistic serving of some of these foods, and it's pretty easy to consume a couple of grams of trans fats. The only sure way to tell is to read those ingredients lists. Remember: If it contains partially hydrogenated or hydrogenated oil of any kind, it's got trans fats, no matter what the sticker claims!

So watch out for packaged foods that normally contain trans fats, even if the package labeling claims they're trans-fat free. Remember that the World Health Organization recommends that we keep our trans fat consumption to less than 1 percent of our daily caloric intake. But those few handfuls of supposedly "trans fat-free" crackers may contain a hidden 5 g of trans fats—that's 40 calories, or 2 percent of your daily calorie intake, and that's just one snack!

If you can't trust the label, what should you do? The best way to ensure that your trans fat intake is low is to avoid foods that have trans fats in them, such as crackers, cookies, chips, and margarine. These foods aren't healthy anyway, and especially not when you're pregnant. So ditch the trans fats for your health and your baby's.

Eating less is a bad idea for your baby. Working out too hard is also a bad idea for your baby, since lifting heavy weights or getting your heart rate above 140 to 160 beats per minute (depending on your age and cardiovascular health) can reduce the amount of oxygen available to your baby. You can't even try to avoid eating fat. Your body can make fat out of anything you eat. Your only defense is to eat a variety of healthy foods and stay active; your body will be back to its prepregnancy appearance soon enough.

WATER

Most of us don't give water much thought. You turn on the tap and water flows out. However, water is one of the most important nutrients for your pregnancy. Your increased needs require you to drink more water. The purity of that water can affect your health and the health of your baby.

Safe Tap Water

In North America, Europe, and many other places around the world, municipal water is carefully regulated and controlled to ensure that it's clean and safe for drinking. It's a real luxury to just be able to turn on the tap and have safe, clean water to drink.

Getting the Lead Out

Heavy metals occur naturally all over the world. Rock formations leach naturally occurring substances like arsenic, cadmium, iron, manganese, and uranium into our water. Pipes and holding tanks can leach copper and lead into the water. These metals can be a cause of concern during pregnancy since your baby is more sensitive to them than you are.

Older homes (pre-1950s in North America) and homes with lead or brass plumbing have been found to contain significant levels of lead in the drinking water. If you have an older home, it may be a good idea to have your water tested. Although the risk of lead poisoning from tap water in most Westernized countries is extremely low, lead can interfere with the health of your unborn child. Letting your tap water run freely for a few minutes prior to consumption can lower the risk of lead intake.

Filtering

Some people like to use a water filtration system at home, since tap water can contain trace amounts of metals, bacteria, and chemicals. There are lots of home filtration systems to choose from, including carbon filters, ultraviolet light filters, and reverse osmosis filtration systems. Fancy water-cleaning products will even alter water pH and oxygen content. You can have one of these water filtration systems installed in your home for added peace of mind. Or you can get water in large jugs from a water depot, your local grocery store, or have them delivered to your house or office.

Untreated Water

If you are considering drinking water from lakes, streams, and rivers during your pregnancy, we have one word for you: don't. These waters may be contaminated with heavy metals, agricultural runoff, or microorganisms such as bacteria, viruses, and protozoa (parasites), none of which you can see from a visual inspection of the water. And the saying "fast-flowing water is safe to drink" is completely wrong.

Let us repeat: Do *not* drink untreated water during your pregnancy! The consequences of drinking or washing in contaminated water are hard to predict, but acute reactions can range from a small rash to severe illness requiring hospitalization. The most common reactions are gastrointestinal problems like diarrhea or respiratory, eye, ear, nose, or throat infections. A gastrointestinal reaction from a microorganism like *Giardia* could result in diarrhea and the risk of developing serious dehydration that could put you and your baby at risk. There are too many safe water sources to risk it—drink safe water for a healthy pregnancy.

WATER TO GO

Buying bottled water is expensive, may not be any better than your tap water, and is hard on the environment with the huge amount of plastic waste it produces. Plus, the soft plastic water bottles can leach chemicals into the water and should not be reused for this reason. So you switch to a hard plastic water bottle and then discover it may contain a harmful chemical called BPA. What should you do? Look for new, BPA-free hard water bottles or use stainless steel for a safe and environmentally friendly way to take your water to go.

Bottled Water

Bottled water used to be considered the purest source of water. This may be true in less-developed countries where tap water is not safe for consumption. But in Westernized countries, research has repeatedly shown that bottled water is not worth the hype it receives. Tap water always comes out the winner in the "what's the purest?" contests.

Some water companies advertise that their water is from the Alps or a natural spring, giving the illusion that it is a pure and untouched water source. But the truth is that untouched ("pure") water does not exist on earth: The world's water is all shared, thanks to underwater tables and rain clouds. The toxins released in the air in China can easily end up in a mountain spring in France. In some cases, the water bottling plants may be in your own community. So you can pay for the bottled water or simply turn on the tap at home and use a filter there.

Hard Water Bottles

Many people have taken the environmental high road when it comes to carrying water around and have switched to using reusable, hard plastic water bottles. This may be a great way to be kind to the environment, but these hard, shatter-proof water bottles may contain a compound called bisphenol-A (BPA). BPA is a synthetic chemical and is the main component of polycarbonate, which is used in many standard plastic products, including food and drink containers as well as baby bottles.

When these plastics are warmed, such as when they are left in a hot car, put in the dishwasher, or filled with warm baby formula, the BPA in the plastic will leach into the food or drink. It is known that our exposure to BPA is probably low, but evidence is lacking about the effects of low levels of exposure, prompting the ban of BPA in some countries, including Canada.

The concern is that BPA can act like a hormone modulator and may lead to adverse effects in humans. Studies have shown that the chemical can imitate the female hormone estrogen, and it has been linked to cancer and infertility in animals.

Herbal Supplements

For most of human history, herbs were our medicines, and using herbs during pregnancy was the only option. Today, synthetic medicines substitute for most natural supplements used for pregnancy. But many still look to natural herbs and vitamins to provide essential nutrition during pregnancy as well as aid in relieving some common discomforts.

Some people believe that herbs offer a less expensive and more natural alternative to medicinal counterparts. But medical professionals do not recommend herbal remedies to pregnant women because the safety of all herbs has not been established to the same degree as pharmaceuticals to date. (One reason for this is that herbs, being natural, are difficult to standardize, unlike synthetics.)

We'll attempt to help guide you through the tricky world of herbs and pregnancy. But we recommend that you consult with your obstetrician or midwife to discuss the safety of herbs during your pregnancy. This information is intended only for educational use.

RECOMMENDED SUPPLEMENTS

Not all supplements are bad for you during pregnancy. Fish oil supplements, probiotics, and vitamins are all thought to offer pregnant women benefits. In particular, vitamin D supplementation is growing in popularity due to new research. A group of Australian researchers reported in 2008 that urban populations are low in vitamin D and that low intakes of vitamin D during pregnancy may have adverse effects on offspring. Minerals are also important during pregnancy. For example, magnesium is an effective laxative for constipation and may work to alleviate leg cramps during pregnancy.

DAILY HERBS

Check out the list of herbs on page 237 that pose some concern during pregnancy, especially if you already take herbal supplements. You may take an herb on a daily basis to help fight off the common cold or improve your health. Be sure to look into every herb you are taking if you become pregnant to ensure that it is not putting you or your baby at any unnecessary risk. We suggest that you stop taking herbal supplements if you're trying to conceive or as soon as you learn that you're pregnant and discuss the safety of any you'd like to continue taking with your obstetrician or midwife before resuming their use.

Culinary Herbs

If you're like most people, your daily herb exposure is in the herbs you use to add flavor to your culinary creations. The herbs you use every day in your cooking, such as basil, rosemary, thyme, cinnamon, tarragon,

garlic, and fennel are safe during pregnancy. That makes these culinary herbs the least tricky of all the foods we've encountered in this chapter.

It's when you start to take herbs for medicinal use or in higher amounts that you need to be cautious. Some medicinal herbs can be dangerous during pregnancy, which is why we suggest that you discuss herbal supplements with your obstetrician or midwife before taking them.

TRADITIONAL PREGNANCY HERBS

Herbalists and midwives have used herbs in pregnancy for centuries as a tool to help induce labor, improve uterine strength, soothe and calm the mother, and more. Some of their most popular herbs include red raspberry leaf, peppermint, ginger, chamomile, and fenugreek, all of which we include in our list of 100 healthiest foods for pregnancy. Let's recap what roles they play in a healthy pregnancy. But first, let's again stress that when we include them in our recommendations, we're talking about using them in moderate amounts, usually in the form of a cup of herb tea, as opposed to taking them in large quantities or in supplement form. Finally, we'll look at three more herbs or herb derivatives that have played an important role in pregnancy: black cohosh, castor oil, and blessed thistle.

Red Raspberry Leaf

Red raspberry leaf is probably the best-known pregnancy herb. Herbalists and midwives recommend red raspberry leaf for morning sickness and to tone the uterus and help ensure a good strong pregnancy. It is also used to stimulate the onset of labor and to promote an easy labor.

Research supports this traditional use. Laboratory studies show that red raspberry induces contractions in uterine smooth muscle cells removed from pregnant women, but it has no effect on strips of cells taken from nonpregnant women. One randomized controlled study found no significant differences in women who used red raspberry and those that didn't, except for a decreased rate in the need for forceps delivery.

The safety of red raspberry is fairly well supported. A small retrospective study of 108 women who took red raspberry or a placebo during pregnancy found no identifiable side effects associated with its use. But it did have noticeable benefits: The women who took red raspberry were less likely to have pre- or postterm gestation, artificial membrane rupture, Cesarean section, or a forceps or vacuum birth.

There is some debate as to the safety of red raspberry consumption during the first trimester because of concern that its uterine effects may increase the risk of miscarriage. So be sure to consult with your obstetrician or midwife before drinking red raspberry leaf tea during pregnancy.

Peppermint and Ginger

Besides labor, the other main misery that pregnant women seek help for is morning sickness. Morning sickness is a term that describes a pregnant woman's problem with nausea and vomiting during the early months of pregnancy. Morning sickness usually occurs during months 2 and 3 of pregnancy, but for some women, it can last longer. Not all women will experience morning sickness, but for those who do, peppermint and ginger can offer some help.

Peppermint is well known for its ability to help relieve nausea from morning sickness. Gingerroot is also well established as a safe way for people to relieve nausea and vomiting. Again, these herbs have traditionally been used in their food forms, and dosages in supplement forms may vary, affecting the degree of safety. Be sure to consult with your obstetrician or midwife about these herbs before using them.

HERBS TO AVOID

This may look like a long list, but it's actually pretty conservative. You may be surprised to find some common culinary herbs on the list (marked with asterisks). We're not suggesting that you stop cooking with these herbs! They're safe for use as culinary herbs; it's their use in high dosages as a medicinal herb that could be a problem.

Aloes	Kava kava
Andrographis	Lavender
Angelica	Lemon balm
Ashwaganda	Licorice
Barberry	Lovage
Black cohosh	Motherwort
Blue cohosh	Oregon grape
Cascara	Parsley* (seed or root only, not leaves)
Castor oil	
Catnip	Passionflower
Cat's claw	Pennyroyal
Cayenne*	Rosemary*
Coltsfoot	Sage*
Comfrey	Senna
Dong quai	Shepherd's purse
Ephedra	St. John's wort
Fennel*	Tansy
Feverfew	Tarragon*
Garlic*	Thuja
Hibiscus	Turmeric*
Horehound	Uva ursi
Juniper	Wild cherry

Chamomile

Chamomile is another popular pregnancy herb. It can help in soothing the digestive system and promoting sleep, treating two common complaints of pregnancy. When consumed in moderation (a cup or two a day), chamomile tea is considered safe during pregnancy. However, some resources suggest that women avoid this herb during pregnancy in large amounts, because it may act as a uterine stimulant and thus has a small risk of leading to a miscarriage. As always, talk to your obstetrician or midwife about chamomile use during your pregnancy.

One reason for chamomile's popularity is that it's a great way to get a hot mug into your hands without the caffeine. As we've seen in the Caffeine entry on page 220, according to the *American Journal of Obstetrics and Gynecology*, caffeine can harm your baby. The study found that consuming more than 200 mg of caffeine daily—about one and half cups of coffee or 7 cups of black or green tea—may double the riskof miscarriage. And like alcohol, caffeine crosses the placenta to the developing fetus.

Fenugreek

In herbal medicine, fenugreek is considered a natural galactagogue. A galactagogue is a substance capable of promoting or stimulating lactation. Natural medicine commonly recommends fenugreek to new mothers who need some help in promoting lactation. See page 256 for more on fenugreek.

Black Cohosh

Used by as many as 45 percent of midwives to induce labor, black cohosh frequently comes up in discussions about pregnancy. There is a lot of traditional evidence for its safety and effectiveness, but there is little clinical evidence to date. You may recall that this herb is on our list of "Herbs to Avoid" on page 237; it should never be taken except under a midwife's or obstetrician's supervision.

Castor Oil

Castor oil is one of the best-documented herbs for stimulating labor. It is used by midwives because it causes muscles to contract in the gastrointestinal tract, which has potential to stimulate the uterus. It may also increase prostaglandin production (a chemical messenger in the body), which stimulates the uterus.

Some clinical research supports the traditional evidence that castor oil works to stimulate labor. A dosage of 60 ml appears in studies to result in labor within 24 hours in about 50 percent or more of pregnant women who are at term. Not much safety data is available, and it is not recommended that castor oil be taken at any other time during pregnancy; it too is on our list of "Herbs to Avoid" on page 237. And of course, even if you are overdue and feeling really uncomfortable, you should never dose yourself with anything to induce labor!

Blessed Thistle

In herbal medicine, blessed thistle—as well as alfalfa, caraway, chasteberry, fenugreek, and goat's rue—are all considered natural galactagogues. As we noted earlier, a galactagogue is a substance capable of promoting or stimulating lactation. Natural medicine commonly recommends blessed thistle to new mothers who need some help in promoting lactation. A lot of traditional evidence supports the use of all these herbs, but little clinical evidence is available. Women interested in this approach should try blessed thistle and the other herbs before they conceive, since this can help eliminate any concerns that they might be allergic to them.

SUPPLEMENTS AND FEMALE COMPLAINTS

The use of supplements during pregnancy may be a tricky area, but many herbs, as well as vitamins and minerals, are well known for their ability to help relieve the discomforts of menopause, premenstrual syndrome, and painful periods. Randomized controlled trial evidence suggests that black cohosh and flaxseed (lignans) are effective for symptoms of menopause. Chasteberry, as well as calcium, magnesium, evening primrose oil, and vitamin B6, are good for premenstrual syndrome. And vitamins B1 and E can provide relief from painful periods and cramping. Some herbs may even help with fertility. (See chapter 8, beginning on page 285, for more on promoting fertility.)

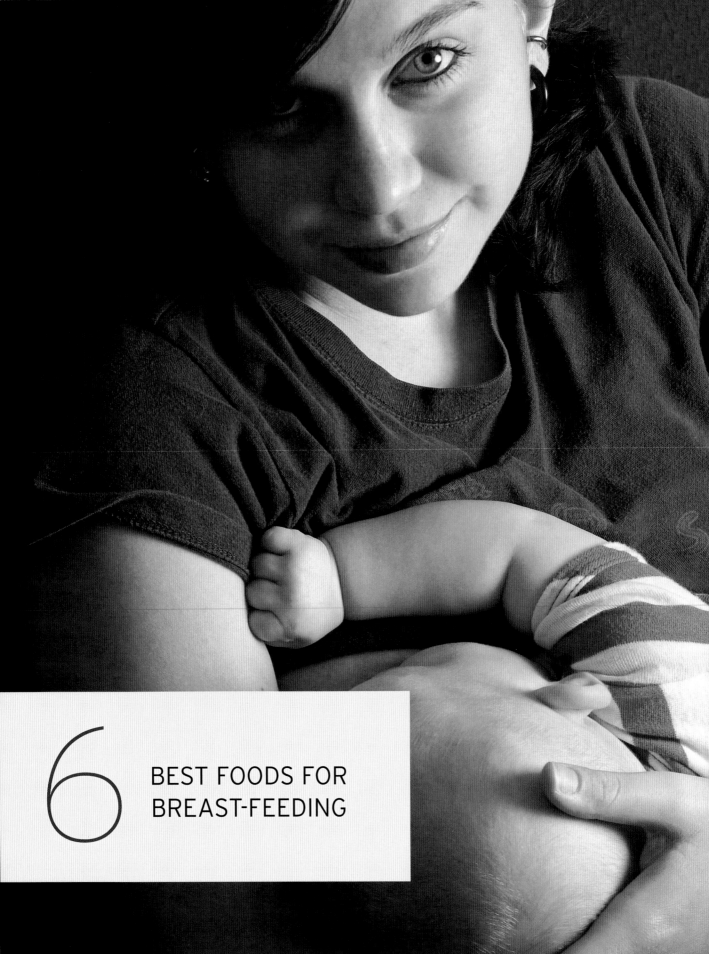

6

BEST FOODS FOR BREAST-FEEDING

BREAST-FEEDING: IT'S FREE, CONVENIENT,

and very healthy for you and your baby—an all-around great choice. It's just doing what comes naturally: At least 99 percent of women who try succeed at breast-feeding. So it's no surprise that breast-feeding is highly recommended to women by health-care professionals and the World Health Organization.

Here's where we come in. Just because you're no longer pregnant does not mean your focus on your diet should change. In fact, now more than ever, your diet is of vital importance to your health and the health of your baby. The process of producing breast milk is almost as taxing on your body as producing a baby. Your body needs more nutrients now than you can imagine. And there are lots of healthy foods to help keep you fueled and your baby growing strong and healthy while you breast-feed. You'll find the best of them in this chapter.

WHY BREAST-FEED?

The benefits of breast-feeding a baby are well known today. The nutritional value of breast milk is superior to that found in infant formulas, plus it is economical, sanitary, and convenient. In addition, breast-fed infants perform better on cognitive-function tests later in life than those fed standard formula.

Breast milk also offers your baby additional immunity. Doctors have long known that infants who are breast-fed contract fewer infections than infants given formula. They presumed that it was because breast milk is more sanitary, as bottles can easily become contaminated by bacteria and viruses. But the truth is that it's what is in breast milk that keeps babies healthy. Breast milk has many components that support your infant's immune response, including antibodies and probiotics.

NUTRITIONAL NEEDS FOR LACTATION AND BREAST-FEEDING

Because every woman's body is different, it's important to work closely with your obstetrician or midwife to develop a nutritional program that's ideal for you. Your nutritional needs change dramatically when you're lactat-ing (breast-feeding). This chart will give you nutritional guidelines for healthy lactation. You'll read about these nutrients in detail later in the chapter.

Key Vitamins

Vitamin B6: 2 mg daily

Folate: 500 mcg daily

Vitamin B12: 2.8 mcg daily

Vitamin C: 120 mg daily

Vitamin A: 4,200 IU daily

Vitamin D: 5 mcg daily

Vitamin E: 19 mg daily

Vitamin K: 90 mcg daily

Key Minerals

Potassium: 5,100 mg daily

Calcium: 1,000 mg daily

Phosphorus: 700 mg daily

Magnesium: 310 mg daily

Iron: 9 mg daily

Zinc: 12 mg daily

PROBIOTICS AS A TUMMY-TUCK?

Researchers from the University of Turky in Finland reported at the European Conference on Obesity in Amsterdam, Netherlands, in 2009 that it is possible that taking probiotic supplements postnatally may help reduce belly fat in new mothers. Involving 256 pregnant women, the study divided them into three groups: one received nutritional counseling and probiotics, another received just nutritional counseling and a placebo pill, and the third received neither. There was a slight reduction in belly fat in the women who received the probiotic. More research in the future will help verify these findings and explain how it works.

During the first few months of life, an infant cannot mount an effective immune response against foreign organisms like bacteria or viruses. In the womb, the placenta passes antibodies to the baby, giving him some advance coverage. But breast-fed infants gain extra protection from the antibodies, immune cells, and probiotics in human milk. These components of breast milk help your baby protect himself or herself against infection, promote healthy levels of probiotics in his or her digestive system (improving gastrointestinal function), and can even help him or her absorb more iron.

BREASTS 101

The anatomy of the breast is more complicated than you'd think. The breast, also called the mammary gland, consists of milk-producing cells and a duct system. The nipple contains fifteen to twenty lactiferous ducts that carry the milk from the cells, where it is produced, to the nipple.

During pregnancy, there is some increase in size and weight of the breasts, most notably in the first and third trimesters. Many women will find they need to move up a bra cup size to accommodate their new breast size. But it's not just your bra size that changes. Suddenly, your modest shirts become racier as your cleavage peeks out the top. You may find you have to make adjustments in your wardrobe throughout pregnancy, and while doing so, get ready for even bigger breasts to come.

During the third trimester, the enlargement of the breasts is caused by milk-producing cells and the formation of early colostrums. In fact, a woman's breast is capable of milk secretion beginning sometime in the second trimester—great news for any women who have a preterm infant.

The placenta has been found to play an important role in breast growth during pregnancy. It secretes ovarian-like hormones in large quantities (lactogen, prolactin, and chorionic gonadotrophin). During pregnancy, the breast can weigh between 400 and 600 grams (0.8 to 1.3 pounds), a possible increase of more than a pound and about two cup sizes. And there is more to come, ladies. During lactation, the breast weighs a lot more—about 600 to 800 grams (1.3 to 1.8 pounds). As you embark on breast-feeding, be prepared: You'll need a wider-strapped bra to support your new breasts.

Making Milk

It's not as simple as your breast just secreting milk, though. A number of processes are carefully synchronized to make sure your baby gets the best mixture of nutrients to help him or her grow big and strong. Some nutrients are created by the milk-producing cells themselves, and others are taken from the mother's plasma. Fat, vitamins, minerals, and water have to be produced and secreted. Proteins, calcium, lactose, phosphate, and other nutrients are also sent into the milk mixture through a process called exocytosis (a process in which cells excrete substances). Immunoglobulins (immune messengers) also must move into the breast milk. These immunoglobulins are what give your baby protection from infections during his or her first few months of life, since a child's own immune system isn't properly formed until about the age of five.

These milk-producing processes happen thanks largely to a hormone called prolactin. This hormone is naturally produced in your body, but your baby's suckling on your nipples stimulates the prolactin levels in your blood to rise, helping your breasts produce more milk.

CAN'T BREAST-FEED?

Some women simply can't breast-feed their babies. This may be due to medical reasons, problems with breast milk flow, lifestyle complications, or it may be their choice. Whatever your reason for not breast-feeding your baby, there's no need to feel guilty. There are still lots of things you can do to ensure that your baby is getting the best food you can offer.

Today infant formulas are vastly improved compared to those offered a few decades ago. Thanks to advances in research in the last few decades, we know the importance of zinc, iron, arachidonic acid (AA, also listed as ARA), docosahexaenoic acid (DHA), probiotics, and many other nutrients in infant development and growth. As a result, you'll find many of these nutrients on the labels of infant formulas available on market shelves today, helping improve the nutritional content of infant formula. In general, there are three types of infant formula: milk based, soy based, and special formulas. Iron-fortified cow's milk is the infant formula most commonly recommended by doctors.

Iron-deficiency anemia is common among formula-fed infants because standard formulas do not contain enough iron, and the iron in infant formula is poorly absorbed by your baby compared to that in breast milk.

If your baby develops an allergy to or intolerance of cow's milk, a soy-based formula is commonly recommended. Nutritionally speaking, look for formulas with key nutrients like iron, DHA (sometimes labeled as omega-3), AA (sometimes labeled as omega-6), and probiotics in them to ensure that your baby is getting lots of these nutrients, since they are still not found in standard infant formulas. The best thing to do is read, ask questions, and use the formula you feel most comfortable with. If your baby has special medical requirements (such as gastrointestinal problems) or is premature, speak with your pediatrician for advice on the right infant formula to choose, as a special formula may be required.

The Let-Down

Once your breasts produce and secrete milk, you'll find breast-feeding easy for you and your baby. The reason for this is a process called the let-down reflex, which is simply the ejection or production of milk by your breasts. Technically speaking, it's the process by which milk is sent into your lactiferous sinuses, which are like holding tanks in your breasts, so it's available for your baby. The let-down is caused by hormones, nerves, and at times, outside stimuli. The primary stimulus for let-down is your baby's suckling. This stimulates your brain to produce the hormone oxytocin, which tells the breast tissue to release or "let down" the milk.

Naturally producing milk when your baby wants to eat is the good news. But milk ejection can also be stimulated by the sound of a crying baby, and since it's hard to go almost anywhere without encountering a baby crying, this can lead to some awkward situations. Before you're embarrassed by leaking breasts in the middle of a dinner party, try putting breast pads in your bra. They'll help catch any escaping milk at less than desirable times.

You will quickly learn to identify the symptoms of the let-down reflex, since they're fairly obvious: milk dripping from the breasts, contraction of the uterus during breast-feeding, or a tingling sensation in the breasts. Once you recognize the signs, you'll be able to use this bodily intuition to help with the timing and length of breast-feeding your baby requires.

Keeping It Going

To keep producing milk, the best technique is to keep a suckling action going on your breasts at regular intervals. This can be done by simply breast-feeding your baby (and be sure to rotate breasts) or by using suckling simulation like manual expression or a breast pump. A breast pump can be very helpful at helping maintain your milk production in the absence of your baby (for example, when you're at work). Drinking enough water and eating foods that fuel your body with the nutrients needed to produce breast milk can also help keep your breasts producing milk.

FOOD AND BREAST-FEEDING

A midwife once told me that she never felt hungrier in her life than when she was breast-feeding. She joked that if it wasn't nailed down or screwed to the wall, she wanted to eat it.

She's not alone. The hunger many women feel during breast-feeding is due to the extra 500 calories your body uses to produce the needed 1 to 2 kilograms (35 to 71 ounces) of milk each day. Interested in getting your figure back before your baby's second birthday? Then make sure those extra calories you are craving are coming from healthy, nutrient-filled foods or you may find it harder to lose that baby fat.

If you find your hunger alarming or you're concerned you may not be eating enough, remember that your body stored an extra 2 to 4 kilograms (71 to 141 ounces) of fat during pregnancy specifically so you would have extra stores of energy available to help you produce breast milk. This stored fat (or as some girlfriends affectionately call it, "back fat") will provide 100 to 200 calories a day for the first 3 months of lactation.

If you breast-feed for longer than 3 months, you may find that your fat stores are disappearing and you'll need to get those essential extra calories from your diet. If your weight falls below the ideal weight (see the chart on page 15 for a guideline or check with your obstetrician), be sure to increase your calorie intake appropriately to ensure that your low body weight doesn't affect your ability to produce sufficient breast milk for your baby.

The Optimal Diet

The optimal diet for lactating women includes eating nutritious foods, very similar to the diet you worked with during pregnancy. The real difference is simply that you need more calories now—500 extra calories a day. Focus on healthy foods that offer your body the nutrients you need for healing and breast-feeding: protein, good fats, calcium, iron, and other minerals, vitamins, and water.

Lots of foods can help you ensure you're armed with all the nutrients your body so badly needs during this time. Water may be the most important since you're producing a lot of liquid for your baby. Protein and fats make up the majority of your breast milk, so you'll need to get plenty of both in your diet now. Plus, your baby needs minerals like calcium, magnesium, zinc, and iron, as well as vitamins to help him or her grow big and strong. Fruits, vegetables, whole grains, nuts, seeds, and fish are great foods to focus on while breastfeeding. And don't skimp! Your body is working really hard to produce all of that milk, and you really do need to eat more.

The Power of Protein

Breast-feeding women are advised to consume more protein (about 12 to 15 g or a quarter- to a half-ounce more per day). This additional protein is thought to cover the extra protein used in milk production. You can meet this increased need for protein, as well as

NATURAL BIRTH CONTROL

During lactation, the production of luteinizing hormone is suppressed. This is the hormone that causes your ovaries to mature and release eggs. It's like natural birth control—your body's way of protecting itself since you're not physically ready to get pregnant again yet. However, it is not foolproof, and some women have become pregnant while breast-feeding. This may be due to the slow increase in your body's levels of luteinizing hormone as you start to wean your baby. With complete weaning, the follicular phase of ovulation is reestablished, increasing your risk of becoming pregnant.

If you're eager to have another baby shortly after this pregnancy, be sure to read chapter 8, beginning on page 285, for tips on foods you can eat to improve your health before another pregnancy. Chapter 8 also has advice on what to eat to boost your fertility.

your energy needs, by drinking three cups of milk each day. But milk will not help you get the vitamin C, vitamin E, iron, zinc, and folic acid you need while breast-feeding. So while breast-feeding, reach for a variety of good-for-you foods like citrus fruits, vegetable oils, leafy green vegetables, nuts, and seeds to help you meet all of your nutrient needs. Many health-care professionals strongly recommend breast-feeding women also continue to take their prenatal multivitamins while breast-feeding to ensure they are getting sufficient nutrients.

DRINK MORE WATER

Breast milk is 90 percent water. All of that water has to come from inside your body. So grab a glass of water—and perhaps a few more—and get hydrated. You'll need this extra water to keep your milk production optimal. If you're suffering from headaches and find that you aren't going to the bathroom frequently enough, you are likely to be dehydrated. Here's a great tip: Many women find that if they drink a glass of water every time they sit down to breast-feed, it's easier to keep up with their increased water needs.

Bone Break

Working hard to ensure that your diet is higher in calcium may not translate into more calcium in your breast milk. Studies have found that increasing calcium consumption in breast-feeding women did not increase the amount of calcium in their breast milk. However, it's still very important to focus on getting plenty of calcium in your diet during breast-feeding. Not having enough calcium in your diet will cause your bones to give up some of their calcium. The result is a loss of bone mass and a weakening of the bones.

If you're an older mom, your calcium needs are even greater. Your bones will continue to increase in bone mass up until your twenties, and then the process starts to slow. Younger mothers have more time to rebuild their bone stores after breast-feeding if they fall short in their calcium intake.

So give your bones a break and be sure to reach for foods that are a good source of calcium while you're breast-feeding. Good sources of calcium include dairy foods, dried fruits, and leafy green vegetables. See the chart on page 12 for a list of foods that are good sources of calcium.

Eat More Good Fats

Are you breast-feeding? Then you need even more essential fatty acids than before. Your breast milk is a source of docosahexaenoic acid (DHA), gamma-linolenic acid (GLA), and arachodonic acid (AA) for your baby. These essential fats help your baby's brain and eyes develop and keep his immune system running optimally. These essential fats are really important after your baby stops breast-feeding too. Human breast milk is 50 percent fat. Make sure your breast milk contains the fats your baby needs by including plant oils and fish oil in your diet. And skip the trans fats hiding in fried and packaged foods. These bad fats can be harmful to your baby.

The Perfect Food

Breast milk has been hailed as the perfect food for an infant. But not all breast milk is created equal. Your diet affects the quality of your breast milk. Ensuring that your diet contains sufficient amounts of essential nutrients like vitamins, minerals, and fats will help you produce the best possible milk for your baby.

One nutrient in breast milk that is proven to be affected by your diet is the essential fatty acid DHA. Experts are finding that babies who don't get enough of these fats from their moms may be at a disadvantage. The long-term consequences of inadequate levels of omega-3 fatty acids are not completely understood, though research shows that infants who don't receive enough omega-3 fatty acids in their diets have lower visual acuity and a great risk for developing attention deficit disorders (ADD and ADHD) and depression later in life.

The amount of DHA and other omega-3s in breast milk varies from population to population. Numerous studies have found that the content of DHA in breast milk depends on the type and quantity of food consumed. Women in Japan have much higher amounts of omega-3s in their breast milk than women living in Canada or the United States. So take a cue from Japanese women and eat more fish to ensure that your breast milk contains enough DHA to meet your baby's needs.

If you don't like fish, you can get omega-3 fatty acids into your diet from fish oil supplements. Fish oil comes in both capsules and liquid form, and some of the newer liquid products are downright delicious and have no fishy taste whatsoever. If you're a vegetarian or can't stomach the thought of fish oil supplements of any kind, you can also get omega-3s from sources like flaxseed, flaxseed oil, or algae. The body will take the omega-3 fatty acid found in flax (called ALA) and turn some of it into DHA (and the other important omega-3 fat, EPA), but it's not a very efficient process. So if you're getting your omega-3s solely from flaxseed oil, for example, you'll need to take at least 2 tablespoons (or more) a day.

Does Your Diet Really Matter?

We know that diet is associated with the quality of your breast milk. And it may keep your milk free of potentially harmful substances too. Some populations of mothers have higher levels of lead in their bodies due to environmental pollution, and this can be transferred to their babies.

Studies done on women in Mexico City have helped raise awareness of this issue and strengthened the importance of a healthy diet during breast-feeding. Researchers from the Harvard School of Public Health reported in 2006 that supplementing the diet with calcium reduced the lead found in the women's breast milk.

DIETING AND BREAST-FEEDING

When you're breast-feeding is not the time to try to lose that extra "baby weight" by dieting! It's important to recognize that moderate to severe restrictions of your caloric intake can affect your ability to produce milk. This is especially important during the first few weeks of lactation, before the process is firmly established. You need to accept that your extra body weight will disappear gradually over the first six months after birth. Rushing this process may not be healthy for you *or* your baby.

There is a myth that breast-feeding speeds the rate of weight loss. This is not entirely true. Yes, your body will use more calories to produce milk than if you feed your baby infant formula. And the calories needed to produce milk are taken from your fat stores, helping reduce your fat stores. However, breast-feeding mothers also need to eat more calories to produce enough milk for their babies.

The sensible approach to weight control right now is to eat a healthy diet packed with nutrient-rich foods. Use the same strategies you used during pregnancy to make sure your diet is adequate but not full of foods that promote weight gain.

SKIP THE BBQ

Based on research from the University of Guelph in Canada, breast-feeding mothers who consume charred meat are passing potentially cancer-causing compounds to their babies. As fat drips onto the coals or hot grill surface, polycyclic aromatic hydrocarbons (PAHs), known carcinogens, are formed and carried back up and onto the meat by smoke. Barbecued meat also contains other known carcinogens, heterocyclic amines (HCAs). Both kinds of carcinogen make their way into breast milk.

In 2008, the researchers reported that fat consumption may also play a role. In the study, 310 women who were one month postpartum were asked dietary questions and had their bone, blood, and breast milk tested for lead levels. The researchers found that a diet higher in polyunsaturated fats, such as omega-3s and omega-6s, limited the transfer of lead from the bones to breast milk. Yet another reason to include fish in your diet during pregnancy and while breast-feeding—it may help protect your baby from toxins in your body, like lead.

Sometimes a woman's diet doesn't appear to affect her breast milk. Some trace minerals, like zinc and iodine, in the diet do not appear to affect breast milk composition. When researchers looked at the effect of mineral supplementation in a group of 32 new moms in Italy, they found that short-term supplementation did not have a significant effect. More research is needed, but this finding suggests that your diet before and during pregnancy may not just be important for your baby in the womb, but it may also play a role in your ability to produce optimally nutritious breast milk. Eating a healthy diet is always important—now more than ever.

Things to Avoid

The rules about what to avoid that applied during pregnancy can be followed during breast-feeding, since anything you expose your body to may end up in your breast milk. There's a bit more leniency now, though. For example, you can indulge in the occasional treat of sushi, deli meat, or hot dogs, now that the risk of damage to your baby if these foods are contaminated by bacteria is lower; your baby is no longer in your body and exposed to your bloodstream. Most drugs are best avoided while breast-feeding, alcohol and cigarettes are still big no-nos, and caffeine is best left off your menu. Talk to your obstetrician or midwife if you have a particular item you would like to add back into your diet now that you're breast-feeding.

What about food? Many myths are circulating that certain foods can cause colic in your baby and the like. Generally, the healthy foods you have been eating for the last nine months are great for breast-feeding too. You may notice that your baby reacts by crying or may experience gas or bloating with certain foods you eat. Some foods may irritate some babies—maybe garlic and spicy foods—but generally, there is no list of foods known to cause gassiness or irritations in babies. Take cues from your baby and he'll tell you when certain foods irritate him. Then you can try avoiding this food for a while and see if this pleases your baby. Remember that gassiness may not be caused by food but could be due to forceful milk let-down, crying, or thrush.

BREAST-FEEDING A PICKY EATER

The rising incidence of obesity in children and their ever-declining acceptance of healthy foods is a major concern today. A review of research in children's food and taste preferences noted that breast-feeding aids food and taste acceptance and that a child's willingness to try new foods is linked to his parents' behavior, which he or she can actually inherit. Eating a healthy diet yourself and breast-feeding may help you ward off having a child who develops into picky eater.

HOW LONG TO BREAST-FEED?

There has been a debate for many years about when to wean your infant from the breast and start him or her on food. In 2001, a World Health Organization Expert Consultation concluded that waiting until 6 months of age to introduce complementary foods to breast-fed infants has several benefits for both mother and infant.

In developing countries, the risks of infant gastrointestinal illnesses are greater, increasing the time in which an infant should be breast-fed. In industrialized countries, there is concern about the potential for exclusively breast-fed infants to become deficient in zinc and iron since breast milk may not provide enough of these minerals. The current expert advice is to start your infant on foods that offer her iron and zinc around 6 months of age.

HITTING THE GYM

Lactating women can certainly go to the gym. But you may need to use some caution if you've had a Cesarean or other medical situations that may affect your ability to get back into an active lifestyle after birth. Your obstetrician or nurse-midwife can help you decide when it's time for you to get back into your regular exercise routine.

Remember to start off slow. You have a new body to work with, and it's been through a lot of changes over the last nine months. Be realistic about your expectations and ease into your workout routine. As for the effect of exercise on breast-feeding, research suggests that exercise does not appear to affect the process of lactation. Breast-feeding women who exercise should be careful to make sure they consume enough fluids, as dehydration can affect lactation, and to ensure that they are still consuming enough calories to make up for their body's increased needs during this time.

FAST FACT

The fats you consume in your diet show up in your breast milk within 6 hours.

IRON AND YOUR BABY

Infant formulas contain more iron than breast milk does, which has lead to rumors that breast milk does not offer sufficient iron. This is not true. Breast milk offers your baby lots of easily absorbed iron. In fact, most babies do not need another source of iron in their diet besides that offered in breast milk until about 6 months of age. So it's generally recommended that solids be introduced at least in part to a baby's diet when they reach 6 months old. Some babies show great interest in grabbing food off your plate by 5 months, and there is no reason not to allow them to start taking the food and playing with it. Any food on your plate that can be mashed with a fork is probably okay for them to play with and even put in their mouths. Your pediatrician can help you assess when your baby is ready for solid foods and which foods to offer first.

Baby's First Foods

Iron and zinc are trace minerals critical for the development and growth of your infant. Exclusive breast-feeding does provide adequate amounts of both of these nutrients for normal-term infants for approximately the first 6 months of life. If your baby was born prematurely or has other health concerns, work with your obstetrician or pediatrician to see if your infant has additional iron and zinc needs.

Currently, recommendations for the introduction of complementary foods when your baby reaches 6 months old do not emphasize an order of foods to offer or specific foods. This is because an infant's gastrointestinal tract is thought to be mature by this age. Your food choices for your baby should focus on meeting his increased needs for iron and zinc since these minerals may not be available in sufficient amounts in your breast milk.

Many baby foods intended to be used in conjunction with breast-feeding, called complementary foods, are typically high in iron but low in zinc, despite recent recognition of the importance of zinc during the second half of the first year of life. Meat is a good food to include in your infant's diet because it contains both iron and zinc. Several studies have investigated the effects of meat as an early complementary food that offers iron and zinc. The conclusions have been that meat is an effective means of providing these essential nutrients.

Top Foods for Breast-Feeding

Good nutrition is essential to help support a successful pregnancy and breast-feeding. During breast-feeding, a mother's needs change. She needs more calories and more protein, and the composition of her diet can affect the quality of her breast milk. Breast-feeding mothers need to eat a diet with sufficient nutrient-rich foods to provide them with enough energy and nutrients to support milk production.

Every food we have discussed in this book is a healthy food and can be added to your breast-feeding menu. However, a few foods offer particular benefits to a breast-feeding woman, like cabbage leaves, dill, fenugreek, mackerel, melon, and milk. Let's take a closer look at some of these foods and the healthy benefits they can offer you and your baby while you're breast-feeding.

HERE ARE THE 6 HEALTHIEST FOODS FOR BREAST-FEEDING:

- CABBAGE
- DILL
- FENUGREEK
- MACKEREL
- MELONS
- MILK

Let's look at each of these healthy foods for breast-feeding and see what makes them tops on our list. By now, you've heard us tell you to be brave and try new or formerly disliked foods. Never come across fenugreek? Can't stand the smell of cooked cabbage? (Actually, if it smells, it's *overcooked*.) Jonny to the rescue once again! "Jonny's Tasty Tips" will give you some great ways to include these foods in your diet.

Cabbage

CABBAGE IS GOOD FOR YOU, YOUR BABY, AND—

believe it or not!—your breasts. Cabbage leaves are packed with healthy nutrients, making cabbage a great choice to keep in your fridge while you're breast-feeding. But you can put those cabbage leaves to a more direct use as well.

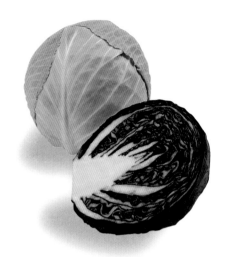

CABBAGE AT A GLANCE

Serving Size: ½ cup (75 g)	Calcium: 4%
Calories: 17	Vitamin A: 1%
Saturated Fat: 0 g	Vitamin C: 47%
Protein: 1 g	Iron: 1%
Fiber: 1 g	

Note: The nutritional facts data provided in this book are approximations based on the foods' nutrient value and a pregnant woman's RDA.

Crunch on Some Cabbage

Cabbage deserves its star status in your diet. Cabbage is a good source of many vitamins and minerals, including thiamin, folate, vitamin B6, vitamin C, vitamin K, calcium, magnesium, manganese, phosphorus, potassium, and fiber. Many of these nutrients are essential to healthy breast-milk production. The B vitamins (thiamin, folate, and vitamin B6) are all vital to proper energy production, which you're really going to need while you try to produce enough breast milk over the next few months. A half-cup of cabbage contains about 23 mcg of folate and about 4 percent of your daily needs of thiamin and vitamin B6.

Vitamin C is super-helpful in promoting a healthy immune system in your body and your baby's, and this vitamin plays a crucial role in skin health—and your skin is trying to quickly spring back into its prepregnancy shape. You'll get about half of your daily needs of vitamin C in just a half-cup of cabbage.

And we can't forget vitamin K. Cabbage is a fantastic source of vitamin K, offering close to your entire day's needs in a half-cup serving (81 mcg per ½ cup of cabbage). Vitamin K is a key nutrient, along with calcium and magnesium, in bone health.

A Good Source of Iron

Your body is most likely a little short on iron, since you have offered so much of your iron to your baby during pregnancy and now are supplying iron in the large amounts of breast milk you are producing daily. Including foods like cabbage in your diet can help: A head of cabbage contains 2 mg of iron. You need 9 mg of iron a day during lactation. We talked about a lot of other great iron-containing foods in the pregnancy chapters, like prune juice, sun-dried tomatoes, artichoke, turmeric, and chickpeas.

Cabbage for Calcium and Magnesium

Cabbage is a great source of calcium and magnesium as well as vitamin K, so you're getting bone-building power in every bite. A half-cup of boiled cabbage contains 36 mg of calcium and 11 mg of magnesium. We'll talk in detail about the importance of calcium when we discuss milk in a few pages, so let's focus on magnesium—the lesser-known mineral—here. Magnesium is as important as calcium for healthy breast-milk production. During lactation, your body is working hard to produce the most nutritious food it can for your baby. Your breasts are demanding minerals like calcium and magnesium from your body to create the breast milk.

If your diet doesn't contain enough magnesium from foods like cabbage, your bones are asked to give up some of their stored magnesium. Giving up nutrients can leave your bones weak. Plus, a deficiency of magnesium in your diet can harm your bones even more since it also affects the cells that create and break down bone. Magnesium is a very important cofactor in bone and muscle health. A deficiency of magnesium can impair your osteoblasts (the cells in your bones that build new bone). And low levels of magnesium in your body will increase the formation and activity of osteoclasts (cells in your bones that break down bone). It's a one-two punch. More important, if you can't produce enough magnesium in your breast milk, your baby's bones may not be getting enough either. Be sure to include foods into your diet that contain magnesium, like cabbage, on a regular basis, as well as plenty of calcium-rich foods to make sure that both your bones and your baby's are strong and healthy.

Jonny's Tasty Tips

If you've ever smelled overcooked cabbage, you've probably never forgotten that sulfurous stink. It may have made you avoid cabbage entirely, and that's a shame, since it's packed with nutrients and cancer-fighting phytochemicals. Purple cabbage is especially rich in the flavonoids called anthocyanins, which pack a really huge antioxidant punch. Cabbage is also high in fiber, and best of all, it's one of the lowest-calorie foods on the planet.

So how do you get the benefits without the stink? It is easy. You can sauté shredded cabbage in a little organic butter or oil with a sprinkling of caraway seeds until it barely wilts and is heated through and then serve it up as a delicious side dish.

But my favorite way to eat cabbage is raw, shredded in coleslaw or mixed in a tossed salad with other greens and veggies. Both green and purple cabbage add great crunch and body to salads. And there are infinite variations on coleslaw. I like to keep mine light rather than weighing it down with goopy mayonnaise and other unhealthy, high-cal dressings. For a pretty, delicious confetti-like coleslaw, add shredded carrots to mixed shredded green and purple cabbage and then mix in finely minced sweet onion (such as Vidalia or WallaWalla). Marinate for at least an hour in a simple vinaigrette: I like to use a little balsamic vinegar and extra-virgin olive oil and enjoy trying different herb combinations. Caraway seeds are great in coleslaw, too. Just before serving, top with sunflower seeds or pepitas (pumpkin seeds) for even more crunch and nutrition.

Dill

YOU MAY THINK DILL IS JUST FOR PICKLING, BUT THIS versatile herb is packed with healthy nutrients to help your body repair itself, produce milk, and keep your baby healthy too. Fresh dill is a good source of fiber, niacin, phosphorus, copper, riboflavin, vitamin B6, folate, iron, and potassium. All of these nutrients support healthy growth and development in your body as well as your baby's. More important right now, fresh dill is a source of four particularly important breast-feeding nutrients: zinc, iron, and vitamins A and C.

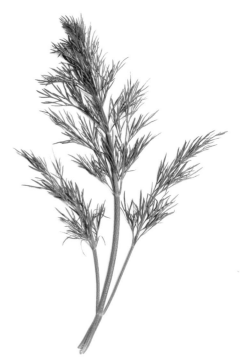

DILL AT A GLANCE

Serving Size: **5 sprigs (1 g)**	Calcium: **0%**
Calories: **0**	Vitamin A: **2%**
Saturated Fat: **0 g**	Vitamin C: **1%**
Protein: **0 g**	Iron: **1%**
Fiber: **1 g**	

FAST FACT

Neither size nor structural composition of the breast significantly influences the success of breast-feeding.

Zinc for Breast-Feeding

Prolactin is the primary hormone regulating milk protein synthesis in new mothers. Dieting and malnutrition have been shown in research to affect plasma prolactin concentrations. Low levels of zinc in your diet may reduce the concentration of prolactin, causing less milk production in your breasts. Including foods in your diet that are a good source of zinc is a great help while breast-feeding. Fresh dill offers you 0.1 mg of zinc per ounce.

An Iron-Rich Herb

Dill is packed with nutrients, including iron. After giving birth, your body's iron stores are likely to be a little low. Just the blood lost during labor can deplete your iron stores, not to mention the immense amount of iron your baby pulled from your body during pregnancy. Eating foods that offer you iron, such as dill (0.1 mg in 5 sprigs), can help you rebuild your iron stores. Iron is needed in your body to carry oxygen from your lungs to your cells, where it initiates energy production. You may find that with more iron in your diet, you have more energy—something you may be lacking until your newborn decides to sleep for a decent length of time at night.

AC Power

Dill is a great source of vitamins A and C, offering about 40 percent of your daily requirement of each in one ounce (28 g). Vitamin C maintains collagen, the scaffolding in your skin that is rapidly trying to repair itself as your belly begins to shrink and your breasts engorge. But this antioxidant does more than keep your skin looking beautiful and youthful. Vitamin C helps heal wounds and strengthens blood vessels, two activities that are going on in your uterus after labor. Plus, the vitamin C in dill will help your body absorb the iron it contains.

While vitamin C is a water-soluble antioxidant, its counterpart, vitamin A, offers antioxidant protection to the fatty parts of your body. Plus, vitamin A is necessary for the repair and growth of the body. Your body is repairing itself and your baby's body is growing, making vitamin A important for both of you.

Jonny's Tasty Tips

Dill is not just for pickles! Those feathery, anise-scented leaves are delicious in a tossed salad or cottage cheese and tomato salad. Or stir the minced leaves into plain yogurt and stir in fresh cucumber slices for a cooling hot-weather salad. Toss some into your next potato or egg salad for a fresh, summery taste. Top sautéed summer squash, cooked carrots, or new potatoes with some minced fresh dill instead of parsley. You'll enjoy the change! Dill also adds a great flavor to herbed bread and rolls, whether baked into the bread or finely minced into softened organic butter and used as a spread. (Dill butter is also delicious on broiled seafood.)

JUST RELAX

For healthy breast-feeding, try to relax before and after breast-feeding. Taking a few minutes to relax can help improve milk production. This is a great rule for eating, too. Relax before and after you eat, and you'll find that you digest your food better, helping you get more nutrients out of your food.

Fenugreek

FENUGREEK IS ONE OF THE MOST POPULAR HERBS for promoting milk production. Many women swear by it, but there is little reliable clinical evidence to date on the use of fenugreek at medicinal dosages. There are no adverse events reported in nursing babies, so there are low risks associated with its use as a medicinal herb (in capsules). But as an ingredient in food, fenugreek is a delicious and very nutritious addition to your spice cupboard. Just one tablespoon of fenugreek contains about 20 percent of your daily needs of iron—an energizing mineral that you'll love to have on your side while trying to keep up with your little one's schedule. Let's dig in!

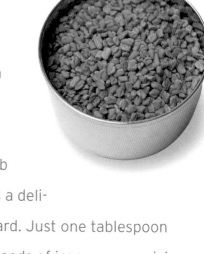

FENUGREEK AT A GLANCE

Serving Size: 1 Tbsp (11 g)	Calcium: 2%
Calories: 36	Vitamin A: 0%
Saturated Fat: 0 g	Vitamin C: 1%
Protein: 3 g	Iron: 20%
Fiber: 3 g	

FAST FACT

A child's immune response does not reach full strength until age five or so.

A Traditional Approach

In herbal medicine, fenugreek is considered a natural galactagogue. A galactagogue is a substance capable of promoting or stimulating lactation. Practitioners of natural medicine commonly recommend fenugreek to new mothers who need some help in promoting lactation since it tends to work quickly, usually within 24 to 72 hours. Typically it's taken in capsule or tea form, though the tea can be rather bitter if brewed too long.

If you haven't eaten food spiced with fenugreek before and are interested in this approach, it's best to try fenugreek before you conceive, since this can help eliminate any concerns that you might be allergic to it. It's not recommended if you have asthma, as it's been known to aggravate the condition, or diabetes, since it's also been shown to lower blood glucose levels. And since fenugreek stimulates the uterus, don't use it at all while you're actually pregnant. Once you've had your baby, it's safe to start flavoring your food with fenugreek again.

That Syrupy Smell

Fenugreek has a warm, lovely maple syrup smell (even though it isn't actually sweet), which can subtly enhance dishes. It's the spice that gives the "maple" flavor to artificially flavored maple syrup. But if you take fenugreek supplements, you might start to smell like maple syrup yourself! (As always, we advise you never to undertake any kind of supplementation regimen except under the direction of your health-care provider.) Simply eating fenugreek-spiced food won't cause this reaction, though, so you can enjoy the maple aroma without worrying that you'll go around smelling like pancakes.

WHAT ABOUT FLAX?

A commonly consumed omega-3 fatty acid called alpha linolenic acid (ALA) is found in plant foods such as canola oil, flax, and walnuts. But ALA is poorly converted to DHA in the human body. Studies have found that despite increasing consumption of ALA in the diet (to 11,000 mg a day from the average 1,300 mg a day) over a four-week period, breast-feeding women could not alter their breast-milk levels of DHA. Your best source of DHA is fish. Serve up some mackerel for dinner and get your breast milk DHA levels up.

Jonny's Tasty Tips

Fenugreek's subtle maple syrup fragrance and warm caramel flavor, which implies sweetness without really being sweet, goes wonderfully in so many foods that if you've never tried it, you're going to be pleasantly surprised. Fenugreek is a natural with chicken—add the whole seeds and a little organic butter next time you bake a chicken breast and you'll see what I mean. Ground fenugreek is delicious in curries and chutneys. Enjoy a sprinkling in applesauce. Sprinkle some on sweet potatoes, winter squash, or pumpkin for a perfect pairing. It's also a staple in Ethiopian and other African cuisines.

Mackerel

MACKEREL MAY NOT SHOW UP OFTEN ON YOUR menu, but now is a good time to change that. Salmon, tuna, mackerel, anchovies, and sardines are among the best sources of omega-3 fatty acids. And omega-3 fatty acids are becoming well known for their ability to improve mood, boost brain power, and more. During breast-feeding, omega-3 fatty acids are as important as they were during your last trimester of pregnancy. In fact, your baby's brain will continue to develop and grow at a rapid rate until the age of five, so be sure that oily fish like mackerel or fish oil is a steady part of your child's diet over the next few years.

MACKEREL AT A GLANCE

Serving Size: **1 fillet (88 g)**	Calcium: **1%**
Calories: **230**	Vitamin A: **3%**
Saturated Fat: **4 g**	Vitamin C: **1%**
Protein: **21 g**	Iron: **8%**
Fiber: **0 g**	

FAST FACT

The amount of DHA in your diet affects the amount of DHA in your breast milk.

Better Brain, Better Vision

DHA (docosahexaenoic acid) is an essential nutrient and a key fat needed in high levels in the brain and retina of the eye. For breast-fed infants, the only source of nutrition, including DHA, for growth and development is their mother's milk. Having enough of this essential fat in your diet as your baby grows and develops during his breast-feeding months can help improve the likelihood of his having higher learning abilities, a better memory, and improved visual acuity.

The amount of DHA in your diet is a major factor that determines how much DHA is in your breast milk. Fatty fish like mackerel are a great source of DHA, with a fillet containing more than 600 mg. Since fish is by far the main food source of DHA, pregnant and breast-feeding women need to eat more of it. In North America, fish is rarely eaten (approximately one serving every ten days), and so not surprisingly the level of DHA in North American breast milk is also very low.

The average Canadian woman only consumes about 80 mg of DHA a day, resulting in only 0.14 percent of the fat in her breast milk being DHA. That's much lower than the DHA level in fortified infant formula. Breast milk is supposed to be the perfect food. These low DHA numbers are alarming, considering the essential effects of DHA in a baby's brain and eye development. To think that it's just a question of eating more fish!

How Much Is Enough?

Experts suggest that getting 300 mg of DHA a day into your diet while breast-feeding can elevate your breast milk levels of DHA. This is based on information from studies where fortified infant formula was given to infants, and the infants showed better mental and visual functioning thanks to the DHA in their diet.

Higher dosages of DHA have also been studied, and it's been found that they have many positive effects on mental development. A Norwegian study found that women who supplemented their diet with 1,183 mg of DHA and 803 mg of EPA per day for a three-month period after delivery (after supplementing at a similar level from week 18 of pregnancy) had children who, at age four, exhibited higher IQ scores.

You can use fish oil supplements or include fish in your diet on a regular basis (at least twice a week). Mackerel is a fatty fish that offers lots of omega-3s. In one fillet of mackerel (about 3 ounces or 90 g), you'll get about 1,250 mg of omega-3 fatty acids. Just remember, not all of that is DHA (or the other important omega-3 fat, EPA).

Help for Preemies

Is your baby premature? He'll benefit from fish oil in his diet. Researchers reported in the *Journal of Pediatrics* in 2004 that when a group of preterm infants (less than thirty-five weeks of gestation) were fed a formula supplemented with long-chain polyunsaturated fatty acids from fish oils (omega-3 fats) and

Jonny's Tasty Tips

Holy mackerel! Mackerel is not only packed with nutrients like DHA, protein, and vitamin B12, it's also low in environmental contaminants, unlike other marine fish. An all-around great choice! There are many types of mackerel, including Pacific, king, Spanish, and cero, but the real star of the show is the Atlantic mackerel, which is on the list of "Best Seafood Choices" on the Oceans Alive website (Oceans Alive is a division of the Environmental Defense Fund). Atlantic mackerel is often used in sashimi, and you can also get it canned, whole, as fillets, and as steaks.

I enjoy mackerel grilled or baked, prepared simply with lemon and organic butter. It also goes well with applesauce or baked in a sauce made from dry apple cider and butter (you can bake small quartered apples with the mackerel in the same sauce). You can even stuff mackerel before baking with a mixture of chopped onion, lemon juice, barley flakes or cubed whole-grain bread, butter or oil, and black pepper or a little chili powder to taste.

borage oils (omega-6 fats), there were improvements in growth and development. The effect was particularly noticeable in boys. Fish oil is a good source of DHA, one of the prominent fats in the brain. Borage oil is a source of arachodonic acid (AA), which helps neuronal development.

Melons

MELONS ARE A GREAT FOOD FOR BREAST- feeding moms. Cantaloupes, honeydew, watermelons—there are so many types of melons you can enjoy. They're full of water, which is a nutrient you really need right now since you're producing close to 2 kilograms (71 ounces) of breast milk every day and breast milk is 90 percent water.

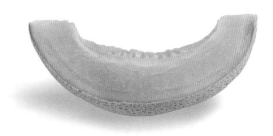

MELONS AT A GLANCE

Serving Size: 1 cup (177 g)	**Calcium:** 1%
Calories: 64	**Vitamin A:** 240%
Saturated Fat: 0 g	**Vitamin C:** 53%
Protein: 1 g	**Iron:** 2%
Fiber: 2 g	

Melons are also good sources of a number of other nutrients, including fiber, niacin, vitamin A, vitamin C, vitamin B6, and folate, all of which work hard to keep you healthy while you're breast-feeding. And they're one of nature's most delicious foods! (Remember, we gave watermelon its own entry on page 76.)

Don't Skip Your Bs

During lactation, your folate needs decrease slightly from the high levels required during pregnancy. This is because your blood volume is decreasing by about 25 percent. But you still need to get your Bs. B vitamins help battle stress and fatigue related to sleep deprivation—a common problem as your newborn tries to settle into a humane sleep schedule. Honeydew melons contain a few B vitamins, including niacin (0.7 mg per cup), folate (34 mcg per cup), and vitamin B6 (0.2 mg per cup). Cantaloupe offers 1.3 mg of niacin, 37 mcg of folate, and 0.1 mg of vitamin B6 per cup.

Enough A for the Two of You

You need more vitamin A than usual—about 4,200 IU per day—when you're breast-feeding. There are so many ways that vitamin A helps your body and your baby's body. Vitamin A is involved in the laying down of new bone, which is rapidly occurring in your growing infant. Vitamin A also helps repair tissues after surgery, an event you may be recovering from after delivery. Vitamin A is an antioxidant and supports a healthy immune system, including the production of immunoglobulins that are transferred from you to your baby in your breast milk. A cup of delicious cantaloupe has about 6,000 IU of vitamin A.

Eat C All Day

Many breast-feeding books discuss the importance of eating healthy foods, including milk, green leafy vegetables, and citrus fruits. The importance of citrus fruits is their vitamin C content. But many other foods are also good sources of vitamin C, including melons. A cup of honeydew melon includes almost half your daily needs of vitamin C, and a cup of cantaloupe has more than 100 percent of your daily needs.

Vitamin C is an antioxidant, so it protects you and your baby from the damaging effects of free radicals. (For more on free radicals, see page 174.) In your skin, vitamin C helps produce collagen, giving the skin structure and strength. Vitamin C also plays a role in the health of the blood vessels and connective tissue in both of your bodies.

The problem with vitamin C is that it is water soluble. That means you can't store it in your body like fat-soluble nutrients such as vitamin A. So you need to eat foods that contain vitamin C throughout the day; just eating one serving of melon in the morning will not cover your vitamin C needs for the entire day. You'll need to toss in some other sources of vitamin C, such as raspberries, kiwi, or red bell pepper.

A Fiber Fix

According to some folks, melons are natural laxatives because of their high water and fiber content. Melon isn't an excellent source of fiber, but it does offer close to 2 g per cup. Fiber is helpful in keeping your bowels moving, which may be a problem after labor, depending on how that all went.

Fiber is also helpful for keeping your blood fat levels low. In your intestinal tract, fiber acts like a sponge to trap fats like cholesterol, reducing the amount your body absorbs. Adding more fiber to your diet on a regular basis can help reduce your absorption of bad fats and improve your cardiovascular health. And healthy blood vessels can transfer nutrients to your mammary glands efficiently, making for optimal breast milk production. Fiber also traps sugar, slowing its absorption into your bloodstream, which can help you feel full longer.

Jonny's Tasty Tips

A slice of ripe cantaloupe or honeydew (or Crenshaw or casaba, for that matter) sprinkled with a little lemon juice is my idea of heaven on earth. Or how about a bowl of multicolored melon balls with a little fresh lemon juice and ginger? But you don't have to keep it simple if you'd rather dress it up. Next time you're grilling, try grilled cantaloupe with a sprinkling of lime juice and chili powder. Or serve ice-cold melon balls or cubes as a cooling counterpoint to a spicy curry.

You can drink your melons, too. Cantaloupe and honeydew make delicious juices. You can mix some cantaloupe juice with watermelon juice and sparkling water for an amazing summer cooler or vary the recipe and add some lemon juice and/or ginger. (If your blender can handle it, you can juice cantaloupe like I do, peel and all.) Honeydew also makes a delicious juice. I love combining it with other melons, sparkling water, and some ginger and mint.

Cantaloupe is delicious in a smoothie too: Blend it with milk and/or yogurt for a sweet, creamy treat. Want to up the fiber ante? Adding a scoop of a high-quality fiber supplement to your smoothie is a great way to get more fiber into your system painlessly. But don't forget: When you add more fiber to your diet, make sure you drink some extra water too!

FAST FACT

Vitamin B6 plays a role in the metabolism of polyunsaturated fats, like DHA, which are needed for the proper development of your baby's rapidly growing brain.

Milk

IT'S TIME TO ORDER SOME MILK WITH YOUR
dinner. While your body is madly trying to produce
milk for your new baby, it's demanding minerals like
calcium, magnesium, and phosphorus from your
bloodstream. If your diet doesn't include enough
of these minerals, your bones will have to give up
some of their stores. Plus, your body needs a lot of
fat and protein to help feed your baby, and milk is a
great source of these nutrients too.

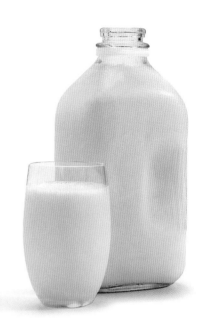

MILK AT A GLANCE

Serving Size: 1 cup (250 ml)	Calcium: 33%
Calories: 102	Vitamin A: 10%
Saturated Fat: 2 g	Vitamin C: 0%
Protein: 8 g	Iron: 0%
Fiber: 0 g	

Make Mine Milk

Researchers from McGill University in Montreal
reported in 2007 that not drinking enough milk during
breast-feeding may result in some nutrient intakes that
are well below those needed for optimal health. The
study involved 175 healthy breast-feeding women who
drank milk throughout the study. They were divided
into two groups; one group drank less than 250 ml
per day, while the others drank more than 250 ml per
day (1 cup or 244 g per day). The researchers found
that drinking less than 250 ml a day compromised
the women's protein and nutrient intakes, and supplements were needed to help their vitamin D and calcium
intakes. The researchers concluded that milk restriction (not drinking enough milk) during pregnancy is not
recommended.

The All-Essential Vitamin D

The first year after birth, a mother's nutritional needs
are great, especially her need for plenty of vitamin D. It
is recommended that all lactating women should take
a supplement that provides 10 mcg of vitamin D per
day, according to the *Journal of Family Health Care*. A
glass of milk offers you about 120 IU of vitamin D, the
equivalent of about 33 percent of an average adult's
daily needs. The current estimate in nutrition textbooks
for the daily needs of vitamin D for a lactating woman
is 5 mcg or 16.5 IU. However, new research is suggesting
that women in the Northern Hemisphere, where sunlight
levels are low, need at least 800 IU per day and most
likely even more. Women who spend little time outside
during the day have even higher needs for vitamin D,
because sunlight is one of the primary sources.

MILK IN YOUR COFFEE DOES *NOT* COUNT!

Caffeine is of less concern during breast-feeding than it was during pregnancy, but it still makes sense not to overdo it. Drinking just one or two caffeine-containing beverages a day during lactation can give your breast milk levels of caffeine that are not considered acceptable. The problem is that too much caffeine in your breast milk can cause your baby to suffer from wakefulness or irritability. It can also cause feeding intolerance and gastrointestinal problems in infants. Choose milk over that espresso for a few more months, and both your baby and your body will thank you.

Crank Up the Calcium

As we've seen, getting too little calcium during pregnancy may limit the amount of calcium available to your baby for growth and bone mineral accumulation. But it's important to get plenty of calcium while you're breast-feeding too. Your diet must contain enough calcium to meet the calcium needs of your breast milk. If your diet does not provide enough calcium in your bloodstream for your lactating needs, your bones will give up some of their precious calcium stores. A cup of milk offers you about a quarter of your daily needs for calcium. You may be wondering if supplements will help fill the gap, but research to date suggests that supplementing your diet with calcium supplements does not appear to increase breast milk concentrations of calcium.

Jonny's Tasty Tips

I'm a big fan of raw milk—it's unmatched for good health. But with doctors recommending that pregnant and lactating women drink pasteurized milk to minimize potential bacterial contamination, I'd suggest that you go for the second-healthiest option: organic milk from grass-fed cows. It's worth heading to the organic aisle if it means protecting your baby from chemicals and added hormones.

What if confronting glass after glass of plain milk isn't your idea of a good time? An easy, delicious way to up the flavor ante is to blend milk with a ripe banana and some crushed ice for a wholesome "shake." Toss in some strawberries for strawberry-banana, a peach for peach-banana, or some mango, ripe cherries—whatever appeals. Yum! Add yogurt if you want a thicker "shake." You can also add milk to creamy soups as a delicious way of getting more. And you can pour it over a bowl of fruit as well as on your oatmeal or other breakfast cereal.

Finally, don't forget my favorite dessert: frozen cherries topped with milk. The milk semifreezes on the cherries to make instant "ice milk." Stir it up and enjoy this healthy homemade version of Cherry Garcia!

VEGETARIANS AND CALCIUM

It can be a challenge for breast-feeding vegetarian women to get the recommended amount of calcium through diet. If you eat eggs and dairy products, you should aim for five to six servings of dairy products and one serving of eggs every day to help you meet your protein and calcium needs. You should also eat more whole grains and legumes, since these contain lots of nutrients found in meat. If you're a vegan or if milk consumption is minimized in your diet for any reason, try to eat more tofu, legumes, nuts, seeds, and leafy green vegetables, which all contain some calcium, and discuss your diet with your health-care provider so he or she can recommend an appropriate supplement.

BOTTLING UP MILK

Heating up a baby's bottle is a task women have done for generations. However, this seemingly natural chore may be putting your baby at risk. Plastic baby bottles contain a compound called bisphenol A (BPA). This chemical is thought to pose a risk to our health, as it may interrupt hormonal action, leading to harmful effects, particularly in developing infants. The main sources of exposure for newborns and infants to BPA are polycarbonate (plastic) baby bottles when they are exposed to high temperatures and cans of infant formula. Consumers can opt for baby bottles that do not contain BPA, including glass bottles.

Bones at Risk

Does breast-feeding put you at a greater risk of developing bone problems like osteoporosis? Studies show that lactation can both benefit and adversely affect bone mass. The research suggests that calcium intake during lactation, duration of lactation, and age at lactation are linked to bone mass. Breast-feeding requires a lot of calcium, which will be drawn from your bones, but never fear—it appears to be fully restored within six months after weaning. Plus, pregnant and lactating women may absorb calcium better than nonpregnant women. And some studies suggest that there may be a link between long-term bone health and breast-feeding. It is recommended that pregnant women make sure that their diet is rich in calcium sources so they and their babies are both getting enough. Milk is a great source of calcium (about 275 mg per cup). See the chart on page 12 for other good food sources of calcium.

Special Proteins

Milk is a great source of protein for your body. Your breast milk also contains protein. All in all, your daily protein needs are now 12 to 15 g more than an average woman of your age needs. A glass of milk can help you get these extra grams—one cup provides 8 g of protein. One particular type of amino acid (the building blocks of proteins) in milk may be particularly beneficial to your growing baby: L-carnitine. L-carnitine is naturally found in breast milk. It is an antioxidant and plays a key role in energy production. You can get L-carnitine into your diet by including red meats and dairy products. Some infants, particularly preterm infants, can have trouble producing L-carnitine, which has resulted in the inclusion of this amino acid in infant formulas.

Many nutritionists—notably Robert Crayton, M.S., author of *The Carnitine Miracle*—consider carnitine an extremely important nutrient for both you and your baby. If you're not a big meat-eater or if you're a vegetarian, you might want to consider carnitine supplements.

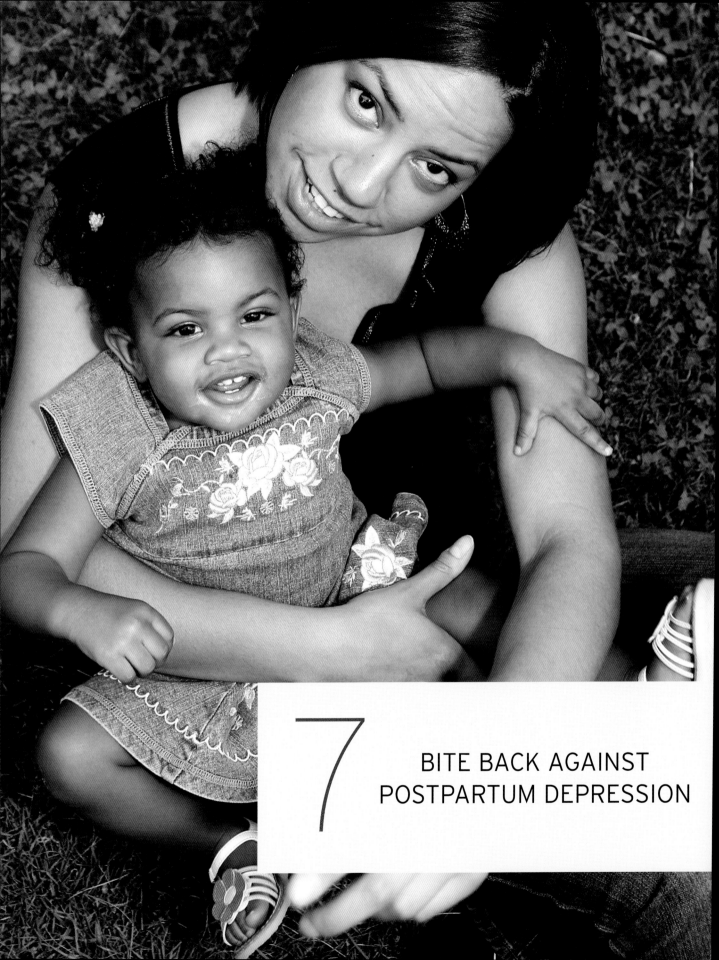

7

BITE BACK AGAINST POSTPARTUM DEPRESSION

MOST PREGNANCY BOOKS WILL HAVE

ended by now. But there is so much going on in your body in the postpartum phase (that's the technical term for the time after birth) that it simply can't be ignored. It took your body forty weeks to create that giant belly and produce a baby. You can't expect to ignore your body now! It has a whole new set of needs: Your belly needs to rebound to its prepregnancy shape, your uterus has to make a drastic recovery, and your muscles and skin need to repair themselves after all the stretching and abuse they have taken.

Your body needs some tender loving care, and you can offer it that by making some healthy food choices during your postpartum months. And we're sure you know that depression is a concern during the postpartum stage. Estimates say that postpartum depression occurs in anywhere from 3 to 20 percent of mothers. There is no known cause of postpartum depression. But considering the major life change you have just endured, wild hormonal fluctuations, and your inevitable fatigue thanks to the irregular sleeping patterns of your baby, it is not surprising that new mothers would have some emotional highs and lows.

BABY BLUES

Having a baby is challenging, both physically and emotionally. It is natural for many new mothers to have mood swings after delivery, feeling joyful one minute and depressed the next. These feelings are sometimes known as the "baby blues," and they often go away within 10 days of delivery. However, some women may experience a deep and ongoing depression that lasts much longer. This is called postpartum depression.

Researchers have identified three types of postpartum depression: baby blues, postpartum depression, and postpartum psychosis. (Make a note: The psychotic part is pretty rare.) The most common—and minor—form of postpartum depression is the baby blues. We know it may not feel "minor" to you while you're in it, but trust us. It's experienced by most new mothers (estimates are 50 to 80 percent of women), and it will pass. It usually starts one to three days after delivery and is characterized by weeping, irritability, lack of sleep, mood changes, and a feeling of vulnerability. These "blues" can last several weeks.

Postpartum Depression

Postpartum depression is more than the occasional crying jag. It is characterized by changing mood, anxiety, fatigue, irritability, depression, panic, and sleep disorders. Physical symptoms include headaches, numbness, chest pain, and hyperventilation. A woman with postpartum depression may regard her child with ambivalence, negativity, or disinterest. Sadly, the result can be a lack of bonding between the mother and her baby. The first symptoms usually appear between the fourth and sixth week after delivery (postpartum). However, postpartum depression can start from the moment of birth or may result from a depression that's evolved continuously since pregnancy began.

Postpartum psychosis is a relatively rare disorder. The symptoms include extreme confusion, fatigue, agitation, alterations in mood, feelings of hopelessness and shame, hallucinations, and rapid speech or mania. Studies indicate that it affects only one in 1,000 women after the birth of their babies. Good news: If you're wondering if you have it, you probably don't.

Risk Factors

There is no single known cause of postpartum depression, but some factors can predispose you to this condition. The changes in hormone levels that occur during pregnancy and immediately after childbirth are almost certainly a factor. The stress of being a new mother, particularly if the experience does not match the mother's expectations, can also be a factor that triggers depression.

But that's not all. Severe premenstrual syndrome (PMS), a difficult relationship, lack of a support network, and stressful events during pregnancy or after delivery can also trigger depression. Having a history of miscarriages or obstetric complications may also be factors. Women who have experienced depression before becoming pregnant or who have experienced postpartum depression in a previous pregnancy appear to have a higher risk of developing it again.

Researchers have looked at age, birthing practices, and many other factors, and no one factor is known to cause postpartum depression. Today, experts believe that postpartum depression is the result of many complex factors. However, it's important to realize that nothing you do will bring on postpartum depression—it's simply not your fault. Listen to your body and take care of yourself, and if you're concerned about postpartum depression, be sure to talk to your obstetrician or health-care provider.

FOOD AND YOUR MOOD

Diet is thought to be at least partially related to risk of developing postpartum depression. Many studies have investigated the dietary intakes of women before labor and their incidence of postpartum depression. A few foods have surfaced as potential factors in the development (or avoidance) of postpartum depression. For example, high-glycemic foods may contribute to the *development* of postpartum depression, while omega-3 fats may help you *avoid* it.

FAST FACT

Rates of postpartum depression are fifty times higher in countries where women do not eat fish. Even homicide, murder, and suicide rates are linked to low intakes of fish.

FAST FACT

Research has shown that women in countries with higher fish consumption, such as Japan, Hong Kong, Sweden, and Chile, have the lowest levels of postpartum depression, while women in countries with the lowest fish consumption, including Brazil, South Africa, West Germany, and Saudi Arabia, have the highest rates of postpartum depression.

Omega-3s for a Happy Me

Omega-3 fatty acids are called "the happy fats" and "the Prozac of the Sea." The brain naturally contains a lot of a type of omega-3 fatty acid called docosahexaenoic acid (DHA). When your brain has lots of this good fat in it, it works optimally, offering you mental clarity and a healthy mood.

Researchers have been able to link our intake of these healthy fats with depression. Experts from the National Institutes of Health found that countries with the highest fish consumption (Japan, Taiwan, and Korea) have the lowest rates of depression. Countries with the lowest fish consumption (New Zealand, Canada, West Germany, France, and the United States) have the highest rates of depression.

As a new mother, you have spent the last forty weeks selectively sending DHA to your growing baby. The fetus and newborn infant depend on their mother for a supply of DHA through the placenta and later from breast milk. This makes your dietary intake of these fats very important during the last trimester of pregnancy and during this postpartum period. It appears that if a mother's diet is lacking in DHA, she is likely to be deficient postpartum, increasing her risks of developing postpartum depression.

There is a growth spurt in your baby's brain during the last trimester of pregnancy and the first postnatal months, so you need certain nutrients, like DHA and another important fat, arachidonic acid (AA), in your diet during pregnancy and breast-feeding to support your baby's needs to make these new brain cells. Eating fish, the best source of the omega-3 fatty acid DHA, is an important part of a healthy postpartum diet. Currently, studies suggest that women consume about 300 mg of DHA a day during pregnancy, lactation, and in the postpartum period to enjoy optimal health.

Low levels of DHA in your diet will not just affect your brain, it will affect your baby's too. In 2001, Norwegian researchers reported a study involving 590 pregnant women who were given either 10 ml of cod liver oil or corn oil to see what effect these fats had on infant brain development and function. Cod liver oil is a good source of DHA, with about 1,183 mg of DHA per 10 ml.

Recently there has been some concern that the vitamin A and vitamin D in cod liver oil are not optimally balanced, which can reduce some of the wonderful health effects of vitamin D. We recommend that you stick with high-quality fish oil or fish oil capsules.

The research findings indicated that the availability of these fats to a growing baby is based on the levels available in the mother via placenta or breast milk. In other words, if there aren't enough good fats in your diet to meet your body's needs, your baby may not be getting enough. The researchers took information from the mothers of 251 of the infants at 3 months of age and discovered that the women who took the fish oil supplement had higher levels of DHA in their breast milk. At age 4, the children were tested to see how the fish oil affected their cognitive function. Only 90 children were tested at age 4, but the results were amazing. The researchers found that the children of mothers who took the fish oil supplement had higher scores for mental processing tasks such as thinking, awareness, and judgment.

Candy's not Dandy after Labor

Researchers from the University of Tokyo suggest that postpartum depression may be due to a sudden fall in insulin levels after delivery. The sudden fall in insulin levels is thought to be caused by a decrease in the level of serotonin (your feel-good hormone) in the brain. This condition may be alleviated by eating foods that have a high glycemic index. Foods with a high glycemic index are foods that send a lot of sugar to your bloodstream quickly. The researchers hypothesized that eating high-glycemic foods would stimulate insulin production.

To test this hypothesis, the researchers conducted a study that involved 865 Japanese women to see if the glycemic index of their diets was related to their risk of developing postpartum depression. If you're already reaching for a candy bar, you'll be disappointed to learn that this study failed to find a convincing link between the two. At first glance, you might think that eating something sweet after labor could help you ward off postpartum depression, but the answer is not likely to be that simple. Remember that a healthy insulin level can be attained (and maintained) with a diet that is rich in vegetables, seeds, nuts, beans, and grains. Foods that are high in fiber and rich in nutrients are always a healthy choice.

OTHER ISSUES

Between adjusting to a new baby in the house and the major disruption it makes in your routines and sleep patterns and experiencing a whole new range of changes in your body, you have plenty to deal with. Worrying about your weight, fighting fatigue, concerns about your parenting abilities—no wonder many new mothers feel overwhelmed and depressed. Let's take a closer look at these issues.

Weight Worries

After the birth of your baby, it's natural to worry about your weight. Some women will find that their body quickly returns to its original appearance, while others will find that the change takes a lot longer. If you remember that it took your body nine months to make the miraculous changes from your normal body to full-term pregnancy, you may start to relax your expectations about getting your prepregnancy body back quickly. In the postpartum, experts say that you may safely lose about four to five pounds each month without reducing your milk supply; however, you need

THE GLYCEMIC IMPACT

The glycemic index and the glycemic load are measures of how fast a food will cause your blood sugar to rise. (The glycemic load is a better measure than the index but is harder to find. For the purposes of this book, we'll use them interchangeably.) Foods with a low glycemic impact (load or index) tend to be high in fiber and cause slow increases in blood sugar levels.

Low-glycemic-impact foods are healthy choices for people with diabetes, because they tend to keep blood sugar levels relatively low, even, and controlled. High-glycemic-impact foods cause a rapid, sharp increase in blood sugar levels (and generally a crash in energy shortly afterward). Sugary cereals, white bread, rice, pasta, and sugar are examples of high-glycemic-impact foods. Vegetables, on the other hand, are almost all low glycemic impact.

to eat at least the minimum number of recommended servings from each food group. Remember: Weight loss should be gradual.

Feeling Sluggish?

If you have had surgery before, you know how tiring it can be. For some women, labor involves surgery, typically a Cesarean section. Imagine being faced with that same level of fatigue you know comes with surgery *and* a newborn to take care of! For some women, the idea of this is so overwhelming that it can lead to feelings of depression.

Even if you don't require surgery, giving birth will leave you feeling drained. Not having a lot of energy can make the best of us feel moody and depressed. And unfortunately, fatigue is a major part of the first weeks of the postpartum stage. Sleep will combat fatigue, but you may not be finding much of that these days, either. An alternative is to eat energizing foods, such as mushrooms, which are packed with B vitamins.

As your baby begins to sleep in a more humane pattern, you'll be able to sleep more yourself. But you'll probably still suffer from some fatigue. This isn't surprising when you consider how much your body has been through. Lingering fatigue may also be caused by low iron levels. Reaching for foods that are high in iron, like apricots, can help. Check out the many energizing foods we've focused on in previous chapters as well.

Your diet postpartum is just as important as your diet during pregnancy. Your body is working hard to produce breast milk, shrink your uterus, realign all of your organs, and repair your stretched and sore muscles and skin. Not to mention that as your baby grows you'll need to build strong muscles to carry him, and you'll also need to develop a new level of endurance to keep up with him!

So rather than obsessing about your weight, focus on continuing to eat a healthy and balanced diet during your postpartum days. In particular, don't let your worries about weight cause you to skip those healthy-fat foods, like avocados, olive oil, and fish. Remember that some fats are good for you, and that fat in your diet helps you absorb fat-soluble vitamins like vitamin A, E, D, and K. You'll need these vitamins over the next few months as your body slowly gets back into shape.

What Should You Feed Them?

With their new babies home and getting bigger by the day, many women find themselves feeling overwhelmed with concerns that they won't be good enough parents. Part of this concern is providing your child with the right nutrition as he or she grows. And yes, your baby is now growing into an infant, and with each stage of growth, his or her dietary needs change.

For the first few months of life, your baby's development follows the same pattern as it did in your last trimester of pregnancy (see chapter 3, beginning on page 124, for the best third-trimester foods). Chapter 6, beginning on page 240, discusses foods to help you with breast-feeding and highlights your baby's nutrient needs as he reaches six months of age. If you're curious about what to feed your growing infant as he gets older, remember that he's continuing to grow and develop as he has all along. His brain is still developing, his bones are growing, and his immune system is developing. The same nutrients that were important for your baby during pregnancy and breast-feeding are important later, too.

This means that the same foods you ate throughout your pregnancy can be the basis of a healthy diet for your growing infant. For example, milk and other dairy products have been an important part of your diet from the first trimester through breast-feeding. It's not surprising that milk is important for infants and kids too. A study of children and teens (ages five through seventeen) found that those who drank milk at noon met or exceeded the recommended daily intake of calcium, compared to the children who drank soft drinks, juice, or fruit drinks at lunchtime. Pack some milk into your child's diet and consider milk for yourself at lunch during your postpartum and breast-feeding months to ensure that you're getting enough calcium too. You can work with your infant and your pediatrician to decide which foods and nutrients are best for your baby's various stages of development.

While your child is an infant, it can be easy to find alternatives that she'll like to eat to ensure that she's still getting enough of the right nutrients. However, as she grows and spends more time at daycare or at school, it can be harder to control her diet. This is when some mothers start to wonder if they should give their children multivitamins. Of course, you should discuss this with your pediatrician, but research suggests that it's a smart move.

A study published in the *Archives of Pediatric & Adolescent Medicine* found that nearly a third of children ages two to seventeen in the United States take a multivitamin or other vitamin or mineral supplement. Sadly, they also found that those in most need are the least likely to take supplements. The data used to create this report was taken from the National Health and Nutrition Examination Survey, which also found that many children and adolescents in the United States fail to consume recommended amounts of vitamins E, C, and A, as well as calcium and magnesium. A daily multivitamin could affordably and safely help fill these nutrient gaps.

HELP FOR PICKY EATERS

If your infant becomes a picky eater, do not fear. In this book, we have identified a wide range of healthy foods you can use to tempt him. For example, if your child develops an aversion to meat, reread the sections on alternative sources of protein such as tahini, lentils, milk, and cheese. You're already armed with lots of options to help you work with your child's changing food preferences.

FAST FACT

The same nutrients that were important for your baby during pregnancy and breast-feeding are also important during infancy and childhood.

Top Foods for the Postpartum Period

The postpartum period is as important a time to eat healthy as pregnancy or conception—so dig in! We've already covered a lot of different foods that offer your body healthy nutrients that will help it work right, and heal quickly after giving birth. There are a few foods that offer you extra nutritional help in the postpartum period, so we saved them for this chapter. But, remember that all 100 healthy foods in this book are good choices for you in this postpartum period.

HERE ARE THE 6 BEST FOODS FOR TO HELP YOU BITE AGAINST POSTPARTUM DEPRESSION:

- APRICOTS
- CRABMEAT
- LENTILS
- QUINOA
- SARDINES
- SHIITAKE MUSHROOMS

Let's look at each of these foods and see what gives them their depression-fighting power. And yes, Jonny's here to help you learn to love sardines and prepare delicious quinoa dishes. Just look for "Jonny's Tasty Tips."

Apricots

NEED A HEALTHY SNACK THAT YOU CAN EAT ON

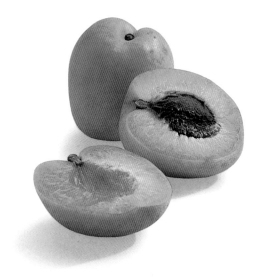

the go? These days, you probably don't have a lot of time to prepare food. In fact, many new moms joke that they're lucky if they can fit a shower into their day. Apricots are the answer! Dried apricots are portable and will even travel well in a diaper bag. They're a great snack choice for you in your postpartum months, since they're packed with fiber, antioxidants, and iron—all of which your body is craving these days.

APRICOTS AT A GLANCE

Serving Size: 1 cup (100 g)	**Calcium:** 7%
Calories: 313	**Vitamin A:** 94%
Saturated Fat: 0 g	**Vitamin C:** 2%
Protein: 4 g	**Iron:** 19%
Fiber: 9 g	

Note: The nutritional facts data provided in this chapter are approximations based on the foods' nutrient value and an adult woman's RDA.

FAST FACT

The iron in animal products is most easily absorbed by your body, so be sure to include the meats featured in other chapters of this book, as well as the crabmeat and sardines in this chapter, to help increase your iron stores.

Adding Iron

If you had a significant amount of blood loss as a result of delivery, you may feel especially weak and tired or short of breath. You may also have a poor appetite. The loss of blood has depleted the iron in your body. Luckily, many foods can help you increase your iron stores, including meat (chicken, fish, and beef), vegetables, beans, and dried fruits. Eating foods that are high in iron can help your body form new red blood cells. Red blood cells are needed to transport oxygen to your cells, so you can get energized and keep up with your new-mom duties. Foods like apricots, crabmeat, sardines, and lentils are great sources of iron.

Jonny's Tasty Tips

An apricot is basically a tasty little low-calorie bundle of nutrients put together in a beautiful, sun-colored package. What's not to like? If you've never tried a raw apricot, get ready for a luscious flavor burst. But make sure you choose ripe fruit!

Look for apricots with a rich orange color. Avoid those that are pale and yellow. Fruits should be slightly soft. If an apricot is too firm, it may not have been tree ripened. Tree-ripened fruits taste better and contain more antioxidants. Research conducted at the University of Innsbruck in Austria suggests that as fruits fully ripen, almost to the point of spoilage, their antioxidant levels actually increase.

Another way I like to eat apricots is stewed. No need to sweeten them; just put the dried fruit in a pan with a little water until they plump up and soften. They're delicious as is or stirred into yogurt, cottage cheese, or oatmeal.

Better Absorption

For optimal iron absorption, be sure to eat a food that contains vitamin C with your iron source. For example, eat some spinach with your fish or some citrus fruit with your crabmeat. The great thing about apricots is that they contain both iron and vitamin C, helping ensure that your body can fully absorb these great nutrients.

Superhero Snack

Apricots are packed with antioxidants. Antioxidants help protect your body from damage by free radicals. Free radicals form in your body when you're stressed, exposed to sunlight, and when you use cleaning and cosmetic products. In other words, they are part of your everyday life. Apricots contain beta-carotene, a type of vitamin A that is a potent antioxidant. Vitamin A is needed for cell growth, development, and repair, making it a very important nutrient for you and your baby at this time. A cup of apricots has almost your full day's needs of vitamin A.

Apricots also contain lycopene, another antioxidant. Lycopene is best known for its ability to support prostate health (share your apricots with your spouse!) and to prevent cholesterol oxidation in your arteries, which can lead to heart disease. Population studies show that eating lots of lycopene can lower your risk of cancer. This powerful antioxidant can help protect your body from a lot of diseases, making it a healthy choice no matter what age you are.

IRON BLOCKERS

Certain foods prevent your body from absorbing iron. Black tea is an example because it contains tannic acid, which can decrease iron absorption. Milk can also affect your ability to absorb iron, so try to drink your milk at a time separate from your iron-rich foods.

Crab Meat

WHILE TAKING CARE OF YOUR NEWBORN, remember to take care of yourself. Good nutrition will provide you with the energy you need to keep up with the demands of your new baby, and it can aid in restoring your prepregnancy shape. Eating foods that contain protein can help. Crabmeat is an easy food to add into your diet during this hectic time. Plus, it contains lots of nutrients to help your body recover after pregnancy.

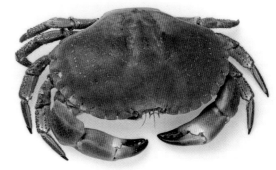

CRABSMEAT AT A GLANCE

Serving Size: 1 cup (135 g)	Calcium: 14%
Calories: 134	Vitamin A: 0%
Saturated Fat: 0 g	Vitamin C: 6%
Protein: 28 g	Iron: 5%
Fiber: 0 g	

More Protein

A cup of crabmeat contains 28 g of protein. That's a lot. Your body really needs protein these days. You need even more protein to breast-feed than you did during pregnancy. Plus, your muscles and skin are trying hard to get back into shape, and they need protein to get there.

Unfortunately, crabmeat is also high in cholesterol, with about 120 mg per cup, making it a fattier meat choice. So it isn't a food that you should eat frequently (once a week is probably enough). But tossing crabmeat into your salad every now and then as an alternative to sardines, tuna, or beans can keep your diet interesting and help keep it simple during these time-strapped days.

Mega Minerals

One of the advantages to including seafood in your diet is that you get to enjoy the benefits of minerals. Crabmeat is a good source of zinc, copper, and selenium. These three minerals are all vital to your health. They are all antioxidants, helping keep your body healthy and free of damage from free radicals. Zinc is also important as your baby's brain continues to grow and develop. Your body will selectively pull zinc from you to ensure that there's enough in your breast milk for your baby's needs. Thus, it's important to get some extra zinc in your own diet, particularly if you're breast-feeding. A cup of crabmeat contains about a third of your daily zinc needs.

You may think of copper in terms of pennies, but your body needs it, too. Copper can help protect your skin and your baby's skin from the harmful effects of sunlight. Copper is part of many enzymes in your body,

Jonny's Tasty Tips

You can eat crabmeat any way you'd prepare lobster or shrimp: grilled with a splash of lime; in a crab "cocktail" with lettuce, lemon juice, and hot sauce; or cold in a salad. (Topping a salad with crabmeat is coauthor Allison's favorite way to enjoy it.) And of course, you can make crab cakes (but, please, bake them, don't fry them!). But crabmeat's flavor is so delicate that I hate to disguise it with heavier seasonings. A splash of lemon juice is just about right!

and enzymes are the key that unlocks the gates of various types of metabolism. Copper also aids in forming red blood cells, and you may need to restock your red blood cell levels if you lost blood during labor. A cup of crabmeat has almost half of your daily needs of copper.

Selenium is one of those minerals we tend to ignore, but it plays crucial roles in our body. In particular, selenium stimulates your immune system's antibody response. A strong immune system will help you stay energized and healthy so you can enjoy every moment of your infant's discovery of the world. Every smile, every laugh, and every surprised look on your little one's face is important! Enjoy them with the help of the 43 mcg of selenium in a cup of crabmeat.

Get Some Get Up and Go

One of the advantages of including meat in your diet postpartum is that it contains vitamin B12. This vitamin is commonly called the energy vitamin. People who have low levels of vitamin B12 in their diet tend to feel sluggish (a common problem for vegetarians). This is because vitamin B12 is involved in energy production. It helps your body use the carbohydrates, protein, and fat in your diet and make energy out of them. A cup of crabmeat can contain anywhere from 10 to 100 percent of your daily vitamin B12 intake, depending on which type of crab you're eating. Blue crab is thought to be one type that offers more vitamin B12.

Happy Fats

Crab is not a great source of omega-3 fatty acids, the happy fats, but it does contain some (about 430 mg per cup). Research supporting the beneficial effects of omega-3 on mood is outstanding and very convincing. Eating more seafood has been found to even help students remain calm and less hostile during exam periods. If it can work on teenagers, imagine its ability to help keep your mood stable as your infant throws another spoonful of tomato sauce off her high chair and across the kitchen.

Evidence supporting the ability of omega-3 fatty acids to help reduce the risk of postpartum depression is also impressive. Crab may be a great alternative for those of you with aversions to fish that have a "fishy" taste, since crabmeat has a deliciously mild, buttery flavor. The best sources of these happy fats are salmon, mackerel, tuna, anchovies, and sardines.

Lentils

WOMEN OFTEN AVOID DRIED LEGUMES LIKE beans and lentils for fear that they will cause embarrassing flatulence. But after being through the increased flatulence associated with pregnancy, you may have learned to deal with the issue. Legumes are one of the healthiest foods on earth. They are packed with minerals, protein, fiber, and vitamins.

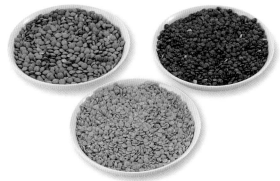

LENTILS AT A GLANCE

Serving Size: 1 cup (198 g)	**Calcium:** 4%
Calories: 230	**Vitamin A:** 0%
Saturated Fat: 0 g	**Vitamin C:** 5%
Protein: 18 g	**Iron:** 65%
Fiber: 16 g	

Lentils in particular are a great food choice during your postpartum months to ensure your diet is packed with the nutrients you need to repair your body, stay happy, and keep up with your new-mom duties. And here's more good news: Unlike beans, lentils don't contain sulfur, so they don't produce gas and won't cause flatulence.

Postpartum Fatigue

Although individuals of all ages and both genders are at risk for developing fatigue, postpartum fatigue is particularly challenging. As a new mother, you have so many demands on you and such important tasks to accomplish during this period of time. Postpartum fatigue may impact your ability to perform your new maternal role and may place you at increased risk for postpartum depression.

Some key nutrients help fight fatigue: vitamin B12, iron, and protein being the main three. Lentils are a poor source of vitamin B12, but they are a great vegetarian source of iron and protein. There are almost 7 mg of iron in a cup of lentils. Fatigue can be caused by low iron levels, and women of childbearing age, particularly new moms, are at a higher risk of having low iron levels in their bodies.

Iron helps your blood cells carry oxygen around your body. Without oxygen your cells can't make energy, and you'd be left dragging your feet to that change table and back. Plus, a lack of energy can add to feelings of depression, so be sure to include foods that contain iron and protein, like lentils, that will help you bite back against postpartum depression.

Keep Going

Lentils are a delicious and filling side dish, but there's no need to push lentils to the side of your plate. They contain enough protein to be your main dish. There are

18 g of protein in a cup of lentils. You can even enjoy that amount of lentils in a lentil soup. Why is protein so important during the postpartum stage? Protein is essential to helping you feel energized and feeling good. Women typically do not eat enough protein, and after birth and during lactation, your body needs more protein than ever. Try adding legumes like lentils to your diet and get the protein you need to keep going.

Crucial Minerals

Recent understanding of infant development during the first year of life has raised awareness about the importance of iron and zinc. These two minerals are essential for proper growth and development in your infant. Fortunately, the breast (mammary gland) has a remarkable ability to adapt if your body is deficient in or has too much iron, copper, and zinc. In fact, the breast can control concentrations of these minerals in breast milk. But eating foods like apricots, crabmeat, and lentils can help ensure that your diet contains sufficient amounts of these minerals. Lentils contain almost 7 mg of iron (over one-third of your daily needs), 2.5 mg of zinc (about 20 percent of your daily needs), and 0.5 mg of copper (about a quarter of your daily needs).

Filling You Up

Getting back to your prepregnancy body is a key priority for many mothers. However, this process needs to occur slowly to allow your body time to heal after pregnancy and ensure you are not lacking any nutrients you need to conduct your duties as a new mom. However, certain foods can help you lose weight sensibly even while you're breast-feeding. These foods are well known to support healthy weight loss. High-fiber foods, especially, are great additions to your diet if you want to naturally shed a few pounds.

Lentils, vegetables, and whole-grain pastas are examples of foods that are naturally high in fiber. In fact, there are 16 g of fiber in a cup of lentils. Fiber has many health benefits, including improving your bowel movement frequency and lowering your blood cholesterol levels and sugar levels too. Fiber also helps make you feel full and satisfied after a meal. Add more high-fiber foods like lentils to your diet and enjoy both satisfaction and some healthy weight loss.

Studies have found that insoluble fiber (cellulose, hemicellulose, and lignin), which are kinds of fiber that can't be dissolved in water, may reduce the risk of obesity. The other type of fiber, soluble fiber, may also help you shed those unwanted pounds. It is thought that fiber reduces the glycemic response in your body. The glycemic response is how much your blood sugar rises after you eat a food. If your blood sugar rises to only moderate levels and does so slowly, you feel more satisfied (full), so you tend to want to eat less food. High-fiber foods can really help you fight cravings, so they can help control how much you eat—a healthy way to lose weight in your postpartum months.

Studies agree. Researchers from Saint Joan University Hospital in Spain reported a study that involved 200 overweight and obese people. They were given a mixture containing fiber or a placebo two or three times daily for four months. The researchers found that weight loss was higher in those that took the fiber (9.9 to 10.1 pounds or 4.5 to 4.6 kg lost) compared to the placebo group (lost 1.76 pounds or 0.8 kg). In addition, satiety (fullness) increased after people consumed the fiber-rich meals. Legumes like lentils are packed with fiber and are a healthy way to help you lose some of that unwanted baby weight.

Lentils for Weight Loss

Data from the National Health and Nutrition Examination survey found that people who included legumes like lentils and beans in their diets weighed an average of 7 pounds (3 kg) less and were 22 percent less likely to be obese than people who didn't eat legumes. The legume-eaters' diets were more nutrient rich, containing more protein, fiber, potassium, niacin, folate, iron, zinc, copper, and magnesium. Their diets also included less fat and sugar. Adding lentils to your postpartum diet can help you shed some unwanted pounds and keep you smiling as you step on the scale.

Quinoa

QUINOA (PRONOUNCED KEEN-WAH) IS AN amino acid-rich seed with a fluffy, creamy texture once cooked. Packed with nutrients that can help your postpartum body recover its shape and fight depression, quinoa is a healthy food for your postpartum months. Plus, it's convenient. You can cook large amounts of quinoa and save the leftovers in the fridge. Then just mix in your favorite raw veggies to make a fast, protein-rich salad any time you need it. With all the spitting up, dirty diaper changing, and games to play, you'll appreciate a healthy, quick, easy lunch that bites back against postpartum depression.

QUINOA AT A GLANCE

Serving Size: 1 cup (185 g), cooked	Calcium: 3%
Calories: 222	Vitamin A: 0%
Saturated Fat: 0 g	Vitamin C: 0%
Protein: 8 g	Iron: 15%
Fiber: 5 g	

Boost Some Super Antioxidants

Quinoa is a very good source of manganese and copper, both of which help your body and your infant through this period of repair and growth. Manganese and copper are cofactor minerals for superoxide dismutase, a potent antioxidant enzyme that protects your body from free-radical damage. In a quarter-cup of uncooked quinoa (which yields three-quarters to one cup cooked), you'll get about half of your daily needs for manganese and 17 percent of your daily requirement for copper.

Zinc Bites Back

Quinoa is an excellent source of zinc. Zinc is an essential mineral involved in more than three hundred different reactions in your body. It can be found in oysters, lean meats, beans, nuts, and whole grains like quinoa. This important antioxidant and anti-inflammatory agent assists your body with the repairs it is working on and is vital to your infant's development.

Most important, zinc is helpful during your postpartum months because it can help bite back against depression. Zinc is involved in the metabolism of omega-3 fatty acids. Omega-3 fatty acids are a major fat in your brain, and having high amounts of omega-3s in your diet is linked to low rates of postpartum depression. Eating fish is a great way to get omega-3s in your diet, but don't forget the zinc. Eat your quinoa!

Jonny's Tasty Tips

Quinoa is one of those foods that's always getting miscategorized—everyone thinks it's a grain and everyone uses it like a grain, but it's actually a seed. Anyway, who really cares? You know how the old saying goes...if it looks like a grain and it acts like a grain...same principle.

So how do you eat quinoa, anyway? You can use quinoa to make flour, soup, or breakfast cereal. Noted natural-foods expert and author Rebecca Wood suggests cooking about 2 cups of stock or water per cup of quinoa, which should yield about 3 cups of cooked grain and take only about 15 minutes to prepare. She reminds us that it's as versatile as rice (and, in my opinion, a good deal better for us) and can be substituted for rice in any recipe or used as a side dish.

Full of Fiber

When grains are processed, they lose precious vitamins and minerals, such as zinc, selenium, and vitamin B6, all of which your body needs right now. Foods made from processed grains (such as white bread) are also devoid of fiber. Fortunately, quinoa is a whole grain, meaning that all of its nutrients—including fiber—are intact. In fact, in just one cup of cooked quinoa, you'll find more than 5 g of fiber, which is about 20 percent of your daily needs.

FOOD AND MOOD

You probably have heard that food affects your mood. It's true! What you eat will affect how you feel—big time! Many people will notice that they can feel moody, irritable, and even depressed when they're hungry. Even eating certain foods can affect your mood. Eating fatty foods can make you feel sluggish and tired. What you eat will affect how you feel. As you are trying to eat to keep your mood positive and avoid postpartum depression, be sure to focus on healthy foods. In particular, fiber is very helpful. High-fiber meals make you feel satisfied and happy. Quinoa and other whole-grain foods are great sources of fiber to help keep you feeling full and keep your mood uplifted.

★ Sardines

FAST, CONVENIENT, AND PACKED WITH nutrients that can help you bite back against postpartum depression, sardines are the ultimate postpartum food. Let's face it: You won't have a lot of time to cook with your new little one at home—particularly if this isn't your first baby and you have older siblings to take care of too. Sardines can be quickly prepared (some by simply opening a can) and added to your favorite dish as a great source of protein, iron, calcium, and the ultimate postpartum nutrient: DHA.

SARDINES AT A GLANCE

Serving Size: 1 can (3.75 oz., 92 g)	Calcium: 35%
Calories: 190	Vitamin A: 2%
Saturated Fat: 1 g	Vitamin C: 0%
Protein: 23 g	Iron: 15%
Fiber: 0 g	

FAST FACT

Studies have found that women who supplement with DHA and eicosapentaenoic acid (EPA) have a lower risk of developing postpartum depression.

DHA and Depression

Your body's levels of DHA may predict your risk of developing depression. When researchers have looked at the amount of DHA in a mother's breast milk and the amount of seafood the mother ate, they discovered that DHA was associated with postpartum depression. Eating little seafood in the diet can lead to low levels of DHA in the mother. And low levels of DHA in the mother is linked to a higher rate of postpartum depression. It's time to order some sardines on your next pizza and bite back against postpartum depression.

Of course, it's more than just your seafood consumption. Pregnant and breast-feeding women, as well as women in their postpartum months, are at the greatest risk for having low DHA levels in their body. This is because a mother's body selectively transfers docosahexaenoic acid (DHA) to the fetus to support optimal development of the baby's neurological system during pregnancy. But if women don't consume enough DHA during their pregnancy, their body's stores can

Jonny's Tasty Tips

I call sardines "health food in a can." I learned to fork them up straight from the can from my friend, the great New York nutritionist and author Dr. Oz Garcia, and they're still one of my favorite pick-me-up snacks.

Look for sardines packed in their own oil. They're harder to find, but worth it. Do *not* be afraid of the fat–it's good stuff! If you can't find them in sardine oil, olive oil is a perfectly fine substitute. Do not–repeat, do *not*–buy the kind that's packed in vegetable oil, which simply loads them up with highly inflammatory omega-6 fats from a heavily processed oil that does nothing good for you. Even sardines packed in tomato or mustard sauce are a better choice than sardines packed in vegetable oil. Put those sardines to work for you today!

THE OTHER HEALTHY FATS

Two other fats are thought to support brain health: arachidonic acid (AA) and eicosapentaenoic acid (EPA). These fats can also be found in fish. However, when consumption of these fats was investigated by the National Institutes of Health, they found that AA and EPA levels of the mother's milk were not related to postpartum depression rates. Still, depression isn't the whole picture, so for healthy brain function and the best shot at mental acuity (aka high IQ), make sure you're getting a rich supply of all the important fatty acids from fish like sardines and wild salmon, fish oil supplements, flaxseeds, and even eggs!

become depleted, and their own brain health can suffer as a result. Low levels of DHA in the body may increase the risk of suffering from major depressive symptoms postpartum. Researchers from the National Institutes of Health found that when diet and postpartum depression rates were compared among various countries, DHA appeared as a major player.

Clinical Trials Agree

Researchers from the Netherlands released a study in 2003 that looked at the blood levels of DHA in 112 women at delivery and then at 32 weeks postpartum. The women were also given a questionnaire to determine their level of depression postpartum. The women who were possibly depressed according to their questionnaire had lower levels of DHA in their blood.

The researchers noted that lactating women were more predisposed to having low DHA levels in their blood, suggesting that they may be at a greater risk of suffering from postpartum depression. In their conclusions, the researchers suggest that increasing dietary DHA intake during pregnancy and postpartum is advisable.

Getting More Sleep

During your postpartum months, you may find yourself craving just a few more minutes of sleep. In fact, some mothers say that craving extra sleep can last for years. If you would like your baby to sleep better, then it's time to start getting more DHA into your diet. Studies have found that supplementing with DHA and EPA during pregnancy and lactation gives rise to infants with improved sleep patterns. And if your baby's sleeping, you can sleep, too.

Shiitake Mushrooms

SHIITAKE MUSHROOMS ARE A VERY flavorful treat to add to your diet postpartum. Shiitake mushrooms are thought to be among the healthiest mushrooms on earth, since they contain significantly higher amounts of vitamins, minerals, and antioxidants compared with their cousins, white button mushrooms.

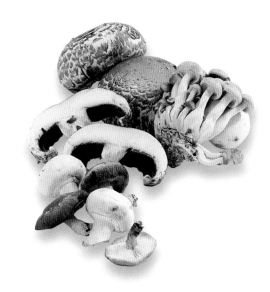

SHIITAKE MUSHROOMS AT A GLANCE

Serving Size: 1 cup (145 g)	Calcium: 0%
Calories: 81	Vitamin A: 0%
Saturated Fat: 0 g	Vitamin C: 1%
Protein: 2 g	Iron: 4%
Fiber: 3 g	

Packed with Bs

B vitamins play a crucial role in energy production in your body. Vitamin B12 is the most popular of the B vitamins for energy production. Niacin, riboflavin, thiamin, and the other B vitamins also play a role in helping your body turn the proteins, carbohydrates, and fats in your diet into energy. Eating mushrooms can help you boost your energy levels and make keeping up with your little one a bit easier. Plus, fighting back against fatigue can help lift your mood.

How much of the B vitamins are in shiitake mushrooms? There is about 0.1 mg of thiamin (about 4 percent of your daily needs), 0.2 mg of riboflavin (about 15 percent of your daily needs), 2.2 mg of niacin (about 11 percent of your daily needs), 0.2 mg of vitamin B6 (about 12 percent of your daily needs), 31 mcg of folate (about 8 percent of your daily needs), and 5.2 mg of pantothenic acid (about 52 percent of your daily needs) in a cup of shiitake mushrooms.

Stressed Out

New mothers may especially appreciate the amount of pantothenic acid in shiitake mushrooms since this B vitamin helps improve your resistance to stress (and your colicky baby or the crash-dive you took into motherhood can be more than a little stressful) Biting back against stress is important since stress is a factor that's thought to trigger depression.

Being Happy

There's still more linking B vitamins and depression. Folate has been linked to depression in scientific studies. Riboflavin has also been linked. A group of Japanese researchers reported the effects of B-vitamin intake on postpartum depression in 2006. The study involved 865 Japanese women who were questioned about their dietary intake and tested for postpartum depression. Postpartum depression developed in 121 of the women between 2 and 9 months postpartum.

Jonny's Tasty Tips

Wondering what to do with that box or bag of shiitake mushrooms? They're a bit chewier and a bit more flavorful than white button mushrooms, so they lend themselves to dishes that could use some added body and oomph. Of course, they're great in Chinese and Japanese dishes like miso soup and stir-fries. Or for a quick pick-me-up, slice some shiitakes and scallions (green onions), grate some fresh peeled ginger, and cook in some tamari or soy sauce while you make some brown rice. For a little crunch, toss in some cashews just before spooning the mushrooms and sauce over the rice.

But though their origins are Oriental, shiitakes are international when it comes to food. I like to add them to Italian dishes like tomato sauce and lasagna or sauté them with portobellos and other mushrooms and some chopped sweet onion in organic butter with a splash of wine and then serve them over whole-grain pasta or brown rice. If you take my advice earlier in this chapter and make yourself a pot of lentil stew, add shiitakes to up the healthy ante. Or brown them in organic butter and stir them into your quinoa. Top with shredded fresh basil and dig in!

The researchers found that lack of sufficient riboflavin (vitamin B2) was associated with postpartum depression, and consuming this vitamin during the postpartum months may be a way to protect against postpartum depression.

Adding vitamin B-rich foods to your diet is a great way to beat postpartum fatigue, and it may also help reduce your risk of developing postpartum depression. Shiitake mushrooms are a great source of B vitamins, as we've seen. You can also enjoy other vitamin B-rich foods like green leafy vegetables, lentils, and fish.

Immune Boosters

Mushrooms are touted as an immune-boosting food. This may be due to the diversity of vitamins they offer. It may also be due to their high antioxidant content. According to researchers at the Pennsylvania State Mushroom Research Laboratory, mushrooms contain significant levels of the antioxidant l-ergothioneine, which acts as a scavenger of free radicals that damage your body. Your body is trying to repair and rebuild itself after having a baby, so it can use all the antioxidants it can get to help it get back into its prepregnancy glory. Plus, mushrooms are a source of selenium, another potent antioxidant (and immune system booster!).

Choose Your 'Shrooms Carefully

While the white button variety is the most popular in the United States, they're not the healthiest choice. Not because they're unhealthy—it's just that so many other kinds of mushrooms are richer in nutrients, not to mention flavor. Besides shiitake mushrooms, coffee-colored crimini mushrooms have a richer flavor and more nutrients than their white button cousins. Oyster, king oyster, and maitake mushrooms also deliver skin-healthy nutrients, and they're larger and have more distinct flavors. Portobello mushrooms are another tasty choice—their large, flat shape and steak-like flavor make them a hit with vegetarians and meat-eaters alike.

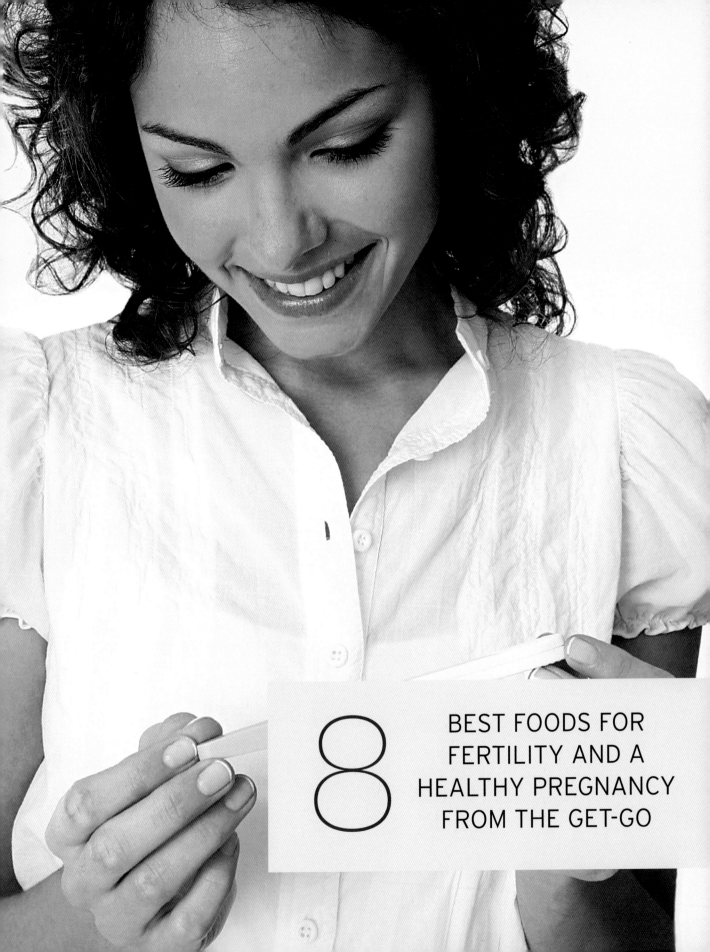

8

BEST FOODS FOR FERTILITY AND A HEALTHY PREGNANCY FROM THE GET-GO

NUTRITIONAL NEEDS FOR FERTILITY

Carving out a perfect diet for everyone is an impossible mission; however, there are some key nutritional rules we can all live by. Below, you'll find the suggested nutritional guidelines for a healthy female of childbearing age. Remember, a healthy diet is one rich in a variety of nutritional foods (and ladies; candy, soda, and fudge are not part of any food group—sorry). A healthy body can not only work right and have a better chance of conceiving, but also it feels good too!

Key Vitamins

Vitamin A: 2,350 IU daily

Folate: 400 mcg daily

Vitamin B12: 2.4 mcg daily

Vitamin C: 75 mg daily

Vitamin D: 400 IU daily

Key Minerals

Calcium: 1,000 mg daily

Iron: 18 mg daily

Sodium: 1,500 mg daily

Zinc: 8 mg daily

Other Key Nutritional Needs

Calories: about 2,400 calories for a woman 19 to 30 yrs, 64 inches (163 cm) tall, 119 pounds (54 kg) (will vary based on height, weight, and energy expenditure)

Protein: about 46 g daily

Fiber: about 25 g daily

Fluids: 2.7 liters daily

WHILE MOST COUPLES MANAGE TO CONCEIVE relatively quickly, others can struggle. Whether you're finding it difficult to conceive, you want to give your first baby the best possible start, or you're getting ready for your next baby, you need the right nutrients on your side. But eating right is not just about increasing your chances of conceiving—a healthy diet before pregnancy is linked to improved health of the baby and lower risks of complications during pregnancy.

WHEN SPROUTS LOOK LIKE SPERM

According to the 1995 National Survey of Family Growth, about 10 percent of Americans suffer from infertility. The rate in Canada is estimated to be between 7 and 8.5 percent. Many couples are struggling with infertility, and some are at the point where the alfalfa sprouts in their sandwiches look like sperm. Despite what your teachers and parents told you as a teenager, an enormous number of factors must be just right in order for you to conceive. In fact, your odds of conceiving in any given menstrual cycle are, at best, 25 percent. Most women ovulate one out of every four months. In addition, uterus conditions, sperm quality and quantity, timing, and many other factors have to be just right.

Many North American couples have problems with infertility, with higher infertility rates in older couples. Unlike some of the household duties, infertility problems are shared equally among both partners: One-third of the time, an infertility problem is traced to the female, one-third to the male, and one-third of the time the cause of infertility is a combination of problems between partners. Sadly, for some couples suffering from infertility the cause will never be known. Many factors affect fertility, including weight and nutrition.

Some couples take a "when it happens, it happens" approach and let nature take its course. However, if you want to get pregnant at a certain time or aren't having any luck conceiving and are becoming a little frustrated, you may want to try to take some control over the situation. You can work to maximize your chances of fertilizing your eggs by measuring your basal temperature or using ovulation kits to determine when you ovulate. Some experts even suggest that the quality of sex can help.

One of the best strategies is to eat right. Proper nutrition not only keeps both you and your partner healthy, but also it may also help boost your ability to conceive. Yes, food may affect fertility. Sure, we've all heard the old wives' tale about oysters being an aphrodisiac, but in this chapter, we'll be sorting through the facts on food and fertility. We'll discuss which nutrients and foods contain the supplies your body needs to conceive.

And, men—you're not free to go yet either! A man's nutritional intake can affect his ability to produce viable and healthy sperm. More emphasis is being put on prepregnancy health, so this chapter is important for all of us. Grab a fork and let's dig into some of the best foods to boost your fertility and improve your prepregnancy health—that goes for both of you!

Chill Out

Stress can also affect infertility. If you're feeling frustrated, remember how hard it is to become pregnant and how low the odds are each month. Some experts suggest that couples shouldn't worry unless they have actively been trying for over one year. Relax: It may help boost fertility. How many times have you heard stories about women who conceived once they gave up worrying about it?

SPREAD THE WORD

Improving women's health before pregnancy is an important strategy for reducing the chances of experiencing problems during pregnancy for both mother and child. In a large, multi-center trial called the Strong Healthy Women Intervention, involving close to seven hundred women, researchers found that when educated about nutrition and exercise, women are more likely to take steps toward a healthier pregnancy, leading to better health for mothers and their babies.

Reducing stress in your lifestyle may also help with fertility. In fact, the *Journal of Human Reproduction* reported that conception was much more likely in couples who reported feeling happy, good, and relaxed. Meanwhile, conception was less likely to occur during the months they reported feeling stressed, tense, or anxious.

So relax, eat right, and give your body all of the nutrients it needs to be strong, healthy, and fertile. And remember, eating right can help prepare your body better for conception.

STRESS LESS

Experts from the University of California in San Diego reported in *Fertility and Sterility 2005* that stress may play a role in the success of fertility treatments, including IVF (in vitro fertilization). After administering a series of questionnaires designed to measure the level of patient stress, researchers found that women with the highest levels of stress had 20 percent fewer eggs available for retrieval in any given cycle compared to women who weren't stressed. Stressed women were also 20 percent less likely to achieve fertilization.

Butts Out!

Ditch those bad lifestyle habits. Smoking, heavy alcohol consumption, and moderate-to-high caffeine consumption are linked to infertility. Plus, these bad habits are unhealthy for your growing baby. For example, smokers tend to be deficient in folic acid, an important nutrient for fetal development. (But don't think you can simply take folic acid and keep smoking—smoking harms your health *and* your baby's in more ways than you can imagine.) Nicotine crosses the placenta, and smoking may increase the risk of the placenta covering the cervix.

Caffeine can interfere with the absorption of iron, a key nutrient needed to help your baby grow and for you to avoid fatigue and anemia. Alcohol is another no-no. Alcohol can harm your baby, affecting his or her development. If you drink, your baby drinks. And remember that your baby's liver isn't functioning very well until after birth, so the effects of alcohol are prolonged.

It's also important for men to kick these bad habits, since they may be associated with low sperm counts and poor sperm health. Ditch these bad habits as early as possible in the baby-making game and give your new baby the best start at life.

Just for Guys

A man's fertility is as important as a woman's when it comes to determining how successful a couple will be in conceiving. In this section, we'll take a look at the state of male fertility in general and how to boost yours in particular.

Getting a Better Sperm Count

In order for conception to occur, viable sperm need to meet an egg. Unfortunately, studies have found that sperm counts are falling worldwide, and male fertility is thought to be declining in general. It has been speculated that environmental factors such as pollutants or pesticides may be contributing to this trend, but no one knows for sure. Lifestyle factors probably have a role in male fertility too.

Hang It Up

Say goodbye and hang up those cell phones, gentlemen. Cell phones may decrease sperm count. At the American Society of Reproductive Medicine conference in 2006, a study was presented that involved 361 men in an infertility clinic. The study found that the more time the men spent on a cell phone each day, the higher number of unhealthy sperm they had. Computers and other electronic equipment were not considered in this study. The research in this area is too preliminary to draw conclusions, but trying to stay off your cell as much as possible can't hurt.

Sperm Food

Some studies have examined the effects of vitamins and minerals in improving male fertility. None of these studies points conclusively to one factor that helps improve fertility in men. Many nutrients, including vitamin B12, E, C, D, selenium, zinc, and magnesium have been investigated. Rather than one "magic bullet," it appears that a healthy diet rich in important nutrients may be what makes the difference in improving a man's fertility.

PINING AWAY

Belgian researchers reported in 2003 that an extract of the bark of seaside or maritime pine (*Pinus maritima*), known as pycnogenol, inhibits one of the main enzymes involved in inflammation, and it is possible that it may offer some benefit to men struggling with infertility.

A POOR RETURN ON INVESTMENT

When a couple is trying to conceive, the spotlight is really on the guy. At this stage, a woman's role is very small: She has to produce one egg. Even though only one sperm is required to fertilize the egg, scientists have discovered that it takes hundreds of sperm working together in order for one to be able to penetrate the membrane of an egg.

This may explain why a man's reproductive system seems so extravagantly wasteful. When a man ejaculates, he deposits approximately 200 million sperm into his partner's vagina. Only 200,000 of these sperm (one out of every thousand) will make it beyond the vagina. And just 400 of these sperm will make it into the Fallopian tube. Talk about a bad return on investment!

A man puts a lot of energy into making sperm, and as we've seen, only a tiny percentage actually make it to their projected destination. Why is there such a drastic death rate of sperm in the vaginal tract? Because a woman's vaginal tract is highly acidic—it has the same pH as a glass of red wine. The acidity of the vaginal tract helps protect it from infection, but it's hell on sperm. Mother Nature's way of helping sperm have a better chance of survival in the vaginal tract is to create highly basic semen. But even so, only a few sperm make it past the cervical mucus, where the environment is more hospitable to them.

Sperm can live in a woman's womb for five days, but to increase your chances of fertility, many experts suggest that a couple have intercourse at least every two days to ensure that there are lots of sperm ready if an egg decides to show up. Doesn't sound too bad, right? But your body needs optimal nourishment to make lots of healthy sperm.

This is one reason why healthy eating is just as important for men as it is for women when trying to conceive. It may be even *more* important for your diet to be as rich in nutritious foods as possible to ensure that your body is producing the most viable sperm it can. Many nutrients are important for male fertility: vitamin A, folic acid, vitamin B12, vitamin C, selenium, zinc, and much more. So fuel up, men—you need it!

FISH, PCBS, AND SPERM

Polychlorinated biphenyls (PCBs) are a potential environmental hazard that may cause a deterioration of male fertility. PCBs can accumulate in foods like fish. In a study of fifty-three men, a group of researchers from India found that when the men's PCB concentrations were compared, those suffering with infertility had detectable levels of PCBs in their seminal fluids, while the fertile men did not. Fish-eating urban dwellers were found to have the highest concentrations of PCBs in their semen.

Go Organic

Researchers in Denmark looked into the possible effect of pesticide consumption on sperm health. The preliminary research found that sperm quality varied among the 256 farmers involved in the study. No firm conclusions could be made as to the difference in eating an organic diet versus conventional foods grown with pesticide use and the effect of sperm quality. However, organic foods have been found to have more potent levels of healthy compounds like vitamins and antioxidants. Go organic whenever possible—it's a healthy choice for all.

FILL UP ON FOLATE

For both men and women, folate plays an important role in fertility. Folate is required for the production of viable and healthy sperm. And a woman's nutrition before pregnancy, particularly during the three months before conception, is thought to be very important both for fertility and the health of the baby. Getting enough folate during this time is key. Folate is linked to proper fetal development, particularly for the prevention of neural tube defects.

Folate, also called folic acid, is a B vitamin that plays an important role in your overall health and the development of the fetus. Current evidence suggests that women of childbearing age should consume between 400 and 1,000 mcg of folic acid daily. Many foods contain folate, but the most abundant amounts can be found in green leafy vegetables. But the folate in food is 40 to 50 percent less bioavailable (available for your body to absorb and use) than synthetic folate found in prenatal vitamins, which is almost 100 percent absorbed. See the chart on page 24 for more foods that contain folate and check out the best foods for fertility in the next few pages, many of which are also sources of folate.

Still Not Enough

Most countries require that foods like breads and cereals be fortified with synthetic folate (folic acid) to ensure that everyone, particularly women of childbearing years, consumes sufficient folate. However, researchers from Harvard University reported in 2006 that in spite of changes to U.S. regulations in 1996, which increased the level of folic acid in foods like enriched breads, cereals, flours, cornmeals, pastas, rice, and other grain products, most women were still not consuming enough folic acid. Even after these increases in folic acid fortification in foods, only half of women were consuming the needed amounts of folate, and some ethnic populations were only consuming a quarter of what they needed.

THE DIRTY DOZEN

When it comes to organic foods, you might be tempted to think that organics are too expensive, too hard to find, and what's the big deal, anyway? If that's the case, you'll be relieved to know that you don't absolutely have to buy organic everything. But how can you tell which organic foods you really should buy?

It's easy, thanks to the Environmental Working Group. They've made up lists of the twelve most contaminated foods (the "dirty dozen") and twelve least contaminated foods to help you prioritize. If you can't find or afford an all-organic menu, it's not all that important to get organic avocados, but organic meat, strawberries, and bell peppers are a different story. Here are their lists to help you prioritize:

12 Most Contaminated	12 Least Contaminated
Peaches	Onions
Apples	Avocados
Bell peppers	Sweet corn (frozen)
Celery	Pineapples
Nectarines	Mangoes
Strawberries	Asparagus
Cherries	Peas (frozen)
Pears	Kiwifruit
Grapes (imported)	Bananas
Spinach	Cabbage
Lettuce	Broccoli
Potatoes	Papaya

Jonny usually adds coffee, milk, eggs, and meat to the "dirty dozen" listed by the Environmental Working Group. Obviously, if you're pregnant, caffeine-containing beverages like coffee won't be an issue, but the added hormones, antibiotics, pesticides, and other contaminants in milk, eggs, and meat make it worth your while (and your baby's) to ante up for organic. You'll be glad you did!

PRECONCEPTION SUPPLEMENTS

More and more women are visiting their doctors or obstetricians for a preconception visit. At such a visit, you can discuss your concerns about pregnancy, and your doctor will check your health, including a pelvic exam, blood work, and a review of both your own and your family's medical history. At such a visit, most obstetricians will recommend that you start taking a prenatal vitamin/mineral supplement. The most important nutrient in this supplement is folate (folic acid).

FAST FACT

Folic acid supplementation is recommended for the prevention of birth defects.

What Folate Does

Folate is of major importance in the beginning stages of fetal development. During the first few days and weeks, the growing fetus requires folate to help set up the basic framework upon which it will grow. Without sufficient folic acid levels, the spinal cord will not form properly, which can lead to spina bifida. How exactly folate helps the spinal cord form and close properly is not fully understood. Scientists do know that folate reduces damage to DNA, the blueprint of cells, and can prevent errors from occurring when a cell is replicating. This is very important since your growing fetus is replicating cells at an amazingly rapid rate.

Depression and Fertility

Certain health conditions are linked to low levels of folate. Women who suffer from depression commonly are deficient in folate and should pay particular attention to their folate intake to ensure that they're getting enough to conceive and carry a healthy baby to term.

Population studies have found that both men and women with low folate levels in their blood are at a higher risk for depression. The link between folate and depression probably lies with folate's role in serotonin production. Serotonin is a neurotransmitter that elicits a happy or feel-good feeling. Omega-3 fatty acids found in fish are also well-known supporters of a healthy mood.

WEIGHING IN

Reaching or maintaining a healthy weight before embarking on your baby journey is a good idea. Now ladies, when it comes to weight, please be careful. We're talking about a *healthy* weight, not a supermodel weight. The few extra pounds on your hips or thighs that drive you nuts may actually be helpful during pregnancy. Research indicates that up to 97 percent of women who think they are overweight are actually a perfect weight.

Going on a fad diet can cause you to deplete your body of the nutrients needed for fertility and to support healthy baby growth. Plus, dieting and being underweight can cause your body to stop ovulating.

At the other end of the scale (pardon the pun), women who are overweight before conception or who gain too much weight during pregnancy, have a higher than average risk of developing preeclampsia (a medical condition in which the mother experiences high blood pressure), requiring labor induction or a

Cesarean section, or of developing gestational diabetes (a form of diabetes that occurs during pregnancy).

To see how your weight measures up, skip the typical measurement techniques such as trying to fit into that tiny pair of pants in your closet we all call our "skinny pants." Instead, calculate your body mass index (BMI). Use the chart on page 15, "Calculating a Healthy Weight," to determine your BMI.

Here's a new breakthrough that you might also want to check out, especially since it's easier to calculate than BMI: your waist-to-hips ratio (W/H ratio). The W/H ratio is turning out to be even more important than your BMI in terms of overall health. To find yours, measure your waist at the thinnest point, and your hips at the widest point. Then divide your waist by hip measurements to get the ratio. A healthy number for women is 0.8 or less.

What's Weight Got to Do with It?

A woman's fertility is highly sensitive to the energy balance of her body. In other words, how well you are nourished will affect your body's ability to conceive. This is because hormones, the chemicals in your body that are involved in communication between various systems, help tell the reproductive system what is happening with a woman's metabolism. When metabolism is abnormal, such as in women who are clinically underweight or obese, your hormone levels are affected. And as you might expect, hormones are a key factor in conception and a healthy pregnancy.

Weighing in for Fertility Treatments

Researchers have been investigating the effects of body weight and diet on fertility treatment outcomes. It is well known that your body weight and nutritional status (how well you eat) are closely related to your fertility. But few studies have investigated the direct effects of diet on the outcome of fertility treatments.

FAST FACT

Prenatal vitamins include the recommended daily dosage of folate in the form of folic acid.

A healthy body weight is connected to healthy hormone levels, and a healthy diet is connected to a healthy body. Despite a lack of evidence to date, a healthy diet is a good idea when trying fertility treatments, especially since it is associated in other ways with conception and a healthy pregnancy.

WHAT ABOUT MEAT?

To eat or not to eat meat—that is the question. At least it's one question when you're trying to get pregnant. Let's look at the issues surrounding meat-eating and conception.

Meatless Conception

Food and fertility are linked. A diet that is low or lacking in certain nutrients could affect a couple's ability to conceive. If you or your partner is a vegetarian, make sure you're making careful decisions about your food to ensure that you aren't deficient in any amino acids, fats, or other nutrients.

Vegetarians can have lower levels of estrogen, a hormone you need in order to conceive. This may be because many vegetarian diets are lower in fat. Low-fat diets can cause women to experience longer menstrual cycles and longer periods, which also can lower fertility. Try adding an avocado to your salad or enjoy another serving of yogurt each day to help increase your daily fat intake. Nuts and seeds are another good source of fats in a vegetarian diet.

If you're a vegetarian, you also need to be sure to include sufficient protein in your diet. For best fertility results, consider increasing your protein consumption by about 10 percent. Why? Well, eating a low-protein diet can negatively affect your menstrual cycle, a cycle that needs to be in top shape for conception to occur.

The Soy Debate

Some Web sites have suggested that vegetarians have a higher intake of soy foods, which may cause a drop in estrogen levels. Soy foods contain phytoestrogens, which may affect natural estrogen levels. But a diet rich in soy and other phytoestrogen-containing foods, such as the diets consumed in Asia, does not affect fertility. So it's unlikely that soy is the cause of lower estrogen levels in vegetarians. It's worth noting that the soy consumed in Asian societies is quite different from many of the highly processed soy foods that line our supermarket shelves. Asians eat healthy, naturally fermented soy like tempeh and miso, not "soy chips," "soy meat," and "soy ice cream." Something to think about!

Debate exists as to soy's role in male fertility as well. Researchers at Harvard University in 2008 reported that a diet high in soy may affect male semen quality. In animal studies, diets high in isoflavones, a compound found in high quantities in soy foods, have been related to a decrease in fertility. The researchers studied the diets of men from couples who were experiencing infertility. They looked at the men's dietary intake over a three-month period. The researchers reported a link between eating more soy-based foods and lower sperm concentration in these men. The strongest link occurred in those who ate the highest amounts of soy-based foods and among overweight or obese men.

A Beefy Question

On the opposite end of the meat-eating scale, what do we know about the effects of a diet rich in red meat? Researchers from the University of Rochester conducted a study in five cities in the United States involving 387 males to see if a mother's beef intake had an effect on her son's semen quality. They reported that men whose mothers consumed high amounts of beef during their pregnancies (over seven beef meals per week) had lower sperm concentrations. It is suggested in this report that xenobiotics (unnatural chemicals like antibiotics) in beef may alter a man's testicular development in utero and adversely affect his reproductive capacity. That sounds scary, but it's important to put this study into perspective. The researchers were using dietary intake from recall. Even the best of us aren't very good at recalling what we ate yesterday, let alone two decades ago when we were pregnant with our son! So don't throw the beef out with the bathwater.

The nutritional value of beef is high. It's a good source of protein, iron, vitamin B12, and many other important nutrients for a healthy pregnancy and improved fertility. But women may want to limit their beef consumption to a few times a week since this study found lower consumption of beef was associated with a lower risk of male fertility problems in the fetus. As with fish, the dietary benefits of beef probably outweigh the negatives, leaving moderation as the safest course of action until further research is done.

PULL THAT SWEET TOOTH

Sweet foods and foods with lots of simple sugars (carbohydrates) are called high-glycemic foods. These foods break down very quickly in your body, causing your blood sugar levels to rise rapidly. A healthy body will work hard to produce insulin, a hormone that can remove sugar from the bloodstream. However, if you frequently eat high-glycemic foods, you place great demands on your body to produce and respond to insulin. Eventually, your body's cells may stop responding to insulin, a condition called insulin resistance.

Insulin resistance results in high blood sugar levels. A high blood sugar level is unhealthy, and it can lead to damage to your small blood vessels, like those in your eyes, fingertips, and kidneys. People with diabetes have an inability to keep their blood sugar levels low, and they commonly experience kidney problems, degenerating eye health, and neuropathy (loss of feeling in the tips of their fingers).

Insulin resistance also impairs fertility. It is unclear exactly how the two are connected; but research has found that there may be a link between low-glycemic foods and better fertility. Some preliminary studies have found that men with diabetes can have infertility problems. And a large study has investigated the link between eating carbohydrates and fertility in women.

In 2007, researchers from the Harvard School of Public Health reported a study involving 18,555 married women to see if the amount or type of carbohydrate eaten affected fertility. They found that women with infertility due to problems with ovulation tended to consume both higher amounts of carbohydrates and more high-glycemic carbohydrates. This suggests that eating better-quality carbohydrates (complex carbohydrates such as vegetables, fruit, and foods that are high in fiber) may be linked to fertility.

Low-glycemic foods such as vegetables and whole grains promote good health. So it makes sense to eat more of these healthy foods if you are a man or a woman trying to achieve optimal health so you can get pregnant and carry a healthy baby to term.

FRUIT FOR CANDY

Skip the candy and satisfy your sweet tooth with fruit instead. Eating sugary foods like candy and other highly processed carbohydrates decreases your body's ability to efficiently send messages (neurotransmission) about the hormone levels you need from your brain to your reproductive organs.

Healthiest Foods for Fertility

There is no single food that is known to improve fertility. No magic berry or foreign mushroom will help you to conceive tomorrow. However, scientists do know that a healthy diet rich in particular nutrients contributes to your overall health and may increase your chances of becoming pregnant.

Your nutrition before pregnancy is very important, because you won't even know you're pregnant until you are a few weeks along. Those first few weeks are very important to your baby's development.

Make sure your body is stocked with the healthy nutrients your baby will need by starting your healthy diet today! A healthy diet includes plenty of vegetables, nuts, seeds, whole grains, beans, and fruit (and all the other 100 healthiest foods in this book). Let's discuss some of the best foods to eat for fertility and a healthy conception.

HERE ARE THE 9 HEALTHIEST FOODS FOR FERTILITY:

- ARUGULA
- ASPARAGUS
- BITTER MELON
- BUCKWHEAT
- ENDIVE
- GUAVA
- OLIVE OIL
- PAPRIKA
- PSYLLIUM

Let's look at each of these foods and see what gives them their fertility-boosting edge. Jonny will help you learn the best ways to prepare and use all the foods on our list in "Jonny's Tasty Tips."

Arugula

BLAST OFF TO GOOD HEALTH WITH THESE
delicious peppery greens. Arugula, also known as
rocket, is a sophisticated change from the usual
lettuce in any favorite salad recipe,and it's packed
with nutrients that may support healthy fertility.

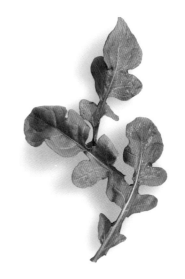

ARUGULA AT A GLANCE

Serving Size: 1.5 cups (28 g)	**Calcium:** 4%
Calories: 7	**Vitamin A:** 13%
Saturated Fat: 0 g	**Vitamin C:** 7%
Protein: 1 g	**Iron:** 2%
Fiber: 1 g	

Note: The nutritional facts data provided in this chapter are
approximations based on the foods' nutrient value and an adult
woman's RDA.

A mother once told me that she raised her children to
eat one green leafy vegetable each day. At first that
made me feel sorry for her kids, but after looking into
these superfoods a little more, I realized that's a rule
we should all use. Green leafy vegetables are the ultimate superfood. One of the most nutrient-packed vegetables, leafy greens contain amino acids, iron, folate,
B vitamins, antioxidants, and countless other nutrients
that not only help your body function properly but also
help fight off disease. So arugula is not just a great
addition to your fertility diet but also a great addition
throughout your pregnancy and postpartum diets.

Leaves of Haute Culture

You'll just love the spicy flavor of arugula as well
as its dark green color and beautiful shape. It makes a
gorgeous salad and goes well with less common salad
ingredients, such as grapefruit or orange sections.
Thanks to the increased interest in haute cuisine in
North America, arugula is now readily available in most
grocery stores.

Always look for the freshest arugula; it should be
dark green and lush. Avoid buying arugula that's even
beginning to turn yellow or limp. For one thing, it's
amazing how a package of baby arugula leaves can
look a little pale one day and be a browned, mushy
mess the next. Not to mention that aging leaves contain few nutrients and simply taste terrible. There is no
need to eat things that might upset your stomach, particularly as you continue to eat arugula into your first
trimester, when morning sickness can occur.

Pretty Manly

A man's ideal meal may not be a pretty salad of
arugula with a few slices of pink grapefruit and some
red onion, but put your masculine pride aside, boys,
and dig in. Arugula is a good source of folate. In one

Jonny's Tasty Tips

Is arugula an aphrodisiac? Well, that's what the ancient Egyptians and Romans thought. I don't know about that, but I do know that it's the überfood of nutritional bargains: Not only is it packed with vitamins, minerals, and carotenoids, one cup contains a whopping 5 calories. (Yes, you read that right: 5 calories.)

If you haven't tasted arugula, you are in for one fabulous treat. Those little leaves pack a big, spicy flavor and a rich, meaty texture that will make your mouth water. (Some of my vegetarian friends get their "meat fix" from arugula.) Arugula's outsized flavor helps it stand up to bold ingredients in a salad, whether you like yours with citrus, almonds, and shaved Parmesan (try a dressing of lemon juice and extra-virgin olive oil on this) or anchovies, feta, and kalamata olives (with a classic Greek dressing or a simple olive oil-balsamic vinegar mix). Or try this favorite: a bed of arugula topped with grilled portobello mushrooms and a drizzle of olive oil and balsamic vinegar or your favorite marinade. (Don't be afraid to experiment; you'd be amazed what ginger or tamari can do here.) And arugula can give a much-needed flavor boost to milder salad greens as well.

But arugula's not just for salads. You can use it any way you'd use spinach: Just wilted in the water it's washed in and served with a splash of balsamic vinegar; sautéed in a little olive oil with minced onion or garlic; or added to omelets, soups, or lentil stew (it's great in black bean soup and as a topping for refried beans, too.)

and a half cups of arugula, there are 30 mcg of folate. Folate is an important nutrient that's needed for male fertility. If masculine pride is on the table, then let's discuss the potential effect folate has on a man's ability to produce sperm with the best genetics.

Masculine Pride

Healthy sperm is vital to conception. Most importantly, the genetic material a sperm contains needs to be perfect. When a sperm does not contain a perfect amount of genetic material (chromosomes), it is called aneuploidy. Little is known about the effect of paternal nutrition on aneuploidy in sperm. Researchers from the University of California reported in 2008 on a study that involved 89 healthy, nonsmoking men to see if what they ate affected the health of their sperm's genetic makeup. They found that the men who consumed more folate had fewer sperm with genetic problems.

Beyond Bs

Arugula is also a good source of vitamins A, C, and K. Plus, arugula contains 15 mg of choline. This nutrient is not well known, but it is vital to your baby's growth and health. Choline is important for early development because it plays a role in brain development. A bone-building bonanza, arugula contains calcium, magnesium, potassium, phosphorus, and manganese. All of these nutrients help ensure that your bones are strong and healthy. This is important as you start your pregnancy since your baby needs a lot of calcium and minerals from your body in order to grow. Stock up now to make sure your bones aren't depleted of these important minerals once your baby starts to grow.

Asparagus

EATING ASPARAGUS MAY GIVE YOUR URINE A FUNNY SMELL, but don't let that scare you away from this healthy, delicious vegetable. These spears are packed with nutrients that may help ensure that your body is working optimally, increasing your chances of fertility.

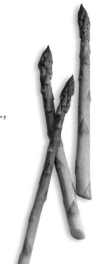

ASPARAGUS AT A GLANCE

Serving Size: ½ cup (90 g)	Calcium: 2%
Calories: 20	Vitamin A: 18%
Saturated Fat: 0 g	Vitamin C: 12%
Protein: 2 g	Iron: 5%
Fiber: 2 g	

Five for Folate

In just five spears of asparagus, your body gets 100 mcg of folate. Twenty spears would offer you 400 mcg. Folate is important to fertility for both men and women. Research has found that folate plays a role in producing healthy sperm in men and may beneficially affect a woman's ability to ovulate. Remember that folate from food sources is not very well absorbed (only about half is absorbed), so next time the side dish of asparagus is being passed around the table, grab it and fill up your plate. Your body will thank you for it.

Spears for Sperm

Researchers in the Netherlands have found that daily consumption of folic acid (5 mg, plus 66 mg of zinc sulfate) can increase sperm count in men who are struggling with fertility. The study involved 212 men. In both the fertile and infertile men, the folic acid and zinc sulfate supplement caused an increase in total sperm count. This research was reported in 2002 in the journal *Fertility and Sterility*; future studies may help us better understand this relationship. In the meantime, folate is important to so many healthy functions that it's a good idea to eat lots of folate-rich foods every day.

Glutathione versus Free Radicals

Asparagus is also packed with some lesser-known nutrients like glutathione. Glutathione is a powerful antioxidant. Antioxidants are helpful compounds found in many fruits and vegetables. Antioxidants can neutralize free radicals, which are harmful compounds that can damage DNA and other parts of your and your baby's cells. Free radicals are always in your body, since they form naturally as a by-product of some of your body's natural processes. However, free radicals also form in your body from chemicals in cosmetics and other body-care products, as well as from sunlight and environmental pollutants. Free radicals can cause damage to sperm. Glutathione is a particularly good antioxidant to have on your side since it can help other antioxidants regenerate, giving you more free radical-fighting power.

Jonny's Tasty Tips

Who doesn't love asparagus, the ultimate springtime vegetable? It's one of the few foods that's equally delicious hot, cold, and at room temperature. I love to steam the spears until they're tender and then chill them and use them any number of ways: drizzled with a little vinaigrette as a salad or side dish; cut into 1-inch (2.5-cm) pieces and added to a tossed salad (I especially love a buttery lettuce like Boston, hard-boiled egg slices, sunflower seeds, and roasted red pepper strips with asparagus); chopped and added to an omelet or stir-fry; or pureed and mixed into hummus or stirred into plain yogurt for a refreshing cold asparagus "soup."

Hot asparagus is delicious, too. Try grilling plump spears with a drizzle of olive oil and lemon juice or vinaigrette. Cream of asparagus soup is a soothing treat when made with organic milk and a dollop of organic butter. A family favorite of my coauthor Allison is to toss asparagus spears in olive oil, rosemary, and garlic before sliding them in the oven on a baking sheet and baking until tender. And simple steamed asparagus with organic butter and lemon juice is the perfect side dish to almost anything. I love it with seafood or chicken and a baked sweet potato!

By the way, like arugula, asparagus has long been touted as an aphrodisiac, probably due to the vegetable's phallic shape. I wouldn't count on that! But there's no question that asparagus is delicious and doesn't fill you up like heavier foods, and as we all know, there's nothing like staggering around with a full belly to put a damper on your sex drive!

Rutin Rush

Asparagus also contains rutin, another lesser-known nutrient that may help with fertility. Antioxidants can help protect sperm, ensuring that the maximum number of healthy sperm is available for ejaculation. Rutin has strong antioxidant properties and can stabilize vitamin C. Vitamin C is also found in asparagus, and if both rutin and vitamin C are taken together, the benefits of vitamin C are intensified. Vitamin C plays an important role in fighting free radicals and wrinkles and in boosting your immunity.

Savvy Shopper

Look for fresh green stalks with tightly closed, compact tips. Stalks should be straight, firm, and about 6 to 8 inches in length. Try to avoid asparagus with white butts, because the white portion is unusable. Note that it's a myth that string-thin asparagus spears taste better than their plump counterparts: the opposite is true. Plump spears are tender, while skinny spears can be fibrous.

Store fresh asparagus by wrapping the bottom of the stalks in a damp paper towel, put them in a plastic bag, and refrigerate. Or stand them upright in a cup or glass with about an inch of water in the bottom until you're ready to use them. However you store them, plan to use those spears within 2 days.

To prepare fresh asparagus, first break off the butt end of each spear where it snaps easily. You can save the woody bases for soup stock if desired. Next, wash the stalks thoroughly and carefully to remove any sand from under the scales. Two healthy ways for pregnant women to prepare their asparagus are to steam or bake them.

Bitter Melon

BITTER? IT MAY SOUND UNAPPEALING, BUT THE bitter melon, also known as the balsam pear, is actually a fun and tasty way to add some excitement to your culinary endeavors as you work toward getting pregnant. And as we'll see, it doesn't have to be bitter at all.

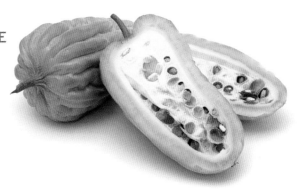

BITTER MELON AT A GLANCE

Serving Size: 1 cup (124 g)	Calcium: 1%
Calories: 24	Vitamin A: 3%
Saturated Fat: 0 g	Vitamin C: 68%
Protein: 1 g	Iron: 3%
Fiber: 2 g	

Bite for Bite

About one cup of bitter melon contains about 90 mcg of folate. That's almost a quarter of your minimal daily needs of folate during conception. And there are just 20 calories in a typical bitter melon! That's the same number of calories you'd get from eating a half a stick of licorice. A common addition to stir-fries in Chinese cooking, the bitter melon or balsam pear is worth a try at home.

Eating foods like bitter melons with high nutritional value and few calories is a great way to help you shed any extra pounds that may be interfering with your fertility. Review the "Weighing In" section beginning on page 292 for a reminder of how a healthy weight is vital to fertility. Plus, bitter melons are packed with fiber. Fiber is really helpful in making you feel full, reducing your cravings for less nutritious and higher-calorie snacks.

Fertility Friend

If you're trying to get pregnant, fiber may be your new best friend. Eating a diet rich in fiber may help boost fertility. Researchers have found that troubles with sugar metabolism, a common problem for people who eat a diet lacking in fiber, may be associated with fertility problems. When the body is fed foods with a high glycemic index (they break down into sugar very quickly), blood sugar levels rise fast, stimulating the production of large amounts of the hormone insulin. Insulin tells the body's cells to gobble up the sugar and help lower the blood sugar level.

However, cells can become intolerant of insulin and can start to ignore it. This is called insulin resistance. And as we saw on page 295, research is suggesting that insulin resistance is associated with infertility (not to mention a host of other health problems, like metabolic syndrome and diabetes). One of the best ways to ensure that your insulin and blood sugar levels are working optimally is to include lots of foods in your diet that are high in fiber (and thus have a low glycemic index). Bitter melons contain a high amount

Jonny's Tasty Tips

When we think of melons, the sweet, delicious flavors of cantaloupe, watermelon, and honeydew typically come to mind. So how could a melon possibly be bitter? The short answer is, it couldn't. Bitter melon isn't really a melon at all, but a cucumber-shaped summer squash grown in tropical areas.

Usually, the bitter-flavored unripe fruit is used as a vegetable. It can be cooked a number of different ways, including stir-fried, steamed, and curried. Some enthusiasts recommend it as part of a vegetable curry with eggplants and onions. It can also be stuffed, pickled, and used in soups. However you prepare it, cooking will mellow its bitter flavor, which is due largely to its quinine content. Just make sure you remove the seeds and the fibrous core before cooking!

of fiber per bite and about 3.5 g of fiber in the whole fruit. Plus, researchers from the Philippines reported in 2007 that bitter melon contains compounds called charantin and p-insulin that may directly affect blood sugar levels, further helping you win the battle against insulin resistance.

Maybe Not for Baby

There are some concerns that medicinal usages of bitter melon in animals has stimulated menstrual bleeding, so bitter melon taken as a supplement is not recommended for use by pregnant women. But as a food, bitter melon is eaten by Asian populations, suggesting that safety concerns for regular consumption of this food are minimal. Nonetheless, experts recommend that bitter melon be eaten moderately, if at all, during pregnancy. Better safe than sorry! Once you get pregnant, it may be time to stop.

Savvy Shopper

Here are some tips for finding the perfect bitter melon. Choose melons that are still green for a more bitter flavor. As they ripen, they turn yellow-orange and have a milder taste, if you prefer that. Bitter melons are available fresh from April to September in most Asian markets and can occasionally be found in larger supermarkets. You can also sometimes find it frozen.

Buckwheat

BUCKWHEAT IS GENERALLY REFERRED TO AS a cereal grain, but it's actually the seed of a broadleaved herbaceous plant, while true grains like corn and wheat are all in the grass family. You can find buckwheat as groats or flour or in pancake mixes at your local food co-op or health food store or at your local market in baked goods and other grain products. Buy it by the bag or in bulk and use it in your baking recipes as a healthy way to improve your fertility. Buckwheat is packed with B vitamins, which are thought to support fertility and can help boost your energy levels.

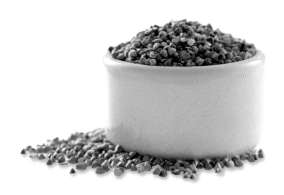

BUCKWHEAT AT A GLANCE

Serving Size: 1 cup (170 g)	**Calcium:** 2%
Calories: 583	**Vitamin A:** 0%
Saturated Fat: 1 g	**Vitamin C:** 0%
Protein: 23 g	**Iron:** 12%
Fiber: 17 g	

B-ing Fertile

There are many B vitamins: thiamin, riboflavin, folate, niacin, vitamin B6, and vitamin B12. We've discussed the role of folate in fertility in great detail earlier in this chapter. Let's take a look at some of the other B vitamins and the role they play in your health and fertility.

CINNAMON TO THE RESCUE!

Controlling your blood sugar levels has been associated with improved fertility. Cinnamon is another food that researchers know supports healthy blood sugar levels. In a study from Beltsville Human Nutrition Research Center, 60 people with type 2 diabetes consumed $\frac{1}{2}$, 1, or $2\frac{1}{2}$ teaspoons of cinnamon daily. After 40 days, all three amounts of cinnamon significantly reduced blood sugar levels, triglycerides, and so-called "bad" cholesterol (LDL). Cinnamon's ability to support healthy blood sugar levels has been called one of the most significant nutritional discoveries in 25 years.

Jonny's Tasty Tips

If you've ever eaten buckwheat, it's probably been in buckwheat pancakes. You may have also sampled the dark, boldly flavored, and prized buckwheat honey. You can find buckwheat pancake and waffle mixes, buckwheat flour, buckwheat cereals, and even buckwheat pasta in health food stores, your local food co-op, online, and even in whole-foods and some mainstream supermarkets. Mixing a little buckwheat flour into your multigrain bread will definitely up the flavor, fiber, and nutrient content.

But bread, cereal, pancakes, and the like aren't my favorite way to enjoy buckwheat. I enjoy the toasted grains in kasha. Make kasha by rinsing buckwheat groats (seeds) with a beaten egg and toasting in a heavy skillet, add water (1½ cups [355 ml] per cup of buckwheat groats), bring to a boil, and then reduce the heat and allow the buckwheat to absorb the water over very low heat. (You can also buy "instant" precooked kasha.) Kasha makes a perfect stuffing for baked winter squash, especially if you stir in onion, garlic, and herbs like winter savory or rosemary, all sautéed in olive oil. It also makes a great side dish if you mix in steamed sliced carrots and/or shredded red cabbage.

Riboflavin is needed to make riboflavin carrier protein. This protein mediates the supply of vitamins to a developing fetus. In other words, without sufficient riboflavin, your fertilized egg will not be able to receive sufficient amounts of vitamins, which could lead to infertility. Niacin can help dilate blood vessels, which can improve a man's ability to reach erection, leading to more successful intercourse. This may also help make intercourse a more pleasurable experience, which is important, particularly if you are feeling pressure about conceiving.

All of the B vitamins play a role in your body's ability to get energy from your food (carbohydrates, fats, and protein). Buckwheat is a great source of B vitamins. A cup of buckwheat (170 g) contains 0.2 mg of thiamin , 0.7 mg of riboflavin, 11.9 mg of niacin, 0.4 mg of vitamin B6, and 51 mcg of folate. But, like other vegetables and grains, it contains no vitamin B12.

Better Insulin Control

Buckwheat has been touted as a healthy food because it can help decrease insulin levels. High insulin levels are associated with infertility. When you eat high-sugar foods, your body has to produce a lot of insulin to get your blood sugar levels back down to a safe level. Fiber is a great way to help your body avoid producing high insulin levels. Fiber in foods like buckwheat can help trap sugar in your intestinal tract, slowing the rate at which your body can absorb it. And buckwheat is a great source of fiber, with one cup offering your body 17 g.

Zinc for Guys

Zinc has been shown to support male fertility. In an interesting article in 2003, researchers from Belgium reported that sperm quality and function improved when food was supplemented with a combination of zinc and folic acid. Buckwheat is a great place to find zinc, with 4.1 mg in one cup (that's about 27 percent of an average person's daily needs).

Endive

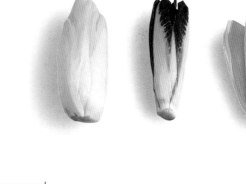

ENDIVE IS A TYPE OF SALAD GREEN YOU

may overlook at the market. It sort of looks

like a tiny yellow-green football. But endive

has a great flavor and is a great way to add

some life to your salads. Plus, endive is

packed with nutrients that are sure to help support

your health and fertility, particularly folate. Two cups of endive contain

142 mcg of folate.

ENDIVE AT A GLANCE

Serving Size: 2 cups (100 g)	**Calcium:** 5%
Calories: 17	**Vitamin A:** 43%
Saturated Fat: 0 g	**Vitamin C:** 11%
Protein: 0 g	**Iron:** 5%
Fiber: 3 g	

FAST FACT

Vitamin B6 plays a role in the metabolism of polyunsaturated fats, like DHA, which are needed for the proper development of your baby's rapidly growing brain.

Folate for Miscarriage Prevention

There are many reasons why a baby may not carry to term. One of the reasons is low folic acid levels in a woman's blood. A study reported in the journal *Obstetrics and Gynecology* in 2000 found that a low level of folic acid is linked to spontaneous pregnancy loss. In the study of 123 women who had more than two consecutive spontaneous early pregnancy losses, the women had low folic acid levels and high homocysteine levels. Homocysteine is a bad fat whose levels are normally kept under control by B vitamins (vitamin B12, folic acid, and vitamin B6). Reach for foods that contain B vitamins to improve your folate levels and your chances of a successful pregnancy. Endive is also a good source of other B vitamins, including thiamin (B1), riboflavin (B2), and pantothenic acid (B5).

Folic Acid for Cleft Palate

A recently observed decrease in the prevalence of cleft lip with or without cleft palate in the United States was associated with the folic acid fortification of enriched cereal grains, which became mandatory in 1998. Several case-control studies have found an inverse association between intakes of folic acid and/or multi-

Jonny's Tasty Tips

You say EN-dive, and I say ahn-DEEV. But however you choose to pronounce this distinctive, delicious yet slightly bitter Continental green, you'll love it. Three kinds of endive are available in most groceries: Belgian endive (also called French endive or witloof), a small, cylindrical head of pale, tightly packed leaves; curly endive or frisee (free-ZAY), with open heads of lacy, green-rimmed, curly leaves; and finally escarole, which is milder and less bitter than either Belgian endive or frisee.

The distinctive flavor of endive makes it a stand-alone green in a salad—it's most enjoyable as the sole green, with other veggies added to enhance it like chopped yellow bell pepper and cherry tomatoes, along with flaked Parmesan or cubed feta cheese in a simple vinaigrette. Endive salads also lend themselves to blue cheese dressing, especially the authentic ones that are basic vinaigrettes with crumbled blue cheese added as opposed to a creamy dressing. My favorite way to enjoy endive is to toss the leaves with some walnuts and sliced pears and maybe a little blue cheese and olives. Olive oil is a nice addition to the mix.

You can also stuff Belgian endive leaves like celery and eat them instead of fatty chips. Try them with homemade pimiento cheese or egg salad stuffing or dip them in your favorite healthy dip or dressing and enjoy the crunch without the calories!

vitamins and the risk of cleft lip. In other words, having good folate levels in your blood will lower your risk of having a baby with a cleft lip or cleft palate.

Experts recommend that all women of childbearing age who aren't taking contraceptives should consume a diet rich in folate (by eating foods like endive) and take an additional daily dose of at least 0.4 mg (or, better, 0.8 mg) of folic acid. Ensuring that your diet contains sufficient folate can help prevent neural tube defects and may reduce the risk of cleft lip with or without cleft palate.

Tossed Goodness

Being a salad green, endive is packed with more than just folate. All greens are a great way to add water and fiber to your diet. Endive is also a good source of vitamins A, C, K, E (in the form of alpha-tocopherol), magnesium, phosphorus, calcium, iron, potassium, zinc, copper, and manganese. In order to have a baby, your body needs be in an exceptional state of health, and all these nutrients are needed to get you there. Be sure to eat lots of healthy foods every day and be active to help get your body ready for having that baby!

Guava

GUAVA IS AN ANTIOXIDANT-RICH FOOD. IT'S
high in vitamin C (377 mg per cup) and contains
other antioxidants like vitamin E (1.2 mg per cup)
and vitamin A (1,030 IU per cup). Antioxidants are
like warriors that protect all parts of your body
from free radicals that cause damage. Free radicals are
everywhere. They're formed when you're exposed to sunlight, use cosmetics, and even
when inflammation occurs in your body. Antioxidants can also help protect sperm
from free-radical damage, which may improve your ability to conceive the healthiest
baby possible.

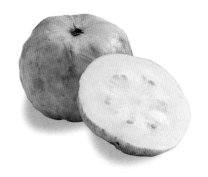

GUAVA AT A GLANCE

Serving Size: 1 cup (165 g)	Calcium: 3%
Calories: 112	Vitamin A: 21%
Saturated Fat: 0 g	Vitamin C: 628%
Protein: 4 g	Iron: 2%
Fiber: 9 g	

Egyptian researchers found that antioxidants such as those found in guava can help improve the quality of semen. An animal study involving 24 male New Zealand rabbits given drinking water with antioxidants (vitamin C in the form of ascorbic acid and vitamin E) found that it reduced the production of free radicals and improved rabbit semen quality. They also noted that a greater improvement was seen from vitamin E alone. This may be because vitamin E is fat soluble, allowing it better access to damaging free radicals in the fat-rich seminal environment.

Warriors for Your Sperm

Oxidative stress, the stress caused by free radicals, is detrimental to sperm function. When a group of researchers from the University of California looked into the association of vitamin C, vitamin E, and beta-carotene (three potent antioxidants) and sperm integrity, they found a slight improvement in sperm health in the men who had higher intakes of beta-carotene.

Manly Mineral

Zinc is another reason guava (which has 0.4 mg of zinc per cup) is a healthy food that helps improve your chances of fertility. Researchers from the University of California, Berkeley, reported that in a study involving 97 healthy men, a high intake of antioxidants (zinc, folate, and vitamins A, C, and E) was associated with

Jonny's Tasty Tips

Guavas are fragrant, delicious tropical fruits that many Americans know only because they're frequently used in jellies. But these red fleshed (and sometimes white fleshed) fruits pack an amazing nutritional wallop. Best of all, you don't have to cook them to get the most from their high antioxidant and nutrient content.

Slice into some guava and enjoy all of its healthy benefits: antioxidants, fiber, and minerals like zinc, manganese, and copper. Eat it fresh as a snack, slice it into your salad for a splash of tropical flavor, or juice it alone or mixed with other fruits and yogurt for a delicious smoothie.

ROYAL JELLY

A study in 2002 showed fertility improvements with the use of 500 mg of royal jelly per day. A more recent study conducted by researchers in Egypt found that applications of a mixture of Egyptian bee honey and royal jelly intravaginally (i.e., applied in the vagina) at the time of intercourse improved fertility rates in a group of women with infertility due to asthenozoospermia (a condition in which many of the sperm have low motility). Royal jelly is a nutrient-rich substance produced by bees to feed the hive's queen and bring her into optimal health and fertility. It's available at health food stores and online.

better semen quality. Vitamin C intake appeared to be associated with sperm number, vitamin E with motility of the sperm, and beta-carotene (a vitamin A precursor) with sperm concentration. In this study, zinc and folate were not found to significantly improve semen quality, but as zinc is involved in healing and folate in so many aspects of fertility, these nutrients are still great additions to your pre-baby diet. All in all, higher antioxidant intake was associated with higher sperm numbers and motility.

More Male Support

The great antioxidant power of guava comes from more than its vitamin A, C, and E content. Guavas include other nutrients that support health: alkaloids, anthocyanins, carotenoids, essential oils, fatty acids, lectins, phenols, saponins, tannins, triterpenes, and quercetin. Quercetin is a powerful antioxidant that may also help improve semen quality. But quercetin does more: It is known to reduce the risk of cancer and improve cardiovascular health. And healthy blood vessels are particularly important for proper penis function.

Olive Oil

WE COULD HAVE FEATURED OLIVE OIL IN ANY trimester of pregnancy or postbirth care since it's a healthy food to include in every type of diet. Olive oil is one of the healthiest fats on earth. Thanks to its versatility in the kitchen and great fatty content, olive oil has become a common food consumed around the world. Eating healthy fats like olive oil is key to having a healthy body and conceiving a healthy baby.

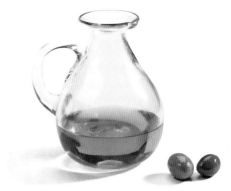

OLIVE OIL AT A GLANCE

Serving Size: 2 Tbsp (28 g)	Calcium: 0%
Calories: 248	Vitamin A: 0%
Saturated Fat: 4 g	Vitamin C: 0%
Protein: 0 g	Iron: 1%
Fiber: 0 g	

Benefits of Fats

There are good fats and bad fats. The worst fats—bad with a capital B—are the man-made trans fats found in processed foods and margarine. (Regardless of what the label says, if the ingredients list "hydrogenated oil" or "partially hydrogenated oil," you're looking at trans fats. Leave it alone!) The monounsaturated and poly-unsaturated fats you find in plant oils like olive oil are good fats. Each oil has a different composition of fats, making some healthier than others. Olive oil, fish oil, and flax oil are among the healthiest oils on earth and are great to include in your pantry—but olive oil is the only one that can handle a little heat.

EAT FOR TODAY AND TOMORROW

One of the leading causes of death around the world is heart disease. Researchers from the Harvard School of Public Health estimate that healthy food choices, together with regular physical activity and not smoking, can prevent over 80 percent of coronary heart disease, 70 percent of strokes, and 90 percent of type 2 diabetes.

So ditch those other sources of fat like margarine and butter. Reach for a healthier alternative like olive oil. It offers your body a wide variety of heart-healthy benefits and is a healthy dietary change you can make today that will help you and your family stay healthy for your lifetimes.

Jonny's Tasty Tips

All olive oil is not created equal. That's why you need to look for extra-virgin olive oil. What does this stuff about virgins really mean? It actually refers to the first pressing of the olives to extract the oil. Extra-virgin olive oil is separated from the olives without heat, hot water, or solvents, and it's left unfiltered, so it retains its antioxidants and other nutrients. Always look for the extra-virgin stuff: It's worth the time and money.

If you're lucky enough to find organic extra-virgin olive oil (which is often a beautiful green, not gold), taste it on a salad, grilled veggies, simple pasta sauce, or in a dip for multigrain bread. I guarantee you'll think you've died and gone to heaven! Your baby—and your heart—will thank you.

SEEDY SPERM

Flaxseed oil, which contains alpha-linolenic acid and lignans, is also thought to help support the production of healthy sperm. According to an article in *Reproductive Biomedicine*, flaxseed oil can help correct deficiencies of omega-3 fatty acid intake (an essential fat that is deficient in a typical Western diet), which is related to impaired sperm motility among men with fertility problems. See page 188 in chapter 4 for the full story on flax.

FAST FACT

Olive oil is part of healthiest diet on earth, the Mediterranean diet. The best kind is extra-virgin olive oil, which has been created without using high temperatures and is therefore richer in all the healthy compounds you want!

Insulin Support

Studies have found that using olive oil in your diet may help decrease your risk of developing insulin resistance. Insulin resistance is a condition in which your body is unable to respond to insulin properly, leaving your blood sugar levels higher than they should be. Unhealthy blood sugar levels are thought to be linked with infertility. Ditch those other fats in your diet and include olive oil more often to improve your health.

Healthy Blood, Healthy Body

The health-promotion properties of olive oil can be explained in part by the presence of plant compounds called phenols. In a study from the University of Cordoba in Spain, twenty-one people with high cholesterol levels consumed either phenol-rich olive oil or olive oil with most of the phenols removed. Only the phenol-rich olive oil significantly increased nitric oxide levels and lowered levels of oxidative stress in the blood. Nitric oxide is important for blood vessel health and dilation. Reducing oxidative stress helps prevent the damage to artery walls that leads to heart disease. Olive oil can help make your body healthier, improving your ability to have a healthy baby.

Paprika

PAPRIKA (*CAPSICUM ANNUUM*) IS A SPICE THAT is packed with nutrients to support health if you're trying to become dads and moms. Paprika is a bright red spice made from powdered hot pepper that is commonly added to cheese, chili powder blends, and sausages for a little heat and a splash of color. And of course, it's famous in the Hungarian dish chicken paprikash. But you can add it to many other dishes, including deviled eggs, rice dishes, cole slaw, and potato or pasta salads.

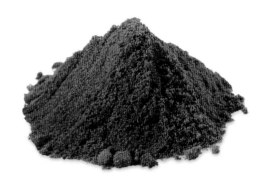

PAPRIKA AT A GLANCE

Serving Size: 1 Tbsp (7 g)	Calcium: 1%
Calories: 20	Vitamin A: 71%
Saturated Fat: 0 g	Vitamin C: 8%
Protein: 1 g	Iron: 9%
Fiber: 3 g	

So now that you have so many ways to use paprika in your diet, why would you want to? Because it's packed with iron, vitamin C, vitamin A, and more nutrients that are helpful in getting mom healthy and dad's sperm healthy too.

C-ing Red

Paprika contains lots of vitamin C and iron. Vitamin C levels are higher in a man's testicles than in his blood. Thus, eating foods that are rich in vitamin C, like paprika, may help ensure that your testicles contain the levels of vitamin C they need to do their job. In fact, animal research studies have found that including foods rich in vitamin C in the diet can increase sperm numbers, motility, and health.

Ironing Out Ovulation Problems

Ladies, paprika's not just good for guys. Having low levels of iron in your diet may put you at higher risk of experiencing problems with ovulation. According to a study by the Harvard University School of Public Health

Jonny's Tasty Tips

The active ingredient in paprika, capsaicin, produces a wealth of health benefits, from boosted metabolism and weight loss to increased production of feel-good endorphins, high vitamin C and A, and even pain relief when applied topically to the skin.

You can find paprika at all levels of heat from sweet and mild to hot. I like to go for Hungarian paprika, and I like mine hot. Chicken paprikash is a classic Hungarian paprika dish, with chicken coated with sour cream and paprika, but I enjoy something simpler even more: roasted chicken with its surface rubbed with organic butter and paprika. Paprika and eggs are also naturals. Besides sprinkling paprika on your deviled eggs, try it on hard-boiled eggs, scrambled eggs, and omelets. Add it to your huevos rancheros and frittatas. Sprinkle some on stuffed peppers, meat loaf, and burgers.

For that matter, you can use hot paprika anywhere you'd normally use chili powder: in refried beans, chili, quesadillas, you name it. Try hot paprika and lime juice on grilled fish, shrimp, scallops, corn on the cob, or grilled sweet potato, zucchini, or summer squash slices. (It's great for perking up baked sweet potato fries, too!) I love the way it balances a creamy cole slaw and have been known to add a sprinkle to slices of cantaloupe and peaches for a delicious counterpoint. Try it and you'll see why!

in 2007, iron levels may significantly impact fertility in women. Of the more than 18,000 women surveyed in the Nurses' Health Study, 483 reported having ovulation problems. Women who ate more free iron (found in fortified foods, legumes, grains, and supplements) appeared to have the greatest protection against infertility. Ensuring that your diet contains sufficient iron levels is important. A sprinkle of paprika is a great way to get a little more iron in your diet.

Go Red for Fertility

A great source of vitamin A is just a sprinkle away. And vitamin A deficiency has dire effects on reproduction. In animal studies, males with low vitamin A levels have trouble making sperm and females tend to have trouble conceiving; in some vitamin A-deficient animals, the sexual cycle will even stop. With a whopping 71 percent of your daily requirements for vitamin A in just one tablespoon of paprika, it may be time to add a little red to your foods.

More in a Pinch

This nutrient-packed spice is a good source of other nutrients too, including vitamin E (2 mg per tablespoon) and vitamin B6 (0.3 mg per tablespoon). Both of these nutrients are key to everyday health and reproductive health as well. Vitamin E is a potent antioxidant needed to keep you healthy, and it's vital to sperm health. Vitamin B6 is an important energy vitamin that keeps you going during the day and night, which matters since it takes a lot of energy to make a baby!

Psyllium

A POPULAR LAXATIVE, PSYLLIUM HAS MORE TO OFFER than a speedy stay on the toilet. In fact, its diversity as a healthy food is better known these days: You'll find psyllium advertised as a beneficial add-in to some common foods like cereal. It's high in fiber, so it's among the healthiest foods you can add to any diet, particularly if you're trying to be the healthiest you can be for your upcoming pregnancy.

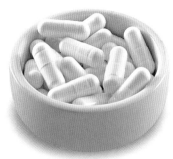

PSYLLIUM AT A GLANCE

Serving Size: 1 oz	Calcium: 8%
Calories: 57	Vitamin A: 0%
Saturated Fat: 0 g	Vitamin C: 0%
Protein: 1 g	Iron: 0%
Fiber: 22 g	

Fullness Factor

Psyllium and the fiber it contains bulks up in the intestines, taking on water, which helps you feel full and encourages proper bowel excretion. The University of London reported that a group of researchers investigating the effects of *Plantago ovata* seed (psyllium) on seventeen female subjects found that it may be useful in weight-control diets because it affects fat intake and may have some effect on feelings of fullness. Adding some psyllium into your diet can help you avoid those less-healthy snacks like cupcakes and chocolate that won't support healthy fertility.

Cleaning Up

Fiber also eliminates the nasty toxins in your body. Did you know that more than eighty thousand toxic chemicals are manufactured in the United States each year? These toxins can be in your water and food supplies and even in your cosmetics. When toxins enter your body, the liver filters them out of your blood and sends them, along with bile, into your intestines, where fiber can trap them and send them out of your body. Without fiber, however, these toxins can become reabsorbed and build up in your system, eventually causing damage, and may reduce your fertility.

Fiber-rich foods like psyllium can help lower your body's toxin levels. Psyllium seed husks are nature's most concentrated source of cholesterol-lowering soluble fiber. The husks (outer seed coats) contain about 60 percent fiber (oats, on the other hand, are only about 5 percent fiber). Just one tablespoon of whole psyllium provides about 9 g of soluble fiber, more than one-third of the recommended daily intake.

Afterword

We want to end this book with an acknowledgment to you, our readers. And here's why: By buying and reading this book, you've shown a tremendous commitment to having a healthy pregnancy and a healthy baby. There's no way to overstate the importance of that commitment and the overwhelming love that created it. You've shown a willingness to partner in your own health care and to create an environment—both in the womb and afterward—that will nurture and support your new family member. We take our collective hats off to you.

Although this book has provided a lot of what we hope are wonderful guidelines and useful information, you should never use it as an inflexible prescription from which you cannot waver! This book should be your helpmate, not your taskmaster, and should never be a source of stress, which is, quite frankly, the absolute last thing you need in your life right now! So the message we want to leave you with can be summed up in one word: Relax.

Wanting to give your baby the best possible start in life may have driven you to try to read as much as you can about pregnancy and health. But the information can be endless, conflicting, and at times confusing. As a pregnant woman experiencing all of the same concerns while writing this book, Allison found that the most important thing is to trust yourself. Your natural instincts will guide you through pregnancy, delivery, and motherhood. You'll do great.

It's worth remembering that people have been having babies for a very long time. Many people reading this book came from families where the information in this book was not available. And even more have come from families where the "rules" were frequently broken, and yet the kids came out great.

(Jonny spends a lot of time in St. Martin with Oliver and Jennifer, dear friends of his from Europe, where having the occasional glass of wine while pregnant is not considered a big deal. Their absolutely beautiful, almost perfect daughter Leslie is "proof" that breaking the occasional rule does not always result in disaster!)

Of course, we're not advocating drinking during pregnancy. But it's really important to remember that it's harder to "screw this up" than you might think, and the fact that you've spent this much time and effort trying to arm yourself with the best information possible shows that you're unlikely to make a mess of things!

This book has been about helping you make the best choices to increase the odds that things turn out really well. Which we're pretty sure they will!

Remember—especially when you feel overwhelmed by all the things you're supposed to know and do—that the guidelines are really simple: Eat good food, move around, take your vitamins, get some sleep, and above all...relax. Stress is probably one of the biggest robbers of health and vitality on the planet. You may not be able to completely avoid it, but to the extent that you can reduce it, you'll be doing yourself and your baby a huge favor.

Finally, remember that the one gift you have to give your baby—both in the womb and for the rest of his life—is something that you can't get out of a book. It's love. That's something you have in plentiful supply, and you don't need any rule book to show you how to give it. Provide your baby with that love—give him/her room to grow, space to fall, and hands to pick him/her back up—and you'll do just fine.

Enjoy the journey.

—Jonny and Allison

About the Authors

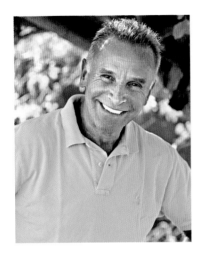

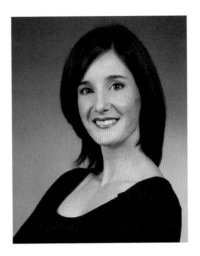

Jonny Bowden, Ph.D., C.N.S., is a nationally known expert on weight loss, nutrition, and health. He's the author of seven acclaimed books, including the bestseller *The 150 Healthiest Foods on Earth* (now in its fourteenth printing), *The Healthiest Meals on Earth*, *The Most Effective Natural Cures on Earth*, and *The 150 Most Effective Ways to Boost Your Energy*. A board-certified nutritionist with a master's degree in psychology and six national certifications in exercise and personal training, he has had his work featured in more than fifty magazines and newspapers, ranging from the *New York Times* to *US Weekly*. He's appeared as a nutrition expert on CNN, Fox News, MSNBC, ABC-TV, NBC-TV, CBS-TV, Martha Stewart Living, and Oprah and Friends. His latest book is *The Most Effective Ways to Live Longer*. Visit Jonny on the Web at www.jonnybowden.com.

Allison Tannis, M.S., R.H.N., is an internationally renowned nutritional expert. She is the author of four books, including the critically acclaimed *Probiotic Rescue* and *Feed Your Skin, Starve Your Wrinkles*. She is a regular contributor to health and fitness magazines, host of radio sensation "Healthy Living," and is a registered holistic nutritionist practicing in southern Ontario. Allison is passionate about making the science of health easy to swallow, so when she discovered that she was pregnant with her first child, she used her own pregnancy experiences and those of the many women she interviewed to motivate and guide her in creating this book, with the goal of helping pregnant women love food rather than fearing it. Visit Allison on the Web at www.allisontannis.com.

Index

Note: Page numbers in italics indicate tables.

100 HEALTHIEST FOODS INDEX

A
acerola cherries, 180-181
aged Cheddar cheese, 182-183
almonds, 31-32
anchovies, 33-34
applesauce, 35-36
apricots, 273-274
artichokes, 184-185
arugula, 297-298
asparagus, 299-300
avocados, 84-85

B
bananas, 38-39
basil, 86-87
bitter melon, 301-302
black beans, 131-132
broth, 40-41
brown rice, 42-43
buckwheat, 303-304

C
cabbage, 252-253
carob, 186-187
carrots, 88-89
celery, 133-134
chamomile, 92-93
cherries, 94-95
chia seeds, 90-91
chickpeas, 96-97
chives, 44-45
chocolate milk, 98-99

coconut oil, 100-101
Coho salmon, 135-136
crabmeat, 275-276
cranberries, 137-138
cream cheese, 46-47
crimini mushrooms, 139-140

D
dill, 254-255

E
eggplant, 143-144
eggs, 141-142
evening primrose oil (EPO), 145-146

F
fenugreek, 256-257
figs, 102-103
flaxseed, 188-189

G
garlic, 149-150
ginger, 48-49
green peas, 151-152
guava, 307-308

H
hemp seeds, 104-105
herring, 153-154

I
ice chips, 50-51

K
kale, 105-106
kefir, 190-191
kiwi, 192-193

L
lamb, 52-53
leeks, 54-55
lemons, 56-57
lentils, 277-278

M
mackerel, 258-259
melons, 301-302
milk, 262-263
molasses, 155-156
multigrain cereal, 60-61
mushrooms, 139-140

N
nori, 108-109
nuts, 157-158

O
oatmeal, 62-63
olive oil, 309-310

P
papaya, 159-160
paprika, 311-312
parsley, 161-162
peanut butter, 64-65
peppermint, 163-164
pinto beans, 66-67
popcorn, 68-69
prune juice, 194-195
psyllium, 313
pumpkin seeds, 196-197

Q
quinoa, 279-280

R
rainbow trout, 198-199
red raspberry leaf tea, 165-166
rhubarb, 167-168
romaine lettuce, 110-111

S
salmon, 135-136
sardines, 281-282
scallions, 112-113
sesame seeds, 169-170
shiitake mushrooms, 283-284
spinach, 200-201
sun-dried tomatoes, 202-203
sweet potatoes, 70-71
Swiss cheese, 171-172

T
tahini, 72-73
tilapia, 74-75
tofu, 114-115
tuna, 118-119
turkey, 120-121
turmeric, 116-117

W
water, 50-51
watercress, 82, 83, 122-123
watermelon, 76-77
wheat germ, 204-205
whole-grain pasta, 206-207

Y
yogurt, 208-209

GENERAL INDEX

A
abortifacients, 49
ACE inhibitors, 212
acerola cherries, 44, 176, 179, 180-181
acetaldehyde, 212
acne, 79, 174, 180, 186-189, 198, 208
aflatoxin, 212
aged Cheddar cheese. See Cheddar cheese
air, swallowing, 177
alcohol, 9, 212, 213, 214, 215-216, 248
alfalfa, 225, 226, 239
alkaloids, 308
allergens, 157, 226
almond/rice beverages, 12
almonds, 12, 30, 31-32, 32, 157, 176
aloes, 237
alpha-linolenic acid (ALA), 90-91, 118, 119, 188, 257, 310
alpha-tocopherol, 306. See also vitamin E
aluminum chloride, 212
amino acids, 104, 142, 176-177, 182, 264, 297
anchovies, 13, 30, 33-34, 230
andrographis, 237
anemia, 86, 102, 195, 204, 243
anencephaly, 10
angelica, 237
angiotensin I-converting enzyme, 200
anthocyanins, 165, 181, 308
anticonvulsants, 212
antidepressants, 212

antioxidants, 13, 24, 32, 35-37, 39, 57, 76, 84-85, 97, 113, 120, 122, 131, 134, 140, 143, 162, 165, 167, 176-177, 180-181, 193, 209, 261, 274, 279, 297, 300, 307-308
apples, 35, 36, 37, 291
applesauce, 30, 35-36, 37
apricots, 10, 270, 272, 273-274
arachidonic acid (AA), 243, 246, 259, 268, 282
areolas, darkening of, 19
arginine, 104
artichokes, 37, 179, 184-185
artificial sweeteners, 214, 216-219
Art of the Nutrition Shift, 7
arugula, 201, 296, 297-298
ashwaganda, 237
asparagus, 10, 20, 25, 168, 291, 296, 299-300
aspartame, 216, 217, 218, 219
asthma, 13
attention deficit disorder (ADD), 246
avocados, 25, 81-85, 232, 270, 291, 293

B
babies, 13
  brain health of, 13
  feeding, 270-271
  introducing foods to, 250
  progression through gestation, 22
baby blues, 266
backaches, 19, 79, 81, 125, 127, 177, 178
bacteria, 87, 137, 190-191, 194, 213, 222, 223, 226, 229, 230, 248. See also specific bacteria

bananas, 30, 38-39, 126, 291
barbeque, 248
barberry, 237
basil, 13, 83, 86-87
beans, 8, 10, 12, 21, 25, 27, 29, 30, 66-67, 130, 131-132, 197, 278. See also specific beans
beef, 294
beef broth, 41
bell peppers, 13, 42, 144, 181, 291
berries, 28, 83, 131. See also specific berries
beta-carotene, 88, 89, 112, 165, 307, 308
beta-sitosterol, 39
beverages. See also alchohol; specific beverages
  caffeinated, 9, 58, 59, 93, 99, 220, 222, 224, 238
  carbonated, 177
  decaffeinated, 222
  sweetened, 9
Bifidobacteria, 190
biotin, 21, 176
birth control, 245
birth defects, 10, 24, 89, 292, 305-306
birth weight, 24, 27, 151-152, 195
bisphenol-A (BPA), 234, 264
bitter melon, 296, 301-302
black beans, 130, 131-132
blackberries, 37
black cohosh, 236, 237, 238, 239
blackstrap molasses, 155, 156, 175
black tea, 224, 226
bladder infections, 82, 137
Blaylock, Russell, 217
blessed thistle, 236, 239

bloating, 177, 183, 190, 193, 194, 206, 208
blood circulation, 81, 82
blood clotting, 149
blood pressure, 39, 45, 149, 200. See also high blood pressure
blood sugar, 27, 39, 43, 45, 152, 294-295, 303
blood volume, 23, 126
blueberries, 37
blue cohosh, 237
body mass index (BMI), 293
bok choy, 12
bone formation, 11, 46
bone health, 99, 118, 163, 168, 171, 208, 246, 264
borage oil, 259
bottles, 264
Bowden, Jonny, 315, 315
brain development, 82, 85, 96, 118, 135, 144, 154, 199, 228, 232, 259, 268, 305
brain health, 13, 55, 63, 75, 199
Braxton-Hicks contractions, 80
Brazil nuts, 157, 158
bread, 25, 28, 83
breast-feeding, 240-264
breast milk, 101, 246-250. See also breast-feeding
breast pumps, 244
breasts, 242-243
  enlargement of, 8, 19, 21, 23, 80, 81
  tenderness of, 19, 79, 174-175
breath, shortness of, 82
broccoli, 10, 12, 25, 105, 181, 291
broth, 30, 40-41
brown rice, 20, 30, 41, 42-43, 139

brown rice pudding, 43
brown sugar, 28
Brussels sprouts, 10, *12*, 105
buckwheat, 296, 303-304
butter, 309
B vitamins, 10, 20, 41-42, 54, 63, 69, 74-76, 123, 139, 161, 163, 169, 176, 191, 203-204, 207, 209, 252, 260, 270, 283-284, 297, 303-305. *See also specific B vitamins*

C
cabbage, 105, 177, 251, 252-253, 291
Caesar dressing, 227
caffeinated beverages, 9, 58, 59, 93, 99, 220, 222, 224, 238
caffeine, 213, 214, 220-221, *221*, 222, 238, 263. *See also* caffeinated beverages
calcium, 11, *12*, 20, 21, 29, 34, 39, 44, 46-47, 80, 85-86, 91, 99, 102, 111, 115, 125, 149, 156, 161, 163, 167, 170-172, 177, 181-183, 186, 225, 241, 243, 245-246, 252-253, 262-264, 270-271, 286, 298, 306
calories, 7, 14, 17, 23, 29, 80, 125, 157, 232, 244-245, 286
Camembert cheese, 47, 182, 230
Campylobacter, 223-224
cancer, 13, 105, 227, 248. *See also* carcinogens
candy, 9
canola oil, 257
cantaloupe, *25*, 229, 260
caraway, 239
carbohydrates, 20, 26-27, 176, 207
complex, 176
carcinogens, 248
cardiovascular health, 96, 149, 309
carob, 179, 186-187
carotenoids, 101, 181, 203, 308
carrots, 83, 88-89
cascara, 237
castor oil, 236, 237, 238
catechins, 165
catfish, 228
catnip, 237
cat's claw, 237
cayenne, 237
celery, 130, 133-134, 168, 291
cell phones, 288
cereals, 62-63
fortified, *24*, *25*
multigrain, 30, 60-61, 176
sugar-coated, 28
cervix, 166
Cesarean sections, 27
chamomile, 82-83, 92-93, 224-225, 236, 238
chasteberry, 239
Cheddar cheese, 11, *12*, 29, 177, 179, 182-183, 230
cheese, 11, *12*, 29, 47, 171-172, 177, 179, 182-183, 213, 214, 229, 230. *See also specific cheeses*
hard cheeses, 230
raw milk cheeses, 229
safe, 230
soft cheeses, 213, 214, 230
cherries, 37, 44, 81, 82, 83, 94-95, 176, 179, 180-181, 237, 291
chévre, 230
chia seeds, 11, 83, 90-91
chicken, 41. *See also* poultry
chicken broth, 40-41
chickpeas, 10, 83, 96-97, 176
The Children of the 90s, 13
chives, 30, 44-45
chlamydia, 212
chloride, 21
chlorogenic acid, 143, 165
chocolate, 220, *221, 222*

chocolate milk, 82, 83, 98-99
cholesterol, 39, 47, 141, 142
choline, 21, 33-34, 55, 64, 65, 66, 74, 75, 85, 96, 298
chorionic gonadotrophin, 242
chromium, 21, 61

chromosomes, 20
cigarette smoking, 212, 248, 288
cinnamon, 303
citrus peel, 224
cleft lip, 26
cleft palate, 305-306
cocaine, 212
cocoa products, *221*, 222
coconut oil, 81, 83, 100-101, 232
coffee, 220, *221*, 222
cognitive ability, 106
Coho salmon, 13, 130, 135-136. *See also* salmon
cola beverages, *221*, 222
cold cuts. *See under* meats
colic, 248
collagen, 57, 95, 134
collards, *12*, 201
coltsfoot, 237
comfrey, 237
complaints, foods that quiet, 173-209
complementary foods, 250
conception, 7, 286, 287, 289, 292, 293, 294, 301
congenital syphilis, 150
congestion, 81
constipation, 45, 50, 79, 80, 81, 155, 159, 170, 172, 175, 177, 183, 184, 187, 189, 190, 193-195, 202, 206, 208, 236
contaminants, 211, 212-213, 248, 291. *See also specific contaminants*
contractions, 80, 161, 165, 166, 169
copper, 21, 44, 53, 66-67, 85-86, 92, 97, 111, 114, 122, 161, 163, 169, 185-187, 203, 254, 275-276, 278, 306
corn, 291
corn syrup, 219
cottage cheese, 230
cowpeas, *25*
crabmeat, 272, 275-276
crackers, 83
cramps, 45, 79, 80, 81, 127, 177, 183, 208, 228, 236
cranberries, 37, 130, 137-138
cravings, 6, 7, 23, 28-29
Crayhon, Robert, 6, 264
cream, 229
cream cheese, 30, 46-47, 230
crimini mushrooms, 130, 139-140
curcumin, 117
custard, 227
cyanocobalamin. *See* vitamin B12
cyclamates, 216, 217-218, 219
cysteine, 104, 120

D
dairy products, 11, 16, 20, 21, 29, 176. *See also specific dairy products*
unpasteurized, 229, 230
dandelion tea, 225
DASH (Dietary Approach to Stop Hypertension), 39
decaffeinated beverages, 222
dehydration, 40, 50, 249
delivery, 11, 24, 153, 166
dental health, 163, 166, 171
depression, 246, 292. *See also* postpartum depression
detoxification, 131-132, 225
diabetes, 13, 27, 152
diarrhea, 228
Dietary Guidelines for Americans, 24
dieting, 29, 207, 225, 233, 247, 292
digestion, 58, 79, 80-81, 125, 128, 159, 164, 170, 172, 177, 183, 187, 190-191, 194-195, 202, 206, 208, 225, 238
dill, 251, 254-255
dioxins, 136
discomfort, 126
diuretics, 58
dizziness, 82
docosahexaenoic acid (DHA), 8, 13, 33, 34, 52, 91, 118-119, 129, 135, 136, 148, 153-154, 188, 198, 243,

246-247, 257-259, 261, 267-268, 281-282, 305
dong quai, 237

E
eating disorders, 16
eclampsia, 39
eczema, 13
eggnog, 227
eggplant, 130, 143-144, 176
eggs, 11, *25*, 130, *139*, 141-142, 176
raw, 214, 227, 229
eicosapentaenoic acid (EPA), 33, 91, 118, 135, 153, 188, 198, 281, 282
electrolytes, 156
ellagitannins, 165
emmenagogues, 49
emotions, 21. *See also* moods
endive, 296, 305-306
energy, 8, 67, 79, 155, 156, 175-177, 184, 189, 193, 196, 204, 209, 252, 270, 277
enzymes, 23, 97, 104, 177, 182, 190, 205
ephedra, 237
Equal. *See* aspartame
erythritol, 217
Escherichia coli (E. coli), 223-224
essential fatty acids, 308. *See also specific essential fatty acids*
essential fatty acids (EFAs), 13, 41, 118-119, 135, 246-247, 308
estrogen, 80, 293, 294
evening primrose oil (EPO), 130, 145-146
excitotoxin, 217
exercise, 67, 79, 98-99, 175, 177, 249
exocytosis, 243
eye development, 135, 228, 232, 259
eyesight, 88, 122, 129, 135, 142

F
fatigue, 19, 36, 50, 195, 196, 204, 270, 277
fats, 8, 9, 13, 14, 20, 29, 33-34, 47, 80-81, 84, 85, 91, 97, 98, 100, 101, 127, 129, 156, 157, 170, 176-177, 226-227, 246, 249. *See also specific kinds of fats*
bad, 309
good, 9, 47, 245, 246, 270, 293, 309-310
fennel, 237
fenugreek, 236, 238, 239, 251, 256-257
fermented foods, 174, 177, 190-191, 208-209. *See also specific foods*
fertility, 8, 19, 245, 285-313
fertility treatments, 293
fetal alcohol syndrome (FAS), 215-216
fetal bone mineralization, 46
fetal death, 224, 226, 230
fetal development, 19, 24, 80-81, 82, 92, 125
fetal infection, 224, 226, 230
fetal movements, 127
fetus, 20
feverfew, 237
fiber, 14, 42, 44, 54, 66, 70, 79, 80, 81, 84, 86, 88, 91, 96, 102, 111, 125, 127, 131, 134, 152, 157, 159, 163, 167, 170, 175, 177, 184, 185, 187, 189, 193-194, 196, 202, 204, 206, 252, 254, 260, 261, 278, 280, 286, 301-302, 306, 313
figs, 11, *12*, 83, 102-103
first trimester, 13, 18-77
fish, 7-9, 11, 13, 29, 108, 128, 129, 174, 177, 179, 213, 229, 230, 232, 245, 247, 267, 270, 290. *See also* seafood; *specific kinds of fish*
selecting, 229-230
fish broth, 41
fish oil, 130, 146, 147-148, 246, 258-259, 309

supplements, 6, 147-148, 236, 247
flatulence, 277
flavonoids, 35, 87, 105, 176
flavonols, 165
flaxseed, 90, 118, 179, 188-189, 232, 239, 247, 257
flaxseed oil, 309, 310
fluids, 80, 125, 126, 134, 175, 202, 286
fluoride, 21
folate (folic acid), 6, 8, 10, 16, 17, 20, 21, 24-*25*, 26, 30-31, 34, 38, 44, 47, 54, 64-66, 80, 84-85, 86, 110-111, 113, 122, 125, 151, 159, 161, 163, 169, 176, 184-185, 200, 205, 211, 241, 245, 252, 254, 260, 283, 284, 286, 289, 290, 292, 297-299, 301, 303-306, 308
folic acid, 25, *25*. *See also* folate (folic acid)
food, heating, 223, 224
food aversions, 29, 73, 74
food cravings, 19
food poisoning, 223-224
food safety, 9, 160, 213, 223, 224, 227, 228, 229
formula. *See* formula
free radicals, 97, 121, 167, 176, 188, 299, 307
frozen yogurt, 28, 29, 39
fruit, 8, 9, 16, 20, 39, 83, 126, 176, 177, 245, 295. *See also specific kinds of fruit*
fruit juice, 28
furans, 136

G
galactagogues, 238, 239
gamma-linolenic acid (GLA), 104, 145, 146, 246
garbanzo beans. *See* chickpeas
garlic, 112, 130, 149-150, 237, 248
gas, 79, 177, 183, 190, 193, 194, 206, 208, 225, 248
"generally recognized as safe" (GRAS) status, 92, 100, 164
genetics, 65, 74, 163
gestation, *22*
gestational diabetes, 27, 43, 61
ginger, 30, 41, 48-49, 178, 224, 225, 236, 237
glutathione, 120, 165, 299
glycemic index, 43, 268-269
glycemic load, 29, 31
goat's rue, 239
gogi berries, 181
grains, 9, 10, 20, 29, 60-61, 83, 176-177. *See also* multigrain cereal; whole grains; whole grains foods; *specific grains*
grapes, 291
Great Nothern beans, *25*
green peas, 130, 151-152. *See also* peas
greens, 105-106, 177, 297. *See also specific greens*
green tea, 224, 226
guava, 296, 307-308
gums, 81

H
halibut, 176
hazelnuts, *12*
HDL cholesterol, 141
headaches, 19, 129
heartburn, 79, 80, 81, 125, 137, 159
heart disease, 10, 13, 23. *See also* cardiovascular health
heart rate, 23
heavy metals, 154, 213, 233
hemoglobin, 92, 176, 184
hemorrhoids, 194
hemp seeds, 82, 83, 104-105, 232
herbs, 236-237, 270
to avoid, 237
herbal supplements, 235-239
herb teas, 58, 82, 214, 224-226
herring, 130, 153-154
heterocyclic amines (HCAs), 248

hibiscus, 237
hiccups, 127
high blood pressure, 38-39, 129, 146, 200
high blood sugar, 294-295, 301-302, 310
high-fructose corn syrup, 219
high-glycemic foods, 43, 268-269, 294-295, 301
high-risk foods, 9
histidine, 104
HIV, 212
Hollandaise sauce, 227
homocysteine, 156
honey, 217
honeydew melon, 260
horehound, 237
hormones, 21, 23, 46, 80, 82, 90, 145, 155, 175, 177, 182-183, 242-243, 245, 293. *See also specific hormones*
hot dogs, 214, 226-227, 228, 248
hydration, 50-51, 58, 82, 99, 123, 134, 165, 246, 249
hydrocephalus, 10
hydrogenated oils, 231, 232
hypercarotenemia, 88
hypertension, 11

I
ice chips, 7, 30, 50-51, 178
ice cream, *12*, 28, 220, 227
immune system, 56, 101, 150, 163, 198, 241-243, 246, 284
immunoglobins, 243
implantation bleeding, 19
indigestion, 159
infant formula, 243
infections, 82. *See also specific kinds of infections*
infertility, 286-287, 308
inflammation, 186, 188, 198, 209, 307
insoluble fiber, 175, 278
insulin, 45, 268, 269, 294-295, 301-302, 304, 310
insulin resistance, 295, 301-302, 310
iodine, 6, 21, 248
IQ, 13
iron, 8, 10-11, 16, 20, 21, 26, 34, 44, 52-54, 62, 66-67, 80, 82, 85, 86, 92, 95-96, 102, 110, 111, 114, 116, 125, 131, 151, 156, 161, 163, 169-170, 175-176, 181, 184-185, 195-196, 200, 204, 207, 225, 241, 242, 245, 249, 250, 252, 254-256, 270, 273-274, 277, 278, 286, 294, 297, 306, 311-312
  absorption of, 11
  iron deficiency, 26, 102, 170, 195, 243
irritable bowel syndrome (IBS), 164
isomalt, 218
itchy skin, 192, 205, 208, 209

J
Jones, K., 215
juniper, 237
junk food, 103

K
kaempferol, 105, 165
kale, 82, 83, 105-106, 201
kava kava, 237
kefir, 82, 174, 177, 179, 190-191
Kegel exercises, 152
kelp supplements, 108
kidney infections, 82
kiwi, 176, 179, 181, 192-193, 291

L
labor, 161, 165, 166, 238
LAC (Live and Active Cultures) seal, 209
lactation. *See* breast-feeding
lactitol, 218
Lactobacilli, 190-191
lactogen, 242
lactose, 191, 243

lamb, 10, 13, 30, 52-53
lauric acid, 101
lavender, 237
L-carnitine, 264
LDL cholesterol, 141
lead, 233, 248
learning disabilities, 24
lecithin, 33
lectins, 308
leeks, 10, 13, 30, 54-55
leg cramps, 45, 79, 80, 81, 177, 208, 236
legumes, 96, 97, 158
lemon balm, 224, 237
lemons, 30, 56-57
lentils, 10, 272, 277-278
L-ergothioneine, 140
let-down reflex, 244
lettuce, *25*, 110-111, 200, 201, 291. *See also specific kinds of lettuce*
licorice, 237
lignans, 90, 239, 310
limb defects, 10
limonin, 57
linoleic acid (LA), 145
Listeria monocytogenes, 47, 223-224, 228, 230
listeriosis, 222, 223, 224, 226, 227
lithium, 212
liver, 24, *25*
Logan, Alan, 188
lovage, 237
lower limb paralysis, 24
low-fat protein, 9
low-glycemic foods, 43, 176, 269, 295
lungs, 82
lutein, 122, 142, 176, 201
luteinizing hormone, 245
luteolin, 162
lycopene, 76, 101, 203, 207, 274

M
macadamia nuts, 157
macaroni and cheese, *12*
mackerel, 13, 228, 228, 230, 251, 258-259
magnesium, 6, 21, 42, 44-45, 55, 85, 86, 92, 102, 109, 111, 114, 122, 131, 155, 161, 163, 167, 169, 176, 185, 195, 196, 203, 225, 236, 241, 245, 252, 253, 262, 271, 289, 298, 306
magnesium oxide, 146
maltitol, 218
mammary glands. *See* breasts
manganese, 21, 42, 44, 53, 55, 64-66, 70, 85-86, 92, 97, 106, 111, 113, 116, 117, 122, 131, 149, 151, 155, 161, 163, 167, 169, 185-186, 203, 252, 298, 306
mangoes, 291
mannitol, 218
margarine, 309
massage therapy, 79
mayonnaise, 227
MCT (medium-chain triglycerides), 101
meat, 20-210, 41, 73, 83, 120, 176, 228, 293, 294. *See also specific kinds of meat*
  deli meats, 120, 213-214, 222-224, 227-228, 248
  pâtés, 228
  processed, 226-227
  raw, 213, 227
  red, 294
  substitutes for, 132, 143
medications, 270
Mediterranean diet, 13
melatonin, 94
melons, 251, 260-261, 296, 301-302. *See also specific kinds of melons*
men, fertility and, 287-290, 297-300, 304, 307, 308, 310-312
meningitis, 150
meningocele, 10
mercury, 7, 74-75, 119, 136, 148, 153, 154, 213, 228, 230
metabolism, 41, 176, 177

methadone, 212
methionine, 74, 104
milk, 8, 11, *12*, 169, 170, 177, 245, 251, 262-263, 264, 270-271. *See also* chocolate milk
  raw milk, 229
  unpasteurized, 213, 230
minerals, 20, 39, 45, 53-54, 66-67, 84, 92, 97, 157, 161, 176, 196, 200, 236, 245-246, 248, 275-276. *See also specific kinds of minerals*
  for the first trimester, 21
  for lactation and breast-feeding, 241
  for the second trimester, 80
  for the third trimester, 125
mint tea, 30, 58-59
miscarriage, 50, 122, 224, 226, 230, 238, 305
molasses, 130, 155-156, 175
molybdenum, 21, 131, 132
monoterpene, 48
monounsaturated fat, 84, 157, 170, 231, 232, 309
mood, 198, 267, 270, 280
  mood disorders, 119
  mood swings, 23, 199
morning sickness, 6, 27, 28, 39, 40, 42, 55, 69, 178, 236
motherwort, 237
mousses, 227
mozzarella cheese, *12*, 230
multigrain cereal, 30, 60-61, 176
multiples, 17
multiple sclerosis, 11
multivitamins, 26, 89, 176, 271
muscles, 182-183, 197, 203
  muscle contractions (See contractions)
  muscle cramps, 208 (See cramps)
  muscle mass, 23
mushrooms, 41, 130, *139*, 139-140, 176, 270, 272, 283-284
myelomeningocele, 10
myricetin, 39

N
nasunin, 144
natural foods, 8
nausea, 8, 13, 19, 23, 27-28, 39, 40-42, 47-48, 225, 237
navy beans, *12*
nectarines, 291
neotame, 217
nerve damage, 24
nervous system, 24, 47, 75, 85, 96, 135, 154, 169-170
nettle tea, 225, 226
neural tube, 24, 84-85
neural-tube defects, 10, 24, 34, 38
newborn pneumonia, 150
newborns, infections in, 150
niacin, 6, 8, 21, 41-42, 44, 53, 63-65, 75, 85, 86, 132, 151, 161, 163, 176, 185, 203, 254, 260, 283, 303-304
nitrates, 227
nitric oxide, 113, 310
nori, 82, 83, 108-109
nosebleeds, 81
NutraSweet. *See* aspartame
nutrients, 8, 85. *See also specific nutrients*
nutrition, 28
nutrition shifts, 28-29
nuts, 20, 21, 27, 83, 130, 157-158, 176, 177, 197, 232, 245, 293. *See also specific nuts*

O
oatmeal, 20, 28, 30, 62-63, 176, 178
obesity, 14, 114-115
oligosaccharides, 206
olive oil, 13, 232, 270, 296, 309-310
omega-3 fatty acids, 7, 33, 90-91, 104, 118, 119, 128, 129, 135, 154, 188, 198-199, 228, 230, 246-247, 248, 258-259, 267-268, 276, 310
omega-6 fatty acids, 72-73, 84, 88, 104, 119, 248, 259

onions, 41, 54, 291. *See also specific kinds of onions*
oral facial cleft, 10
orange juice, *12, 25*
orange peel, 224
oranges, *12, 25,* 181
Oregon grape, 237
organic foods, 35, 37, 209, 290, 291
ovarian cancer, 105
ovaries, 105
overeating, 207
overweight, 14. *See also* weight
ovulation, 245, 311-312
oxidative stress, 113, 122, 310
oxygen, 82, 176, 204

P
pantothenic acid, 21, 44, 53, 96-97, 123, 161, 283, 305
papain, 159
papaya, *25*, 130, 159-160, 291
paprika, 13, 296, 311-312
parasites, 223, 226, 229
parsley, 130, 161-162
parsley oil, 162
parsley root, 237
parsley seed, 237
passionflower, 237
pasta, 83
  whole-grain, 179, 206-207
peaches, 291
peanut butter, 30, 39, 64-65
peanuts, *25*, 157, 158
pears, 291
peas, 10, *25,* 151-152, 291
pecans, 157
penicillin, 212
pennyroyal, 237
pepitas. *See* pumpkin seeds
peppermint, 130, 163-164, 224, 236, 237
peppermint oil, 164
peppermint tea, 58-59, 82, 163, 164, 225
peppers. *See* bell peppers
periods, 19, 26
  missed, 19
pesticides, 35, 37, 212, 288, 291
pet treats, 229
phenols, 143, 165, 308
phosphate, 243
phosphatidylcholine, 33
phosphorus, 21, 42, 44, 47, 53, 66-67, 85-86, 102, 111, 114, 122, 131, 149, 151, 156, 161, 163, 169, 185, 203, 241, 252, 254, 262, 298, 306
phytonutrients, 39, 105. *See also specific nutrients*
picky eaters, 271
  breast-feeding, 249
pineapples, 291
pine nuts, 157

pinto beans, 10, *12*, 30, 66-67
placenta, 140, 150, 242
placental abruption, 140
plant oils, 9, 246
plums, 37, 194
pneumonia, 150
pollock, 228
pollutants, 288
polychlorinated biphenyls (PCBs), 136, 148, 154, 212, 228, 290
polycyclic aromatic hydrocarbons (PAHs), 248
polyunsaturated fats, 65, 84, 170, 231, 232, 248, 309
popcorn, 28, 30, 68-69
Portabella mushrooms, *139*
postpartum depression, 6, 8, 13, 119, 154, 199, 265-284
postpartum period, 265-284
postpartum psychosis, 266
potassium, 21, 38-39, 40, 44, 82, 85-86, 92, 102, 111, 113, 122, 126, 134, 159, 161, 163, 167, 185-186, 193, 195, 200, 202, 241, 252, 254, 298, 306
potato chips, 28

potatoes, 37, 291
poultry, *229. See also specific kinds of poultry*
preeclampsia, 11, 24, 129, 146, 150, 158, 171, 172, 200
pregnancy, 21
optimum diet for a healthy, 285-313
signs of, 19
"pregnancy glow," 81
premature delivery, 224, 226, 230
prenatal vitamins, 11, 14, 89, 111, 171, 245, 293
preservatives, 227
preterm delivery, 11, 24, 153
preterm labor, 50, 82, 153
proanthocyanidins, 181
probiotics, 82, 177, 183, 190-191, 206, 208-209, 236, 242-243
progesterone, 80, 175
prolactin, 242, 243
prostaglandins, 145
protein, 6, 9, 14, 16, 20-21, 23, 41, 52, 60-61, 63-66, 70, 80, 82, 86, 91, 96, 98, 114-115, 122, 125, 135, 139, 142, 151, 156-157, 169, 176-178, 182-183, 189, 196-197, 205, 207, 243, 245, 264, 271, 275, 286, 294
protein deficiency, 52
prune juice, 179, 194-195
prunes, 37
psyllium, 296, 313
pudding, 43
pumpkin seeds, 10, 179, 196-197
pycnogenol, 289
pyroxidine. See vitamin B6

Q

quercetin, 36, 165, 308
quinoa, 272, 279-280

R

radioactivity, 212
Raffelock, Dean, 6
rainbow trout, 179, 198-199
raspberries, 37
reactive carbonyls, 219
recommended daily allowance (RDA), 33
red raspberry leaf, 236-237
red raspberry leaf tea, 130, 165-166, 224
retinol, 89, 212
rhubarb, 130, 167-168
riboflavin, 6, 8, 21, 41, 44, 47, 53, 63, 85-86, 109, 111, 123, 161, 163, 176, 186, 203, 209, 254, 283-284, 303-305
ribosomes, 176
rice, 25, 39
brown, 20, 30, 41, 42-43, *139*
white, 43
ricotta cheese, 230
romaine lettuce, 83, 110-111
rose hips, 224, 225
rosemary, 237
Rountree, Robert, 6
royal jelly, 308
rubella, 150, 212
rutin, 300

S

saccharin, 216, 217-218, 219
sage, 237
salad dressings, 229
salads, 83
salmon, 11, *12*, 13, 20, 130, 135-136, 228
Salmonella, 223-224, 228, 229
salt, 8, 126, 226-227. See also sodium
saponins, 308
sardines, 11, *12*, 13, 230, 272, 281-282
saturated fat, 9, 47, 84, 100, 101, 231
sauces, 229
scallions, 83, 112-113
seafood, 214, 228-229. See also fish; shellfish; specific kinds of seafood

smoked, 213, 229
seaweed, 108-109
second trimester, 78-123
seeds, 20, 21, 82, 83, 169-170, 176, 177, 196-197, 232, 245, 293. See also specific kinds of seeds
selenium, 6, 14, 21, 41-42, 53, 66, 74, 75, 85, 97, 114, 120, *139*, 139-140, 149, 158, 176, 181, 275-276, 289
senna, 237
sepsis, 150
serotonin, 121, 132
sesame seeds, *12*, 130, 169-170
sesquiterpene, 48
shark, 228
shellfish, 228-229, 275-276. See also specific kinds of shellfish
raw, 213, 229
shepherd's purse, 237
shiitake mushrooms, 272, 283-284
shogaol, 48
shrimp, 228, 229
silica, 127, 133, 134, 167, 168
skeletal development, 97
skin health, 57, 75, 79, 81, 84, 88, 126, 133, 134, 163, 167, 174, 187, 188-189, 192-193, 198, 205, 208-209
sleep, 136, 282
sleep aids, 93, 94, 238
smoothies, 39
snoring, 81
soda, 28, 220
sodium, 21, 29, 40, 80, 82, 85, 125, 126, 134, 156, 202, 286
soluble fiber, 175, 206, 278
sorbitol, 218
soy, 115, 294
soybeans, *12*, 176
soy beverage, *12*
soynuts, *12*
sperm, 288, 289-290, 298-300, 307-308, 310-311
sphingomyelin, 33
spicy foods, 248
spider veins, 126
spina bifida, 24, 34, 150, 205
spinach, 10, 24, *25*, 82, 176, 179, 200-201, 291
Splenda. See sucralose
sprouts, 229
Stevens, Melissa, 158
stevia, 217
Stilton cheese, 47, 230
St. John's wort, 237
strawberries, 37, 181, 291
strep B, 150
stress, 283, 287, 288
stretch marks, 126, 174-175
structural heart disease, 10
sucralose, 216, 218, 219
sucrose, 217, 219
sugar, 27, 43, 151-152, 186, 195, 217, 219, 295
sugar alcohols, 219
SugarTwin. See cyclamate
sulfates, 222
sulfite oxidase, 131
sulphoraphane, 105
sundaes, 28
sun-dried tomatoes, 179, 202-203
sunflower seeds, 42
sunlight, 11
superfoods, 17
superoxide dismutase (SOD), 106
supplements, 235-239, 292. See also specific kinds of supplements
recommended, 236-237
sushi, 108, 229, 248
sweetened beverages, 9
Sweet'N Low. See saccharin
sweet peppers. See bell peppers
sweet potatoes, 30, 70-71
sweets, 9, 294-295
swelling, 19, 81, 125, 126, 129, 156, 159, 193
Swiss chard, 201
Swiss cheese, *12*, 130, 171-172, 230
swordfish, 228
syphilis, 150, 212

T

tahini, 10, 11, *12*, 30, 72-73, 170
tannins, 308
Tannis, Allison, 315, *315*
tansy, 237
tarragon, 237
taste buds, 112
tea, 30, 58-59, 130, 163-164, 165-166, 220, *221*, 222, 224-226. See also specific kinds of tea
teratogens, 212
tetracycline, 212
thalidomide, 212
thaumatin, 218
thiamin, 6, 21, 44, 63, 77, 85, 111, 131, 143, 151, 161, 169, 176, 203, 252, 283, 303-305.
third trimester, 124-172
thuja, 237
tilapia, 30, 74-75
tilefish, 228
tofu, 11, *12*, 41, 83, 114-115
tomatoes, 144
sun-dried, 179, 202-203
tomato juice, *25*
Toxoplasma gondii, 212, 223-224
toxoplasmosis, 212, 222, 223
trans fats, 9, 214, 231-232, 246, 309
tricky foods, 210-239
tricyclic antidepressants, 212
triplets, 17
triterpenes, 308
trout, 177, 179, 198-199
tryptophan, 121, 132
tuna, 13, 83, 118-119, 228, 230
turbinado sugar, 217
turkey, 83, 120-121, *139*. See also poultry
turmeric, 83, 116-117, 237
turnip greens, *12*, *25*
twins, 17
type 2 diabetes, 152

U

undercooked foods, 223-224, 227-229. See also food, heating
unpasteurized dairy products, 229, 230
unprocessed foods, 8
urinary tract, 137
urinary tract anomaly, 10
urinary tract infections, 82, 137
urination, frequent, 19, 125
uterus, 21, 80, 82, 125-127, 137, 159, 165, 197
uva ursi, 237

V

vaginal discharge, 82
vaginal infections, 82
valium, 212
varicose veins, 81, 126
vasodilation, 165
vegetables, 8, 9, 13, 16, 20, 27, 29, 83, 126, 176, 177, 245. See also specific vegetables
unwashed, 213
vegetarian baked beans, *25*
vegetarians, 10-11, 176, 264, 293, 294
viruses, 229
vision. See eyesight
Vital Choice, 119
vitamin A, 8, 14, 20-21, 24, 29, 44, 54, 63, 70-71, 76, 80, 85-86, 88-89, 92, 109-113, 122, 125, 151, 159, 161, 163, 165, 200, 225, 232, 241, 254-255, 260-261, 268, 270-271, 274, 286, 289, 298, 306-308, 311-312
vitamin B1. See thiamin
vitamin B2. See riboflavin
vitamin B3. See niacin
vitamin B6, 6, 8, 13, 21, 38, 42, 44, 49, 52-55, 63, 70-71, 77, 86, 96, 109, 111, 113, 123, 143, 149, 156, 161, 169, 176, 195, 241, 252, 254, 260, 261, 283, 303-305, 312
vitamin B7. See biotin

vitamin B9. See folate (folic acid)
vitamin B12, 6, 8, 21, 47, 53, 75, 80, 109, 125, 176, 241, 276, 277, 286, 289, 294, 303-305
vitamin C, 6, 8, 21, 26, 38, 44, 54, 56-57, 70, 76, 80-81, 85-86, 88, 95, 110-113, 116, 122, 125, 127, 134, 137-138, 149, 151, 159, 161, 163, 167, 176, 180, 181, 185, 192-193, 203, 225, 241, 245, 252, 254-255, 260-261, 271, 274, 286, 289, 298, 300, 306-308, 311
vitamin D, 11, 21, 80, 118, 125, 232, 236, 241, 262, 268, 270, 286, 289
vitamin E, 6, 21, 24, 29, 75, 86, 122, 127, 161, 165, 193, 205, 232, 241, 245, 270-271, 289, 306-308, 312
vitamin K, 21, 44, 55, 85-86, 88, 102, 110-111, 122, 143, 151, 161, 167, 185, 200, 203, 241, 252, 253, 270, 298, 306vitamins, 11, 20, 21, 24-25, 26, 29, 84, 101, 135, 157, 161, 162, 196, 236, 245, 246. See also multivitamins; prenatal vitamins; specific vitamins
fat-soluble, 232, 270
for the first trimester, 21
for lactation and breast-feeding, 241
for the second trimester, 80
for the third trimester, 125
volatile oils, 87
vomiting, 13, 19, 27, 28, 39, 40, 42, 48, 50, 178, 237

W

waffles, *12*
walnuts, 257
warfarin, 212
water, 7, 30, 50-51, 82, 126, 127, 134, 175, 177, 214, 233-234, 244-246, 261, 306
mineral water, 28
tap, 233, 233, 234, 234
untreated, 233
water filtration systems, 233
watercress, 82, 83, 122-123
watermelons, 30, 76-77, 260
weight, 14, *15*, 16, 23, 29, 232, 269, 270, 292-293, 301. See also birth weight
weight gain, 7, 14, 126-127, 129, 178
weight loss, 7, 63, 128, 247, 278
wheat bran, 42
wheat germ, *25*, 179, 204-205
white button mushrooms, *139*, 140
white tea, 226
whole-grain foods, 60-61
whole-grain bread, 28, 83
whole-grain pasta, 179, 206-207
whole grains, 8, 9, 176, 206-207, 245. See also whole-grain foods
wild cherry, 237

X

X-rays, 212
xylitol, 217, 218

Y

yams. See sweet potatoes
yeast infections, 82
yellow dock tea, 225, 226
yerba mate, 220
yogurt, 11, *12*, 39, 82, 174, 177, 179, 208-209

Z

zeaxanthin, 122, 201
zinc, 6, 14, 21, 44, 53, 65, 80, 86, 92, 97, 109, 125, 161, 163, 181, 197, 241, 243, 245, 248-250, 254, 275, 278-279, 286, 289, 304, 306-308
zinc deficiency, 109, 197
zygote, 20

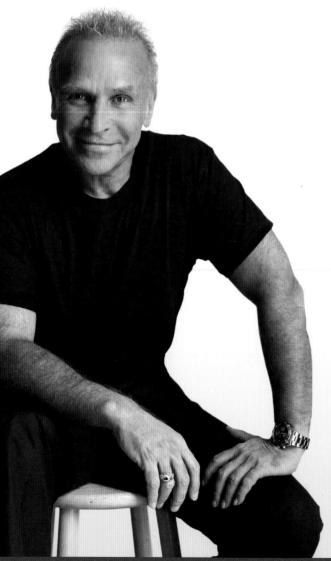